Spectroscopic Techniques for Cancer Diagnostics

Online at: https://doi.org/10.1088/978-0-7503-5949-8

About the Series

The Biophysical Society and IOP Publishing have forged a new publishing partnership in biophysics, bringing the world-leading expertise and domain knowledge of the Biophysical Society into the rapidly developing IOP ebooks program.

The program publishes textbooks, monographs, reviews, and handbooks covering all areas of biophysics research, applications, education, methods, computational tools, and techniques. Subjects of the collection will include: bioenergetics; bioengineering; biological fluorescence; biopolymers *in vivo*; cryo-electron microscopy; exocytosis and endocytosis; intrinsically disordered proteins; mechanobiology; membrane biophysics; membrane structure and assembly; molecular biophysics; motility and cytoskeleton; nanoscale biophysics; and permeation and transport.

A list of recently published title in this series can be found here: https://iopscience.iop.org/bookListInfo/iop-series-in-biophysical-society.

Spectroscopic Techniques for Cancer Diagnostics

Edited by
Inbarasan Muniraj
Department of Electronic Engineering, Maynooth International Engineering College, Maynooth University, Maynooth, Co. Kildare, Ireland

Bryan Hennelly
Department of Electronic Engineering and Department of Computer Science, Maynooth University, Maynooth, Co. Kildare, Ireland

IOP Publishing, Bristol, UK

ISBN 978-0-7503-5949-8 (ebook)
ISBN 978-0-7503-5947-4 (print)
ISBN 978-0-7503-5950-4 (myPrint)
ISBN 978-0-7503-5948-1 (mobi)

DOI 10.1088/978-0-7503-5949-8

Version: 20251201

IOP ebooks

British Library Cataloguing-in-Publication Data: A catalogue record for this book is available from the British Library.

Published by IOP Publishing, wholly owned by The Institute of Physics, London

IOP Publishing, No.2 The Distillery, Glassfields, Avon Street, Bristol, BS2 0GR, UK

US Office: IOP Publishing, Inc., 190 North Independence Mall West, Suite 601, Philadelphia, PA 19106, USA

The editors dedicate this book to the late Professor John T Sheridan who was involved in the inception of the book.

Contents

Preface

The big picture

Cancer remains one of the most formidable challenges in modern medicine, with its complexity and heterogeneity demanding innovative approaches for early detection, accurate diagnosis, and effective treatment. Spectroscopy has emerged as a powerful tool to examine the molecular and biochemical alterations that characterize cancerous tissues, and the effort to advance this approach has brought together a collaboration between physicists, engineers, chemists, biologists, clinicians, and data scientists. This book, *Spectroscopic Techniques for Cancer Diagnostics*, brings together a comprehensive exploration of some of the latest spectroscopic techniques and their transformative applications in oncology.

A criticism of vibrational spectroscopy in previous decades has been the lack of penetration into the clinic. While research funding produced exciting results in the laboratory, translation to clinical practice seemed elusive. However, as evidenced by the contributions in this book, the journey into the clinic is now well underway. The gap between the lab and the clinic has been narrowed—and in many cases, bridged—demonstrating the growing impact of spectroscopic technologies in real-world cancer diagnostics and treatment.

At its core, vibrational spectroscopy studies the interaction between matter and electromagnetic radiation. In cancer research, these techniques provide a non-invasive or minimally invasive means to probe the molecular composition of tissues, cells, and biofluids. They enable the detection of subtle biochemical changes that often precede morphological alterations, offering the potential for earlier and more accurate diagnosis. From visible and near-infrared (NIR) absorption spectroscopy to Fourier transform infrared (FTIR) spectroscopy, quantum cascade laser (QCL)-based infrared absorption, and Raman spectroscopy—including advanced forms such as stimulated Raman scattering (SRS) and surface-enhanced Raman spectroscopy (SERS)—each technique brings unique capabilities to the table. This book covers all of these vibrational spectroscopic methods, highlighting their strengths, limitations, and applications in cancer diagnostics and research.

Key spectroscopic methods covered

At their core, both **absorption spectroscopy** and **Raman spectroscopy** are vibrational spectroscopic techniques, meaning they probe the molecular vibrations of a sample to reveal its chemical composition. However, they differ fundamentally in their underlying mechanisms and the type of information they provide.

Absorption spectroscopy (including visible, NIR, and IR) measures the absorption of light by a sample at specific wavelengths, corresponding to the energy required to excite molecular vibrations. This results in a spectrum that reflects the characteristic vibrational modes of the sample's molecules. Absorption spectroscopy is particularly sensitive to functional groups such as C–H, O–H, and N–H bonds, making it highly effective for identifying biochemical changes in tissues.

Raman spectroscopy, on the other hand, relies on the inelastic scattering of light. When a sample is illuminated with a laser, a small fraction of the scattered light shifts in energy due to interactions with molecular vibrations. This shift, known as the Raman effect, provides a 'molecular fingerprint' of the sample. Unlike absorption spectroscopy, Raman is less affected by water, making it ideal for studying biological samples. Additionally, advanced techniques like SERS enables the detection of trace amounts of biomarkers with high specificity, and CARS and stimulated Raman enable high-speed detection of Raman susceptibility.

Together, these complementary techniques offer a comprehensive toolkit for cancer research. Absorption spectroscopy excels in rapid, high-throughput screening and is well-suited for analysing bulk tissue properties, while Raman spectroscopy provides detailed molecular insights at the cellular and subcellular levels.

Our three themes

The chapters in this book are organised around three major themes: **visible and NIR absorption spectroscopy, IR absorption spectroscopy**, and **Raman spectroscopy** (and its many variants!). Each section explores the principles, instrumentation, and clinical applications of these techniques, with a particular focus on their role in cancer detection and analysis.

1. **Visible and NIR absorption spectroscopy:**
   The first section introduces hyperspectral imaging (HSI), a technique that captures detailed spectral data across a wide range of wavelengths, from ultraviolet to mid-infrared. HSI has shown remarkable promise in cancer research, particularly in histopathological applications, where it enhances the differentiation between healthy and cancerous tissues. One of the features of this spectroscopy is the relatively low cost, the main requirement being the hyperspectral camera or a tunable filter. Chapters in this section discuss the integration of HSI with machine learning for automated diagnostics, as well as its use in generating synthetic datasets for training advanced diagnostic models.
   - *Chapter 1* by Ling Ma and Baowei Fei introduces HSI as a transformative tool in cancer research, particularly in histopathology. The chapter highlights how HSI captures detailed spectral data across a wide range of wavelengths, enabling the differentiation between healthy and cancerous tissues. The integration of HSI with machine learning for automated diagnostics is also discussed, showcasing its potential to improve reproducibility and reduce diagnosis times.
   - *Chapter 2* by Valluri Ayyappa *et al* focuses on the application of HSI in oral cancer detection. The authors present a novel approach using synthetic hyperspectral datasets and advanced unmixing algorithms to improve diagnostic accuracy. This chapter emphasizes the importance of robust datasets and computational methods in advancing cancer diagnostics.
2. **IR absorption spectroscopy:**
   The second section focuses on infrared spectroscopy, particularly FTIR and QCL-based methods. FTIR spectroscopy has proven to be a powerful tool in

cancer diagnostics due to its ability to detect molecular vibrations associated with nucleic acids, proteins, and lipids, which are often altered in cancerous tissues. The section also explores the use of infrared imaging for virtual staining in histopathology, a groundbreaking approach that eliminates the need for chemical staining and enables rapid, label-free tissue analysis.

- *Chapter 3* by Neha Sylvia Walter and Shalmoli Bhattacharyya provides a comprehensive review of FTIR spectroscopy in cancer diagnosis. The chapter explores how FTIR detects molecular vibrations associated with nucleic acids, proteins, and lipids, which are often altered in cancerous tissues. Case studies across various cancer types, including lung, breast, and colorectal cancers, demonstrate the clinical potential of FTIR.
- *Chapter 4* by Kianoush Falahkheirkhah, Jihun Oh, and Rohit Bhargava introduces QCL-based infrared imaging for virtual staining in histopathology. This groundbreaking approach eliminates the need for chemical staining, enabling rapid, label-free tissue analysis. The chapter also discusses the integration of QCL imaging with machine learning to enhance diagnostic accuracy and reduce uncertainties in virtual staining.
- *Chapter 5* by Panchali Saha and Murali Krishna Chilakapati explores blood-based diagnostics using infrared spectroscopy. The chapter reviews studies on serum and plasma analysis, highlighting the potential of FTIR for early cancer detection and monitoring. The integration of machine learning for spectral data analysis is also emphasized, showcasing its role in improving diagnostic precision. This chapter is not limited to FTIR but also reviews the use of fluorescence and Raman spectroscopy for blood diagnostics. This brings us seamlessly into the next section.

3. **Raman spectroscopy:**
The final section deals with Raman spectroscopy and its enhanced variants, such as SERS, CARS, and SRS. These techniques provide detailed molecular fingerprints of tissues, enabling the identification of cancer biomarkers with high sensitivity and specificity. The section also highlights the integration of Raman spectroscopy with machine learning for real-time, *in vivo* optical biopsy, as well as its application in blood-based diagnostics.

- *Chapter 6* by Phularida Amulraj *et al* provides an in-depth overview of Raman spectroscopy and its enhanced variants, such as SERS, for cancer analysis. The chapter discusses the use of Raman spectroscopy to detect molecular changes in various cancers, including breast, lung, and prostate cancer. The development of novel SERS substrates for improved sensitivity is highlighted.
- *Chapter 7* by Yulia A Khristoforova *et al* focuses on the application of Raman spectroscopy for skin cancer diagnostics. The authors present a portable Raman system for *in vivo* analysis of skin lesions, demonstrating its potential for real-time, non-invasive diagnostics. The integration

of chemometric methods, such as partial least squares discriminant analysis (PLS-DA), is discussed to achieve high levels of diagnostic accuracy.

- *Chapter 8* by Tim McNamara and Bryan M Hennelly explores the integration of hyperspectral imaging and Raman spectroscopy in histology. The chapter highlights the use of SRS microscopy for real-time tissue diagnosis during surgical procedures, with case studies demonstrating its impact on tumor margin assessment.
- *Chapter 9* by Piyush Kumar and Aditi Sahu delves into serum Raman spectroscopy for biomedical diagnostics. The chapter reviews advancements in using Raman spectroscopy to analyse blood serum for the detection of both cancerous and non-cancerous conditions. The potential of Raman spectroscopy for early cancer detection and patient monitoring is emphasized.
- *Chapter 10* by Sanoop P *et al* concludes the book with a discussion on innovative phototherapy approaches guided by SERS. The chapter explores the use of multifunctional nanoparticles for combined diagnostics and therapy, highlighting the potential of SERS-guided photodynamic therapy (PDT) and photothermal therapy (PTT) to improve cancer treatment outcomes.

Sample types and hyperspectral imaging

A recurring theme across the chapters is the diversity of sample types analysed using spectroscopic techniques. While traditional methods often rely on excised tissue samples transported to laboratory equipment, there is a growing emphasis on *in vivo* optical biopsy and the use of blood-based samples. Blood serum and plasma, in particular, have gained attention due to their ease of collection, minimal invasiveness, and potential for repeated monitoring. Several chapters in this book explore the use of spectroscopic techniques to analyse blood samples, offering new avenues for early cancer detection and patient monitoring. Indeed at the time of writing this preface, there are several companies engaged in blood-based spectroscopic diagnostics.

Another area of significant commercial interest and rapid advancement is the application of hyperspectral imaging in cancer research. Hyperspectral imaging combines spatial and spectral information, enabling the creation of detailed molecular maps of tissues. This technique has been successfully applied in various contexts, from whole-slide imaging in histopathology to real-time tumor margin assessment during surgery. The integration of hyperspectral imaging with machine learning algorithms further enhances its diagnostic capabilities, paving the way for automated and high-throughput cancer diagnostics.

Machine learning and data analysis

The role of machine learning in spectroscopic cancer research cannot be overstated. Across the chapters, authors highlight the use of advanced computational methods, such as principal component analysis (PCA), support vector machines (SVMs), convolutional neural networks (CNNs), and deep learning ensembles, to analyse complex spectral data. These techniques enable the classification and segmentation of hyperspectral images, improve diagnostic accuracy, and provide insights into the molecular composition of tissues. The integration of machine learning with spectroscopic methods is not only enhancing the precision of cancer diagnostics but also driving the development of personalized treatment strategies.

The future of spectroscopy in cancer research

As we look to the future, the potential of spectroscopy in cancer research is boundless. Advances in instrumentation, such as portable Raman systems, rapid coherent Raman systems, and QCL-based IR imaging devices, are making these technologies more accessible for clinical use. The integration of spectroscopic techniques with artificial intelligence and machine learning is expected to further enhance their diagnostic accuracy and efficiency. Additionally, the development of multifunctional nanoparticles for combined diagnostics and therapy, as discussed in the final chapter, represents a promising direction for the field.

This book aims to serve as a comprehensive resource for researchers and clinicians alike, providing a detailed overview of the current state of spectroscopic techniques in cancer research while also highlighting emerging trends and future directions. It is a deep-felt hope of all of the authors of this book that our work will contribute to the ongoing efforts to improve cancer diagnostics and treatment, ultimately leading to better outcomes for patients worldwide.

Editor biograpies

Inbarasan Muniraj

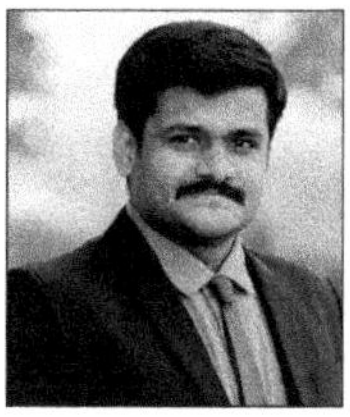

Inbarasan Muniraj received his BE degree in Electronics and Communication Engineering from St. Peter's Engineering College (affiliated with Anna University, Chennai, India) in 2009, and his ME degree in Computer Engineering from Chosun University, Gwangju, South Korea, in 2013. Upon completing his postgraduate studies, he worked as a Research Scientist at the Gwangju Institute of Science and Technology, South Korea. With financial support from the Government of Ireland under the Irish Research Council's Early Career Postgraduate Scholarship Programme (2014–2017), he completed his PhD in Optical Engineering from University College Dublin (UCD), Ireland. Following a postdoctoral fellowship at UCD, he joined Intel Corporation, Ireland, where he held several technical and research-oriented roles between 2018 and 2020. From 2020 to 2024, Dr Muniraj served as an Assistant Professor at SRM University-AP and later at Alliance University, Bengaluru, India. During this period, he successfully led two research projects funded by the Department of Science and Technology (DST), including the SERB Start-Up Research Grant (SRG) and the DST–JSPS Collaborative Research Programme. In 2024, he also received International Travel Support from DST. Dr Muniraj's research expertise lies in optical and computational imaging, with interdisciplinary applications in biophotonics and Industry 4.0. He has authored over 75 publications, 1 technical eBook, and co-invented one US and three Indian patents at the time of writing.

Bryan Hennelly

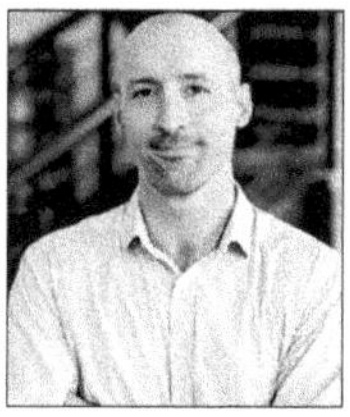

Bryan Hennelly received his BE in Electronic Engineering from University College Dublin in 2001 and his PhD, also from UCD, in 2005 in optical engineering and computational imaging. Following a postdoctoral fellowship at Maynooth University funded by the Irish Research Council, he became a joint staff member of the Department of Electronic Engineering and the Department of Computer Science, where he teaches several modules and has established two biophotonics laboratories. His research interests include wave theory, nonlinear optics, coherent and statistical optics, vibrational spectroscopy, and general relativity. He has received extensive funding through numerous grants from Research Ireland and the European Union for projects relating to advanced imaging and the application of vibrational spectroscopy in biomedicine. At the time of writing, his current focus is the development of a label-free flow cytometry system capable of classifying cells using broadband CARS with a 5 ms acquisition time. He has authored over 100 publications, collaborates widely with partners in industry, academia, and health service institutions, and has just graduated his tenth PhD student at the time of writing.

List of contributors

Suresh Aala
Department of Electronics and Communication Engineering, School of Engineering and Science, SRM University-AP, 522502, India

Phularida Amulraj
RAman REsearch Laboratory (RARE Lab), Department of Chemistry, SRM University-AP Amaravati, Andhra Pradesh, 522240, India

Valluri Ayyappa
Department of Electronics and Communication Engineering, School of Engineering and Science, SRM University-AP, 522502, India

Rohit Bhargava
Beckman Institute for Advanced Science and Technology, Departments of Electrical and Computer Engineering, Chemical and Biomolecular Engineering, and Chemistry, Bioengineering, Mechanical Science and Engineering, Cancer Center at Illinois, University of Illinois at Urbana-Champaign, Urbana, Illinois, United States

Shalmoli Bhattacharyya
Department of Biophysics, Postgraduate Insitute of Medical Education and Research (PGIMER), Chandigarh, 160012, India

Ivan A Bratchenko
Samara university, Samara, Russia

Lyudmila A Bratchenko
Samara university, Samara, Russia

Murali Krishna Chilakapati
Advanced Centre for Treatment, Research and Education in Cancer (ACTREC), Training School Complex, Homi Bhabha National Institute, Anushakti Nagar, Maharashtra, India.

Sunil Chinnadurai
Department of Electronics and Communication Engineering, School of Engineering and Science, SRM University-AP, 522502, India

Kianoush Falahkheirkhah
Beckman Institute for Advanced Science and Technology, University of Illinois at Urbana-Champaign, Urbana, IL, United States

Baowei Fei
Department of Bioengineering, and Center for Imaging and Surgical Innovation, and Department of Radiology, University of Texas at Dallas, Richardson, TX, United States

Bryan M Hennelly
Department of Electronic Engineering and Department of Computer Science, Maynooth University, Maynooth, Co. Kildare, Ireland

Manu M Joseph
Department of Life Sciences, CHRIST University, Bengaluru – 560029, Karnataka, India

Oleg I Kaganov
Samara State Medical University, Samara, Russia

Yulia A Khristoforova
Samara University, Samara, Russia

Sergey V Kozlov
Samara State Medical University, Samara, Russia

Jayasree Kumar
RAman REsearch Laboratory (RARE Lab), Department of Chemistry, SRM University-AP Amaravati, Andhra Pradesh, 522240, India

Piyush Kumar
Icahn School of Medicine at Mount Sinai, New York, USA

Ling Ma
Department of Bioengineering, and Center for Imaging and Surgical Innovation, University of Texas at Dallas, Richardson, TX, United States

Irina A Matveeva
Samara University, Samara, Russia

Tim McNamara
Department of Electronic Engineering, Maynooth University, Maynooth, Co. Kildare, Ireland

Alexandr A Moryatov
Samara State Medical University, Samara, Russia

Prasanna Kumar Mukkara
Department of Electronics and Communication Engineering, School of Engineering and Science, SRM University-AP, 522502, India

Jyothi B Nair
Leibniz Institute of Photonic Technology, Jena, Germany

Hemanth Noothalapati
Department of Biomedical Engineering, Chennai Institute of Technology, Chennai, Tamil Nadu, India, Department of Chemical Engineering, Indian Institute of Technology Hyderabad, Kandi, Sangareddy, Telangana, India, Faculty of Life and Environmental Sciences, Shimane University, Matsue, Japan

Jihun Oh
Mechanical Science and Engineering, University of Illinois at Urbana-Champaign, Urbana, IL, United States

Andrey E Orlov
Samara regional oncological dispensary, Samara, Russia

Rajapandiyan Panneerselvam
RAman REsearch Laboratory (RARE Lab), Department of Chemistry, SRM University-AP Amaravati, Andhra Pradesh, 522240, India

Panchali Saha
Advanced Centre for Treatment, Research and Education in Cancer (ACTREC), Training School Complex, Homi Bhabha National Institute, Anushakti Nagar, Maharashtra, India

Aditi Sahu
Memorial Sloan Kettering Cancer Center, New York, USA

P Sanoop
Madanapalle Institute of Technology & Sciences (MITS) Madanapalle, Andhra Pradesh, 517326, India

Neha Sylvia Walter
Department of Biophysics, Postgraduate Insitute of Medical Education and Research (PGIMER), Chandigarh, 160012 India

Valery P Zakharov
Samara University, Samara, Russia

IOP Publishing

Spectroscopic Techniques for Cancer Diagnostics

Inbarasan Muniraj and Bryan Hennelly

Chapter 1

Hyperspectral microscopic imaging in cancer research

Ling Ma and Baowei Fei

Digital and computational pathology is an active research area that aims to improve the reproducibility and objectivity of pathological diagnosis and save time in routine examination [1]. Machine learning techniques, particularly deep learning models, have played an essential role in digital pathology [2]. Various studies of deep learning-based cancer detection in whole-slide digitized histological images have been investigated, and most of them were carried out in RGB images. Hyperspectral imaging (HSI) and multispectral imaging (MSI) are emerging optical imaging techniques, which are noncontact, noninvasive, nonionizing, and label-free [3]. HSI generates a three-dimensional (3D) data cube, also known as hypercube, which contains a series of 2D grayscale images across a wide electromagnetic spectrum from UV to mid-infrared (MIR) [3, 4]. The main difference between HSI and MSI is the number of spectral bands within the data cube. A data cube acquired by MSI usually contains 3–10 bands, while that acquired by HSI has tens or even hundreds of narrow spectral bands [5]. HSI was originally developed for remote sensing, but it has been gaining attention in the medical imaging field [3]. In histopathology, HSI utilizes the optical properties of human tissue such as transmittance and fluorescence, which are related to tissue microenvironment or biochemical constitutents [3, 4], and it can provide tissue pathophysiology through spectral characteristics. Therefore, it is promising for disease diagnosis and histology research.

Studies have proven the usefulness of HSI in microscopy applications [6–14]. One of the promising applications for this technology is employing HSI for whole-slide imaging (WSI) to aid the histopathological cancer detection of tissue samples because HSI not only provides a reproducible and quantitative diagnosis of the slides but also improves the classification results compared with RGB [11, 12, 15, 16]. Although various steps such as fixation and embedding during the preparation of the histological samples may alter a few tissue features, such as the texture and the water content, lots of important molecules such as proteins are preserved in the

doi:10.1088/978-0-7503-5949-8ch1

tissue slides. The light absorption, scattering, and autofluorescence of these molecular components all contribute to the spectral characteristics in hyperspectral histological images [17, 18], which provide a different perspective from the traditional gross-level reflectance HSI. Even for the dyes, HSI can expand the three-channel color information into a much wider spectral dimension, which might increase the discriminability.

1.1 Hyperspectral microscopic imaging mechanisms

HSI can be classified into four types according to its acquisition mode, namely whiskbroom (point-scanning), spectral-scanning (wavelength-scanning), push-broom (line-scanning), and snapshot [3, 5]. The point-scanning mode is to scan the object point-by-point, which is very slow and not commonly used anymore.

Line-scanning hyperspectral imaging systems, in other words, push-broom systems, tend to have a good spatial and spectral resolution. It is a popular hyperspectral image acquisition method for its high resolution and large availability. However, it requires relative motion between the camera and the object (histologic slide) [14, 19]. The camera captures one line of pixels of the scene (y-axis) at one time. The other spatial dimension (x-axis) is obtained by moving the field of view (FOV) of the camera in that direction. Push-broom cameras are the most common systems in remote sensing field and other industrial sectors due to their high spectral resolution, showing reduced capturing times with respect to the whiskbroom cameras [5, 20]. When using push-broom cameras in microscopy, the relative motion between the camera and the object, which is the histology slide, is usually achieved by employing a motorized stage that is synchronized to the camera acquisition [6, 19]. If movement artifacts occur during the acquisition period, the spatial aliasing can cause an issue and significantly reduce the image quality [20]. Meanwhile, due to the intrinsic of push-broom cameras, each frame only contains the spatial information of a line in the object. Therefore, it can be slightly difficult to focus the camera by evaluating the sharpness of limited spatial components.

Based on the mechanism of line-scanning, some cameras move the translational mechanism inside. So, instead of moving the motorized stage, a servo motor drives the imaging sensor behind the diffraction grating to finish the scanning process internally [21, 22]. In addition, a type of commercial hyperspectral device called a 'snapscan' camera was developed [23] and actively used in hyperspectral microscopy [10, 12, 16, 24–29]. The image sensor, which is overlaid by Fabry–Pérot filters, moves inside of the camera along one spatial dimension. The bandpass values of the filters varied across the translation direction, so by moving the sensor, both spatial and spectral components are sampled. The significant improvement of both cameras is that users no longer need to manage the synchronization of camera acquisition and motorized stage.

The spectral-scanning method steps through the wavelength range and captures one grayscale image of the whole FOV at each step. Similar to line-scanning, it also takes good care of both the spatial resolution and spectral resolution [3, 5, 30]. Among the published studies, we found the spectral-scanning microscope systems being mostly employed, due to the fact that they have a good image resolution and spectral resolution without the need of providing relative motion between the camera and the slides, made them relatively easy to implement. Spectral-scanning HSI systems are made of a monochromatic sensor and a spectral-scanning component, which can be an electrical tunable filter, a filter wheel, or others. For tunable filters, liquid crystal tunable filter (LCTF) [31–34] and acousto-optic tunable filter (AOTF) [35–38] are two popular choices. When a relatively small number of wavelength bands are needed, such as for fluorescence imaging, a set of filters on a filter wheel [39, 40] would be sufficient and more cost effective. When a tunable filter is used, the imaging system (tunable filter and monochromatic sensor) is mounted on the microscope optical ports via a video adapter. For comparison, the tunable filter is faster and easier for adaptation than a filter wheel, and it is capable of scanning more spectral bands.

Snapshot hyperspectral cameras are able to capture the spatial and spectral information simultaneously [5, 14, 30]. They are well-known for the small size, light weight, and the lowest acquisition time. Commercial snapshot cameras usually have filters integrated on the imaging sensor and they can be easily adapted to the microscope simply through a video adapter [25]. In addition, Yu *et al* [41] developed a snapshot hyperspectral microscopy system based on microlens array. Hedde *et al* [42] developed an ultrafast phasor-based hyperspectral snapshot microscopy based on sine/cosine interference filters for biomedical imaging not feasible with conventional hyperspectral imaging methods.

The resolution of hyperspectral images depends on the specific imaging system, but generally, spectral-scanning and line-scanning methods achieve better spatial and spectral resolution than snapshot. Despite the fact that the video-rate acquisition speed of snapshot cameras is beneficial for some intraoperative applications such as hemodynamic assessment; the compromised spectral and spatial resolution might limit their use in cancer histology studies at this stage. Nevertheless, all three acquisition methods are applicable for adaptation with microscopes for histology analysis.

1.2 Automated whole-slide hyperspectral microscopic imaging systems

Digital pathology is becoming a standard practice to analyze histological slides. WSI, the process of scanning and digitizing the entire slide at 40× magnification for later analysis, is an important part of the process. WSI uses a specialized scanner to generates a large digital slide and specialized software to view, analyze, and annotate the resulting image. A wide range of commercialized hardware and software have been introduced in the last decade [1–4]. Researchers at large clinical institutions created and published large histological whole-slide datasets publicly, such as CAMELYON and BreaKHis [5, 6]. These datasets helped advancing research in the area, especially in automating diagnostic methods. Computer-aided diagnosis (CAD) relies on many of these datasets to train and validate their results.

There are challenges for training networks with hyperspectral histological images, one of them being the lack of whole-slide hyperspectral data. The majority of histological HSI dataset were acquired manually. In order to promote HSI in histology, it is very important to develop automated whole-slide hyperspectral imaging microscope system.

1.2.1 Automated hyperspectral whole-slide imaging systems

With hyperspectral microscopy gaining popularity in recent years, there have been a few studies developing and employing whole-slide hyperspectral microscopes. Enfield *et al* [43] developed an in-house automated whole-slide hyperspectral microscope system based on spectral-scanning imaging and used it to study the spatial tumor-immune cell interactions associated with lung cancer recurrence. The system consisted of a Zeiss microscope, a motorized *x–y* translational stage, a CRI light filter, and an RGB camera. With a 20× objective lens, the microscope had a spatial resolution of 0.33 μm pixel^{-1}. The system used a continuously active focus and was able to collect up to 16 spectral bands per hypercube within the wavelength range of 420–720 nm. Once the area was imaged, the system stitched all overlapping camera fields together to make a seamless hyperspectral image.

Ishikawa *et al* [21] built a whole-slide HSI acquisition system for cancer detection in H&E-stained human pancreatic tumor tissue microarray (TMA) slides. Similarly, this system contains an upright light microscope, a hyperspectral camera, and a motorized *x–y* stage for the scanning of the slides. Different from the previous spectral-scanning HSI, this setup employed a push-broom hyperspectral camera that has an internal mechanical/optical shifting system. The camera takes 3$\sim$7 s to acquire a single hypercube with 480 × 752 pixels. It achieves about 5 nm spectral resolution within the 400–800 nm wavelength range, which is determined by the halogen light source. With a 20 × objective magnification, the system has a spatial resolution of 0.25 μm pixel^{-1}. During whole-slide scanning, the XY stage moves in a serpentine fashion while *Z* focus with 2 μm increments was actively carried out. The autofocus methods will be discussed in the next section.

Tran *et al* [26] employed a snapscan hyperspectral camera and developed a customized automatic hyperspectral imaging microscopic system for whole-slide scanning of head and neck cancer histological slides. Specifically, the snapscan camera can capture the entire hyperspectral cube without camera movements. It captured hyperspectral images with up to 150 wavelengths in the range 470–900 nm with an image size of 2000 × 2000 spatial pixels. The camera had a full-width half maximum value (spectral resolution) ranging from 3.1 nm at 487 nm to 11 nm at 900 nm. A commercial *X–Y* motorized stage was used for motion of the stage in the *X–Y*-direction, in order to fulfill the whole-slide scanning. And a high-precision encoded stepper motor focus drive was used for the motion in the *Z*-direction to achieve automatic focus. In addition to the three main components (microscope, camera, stage), this system also included a commercially available high-resolution RGB camera, which was synchronized with the snapscan hyperspectral camera and used to acquire standard histological images for visualization purpose. Not only does the system carried out autofocus, but also reconstructed the whole-slide hyperspectral image using a phase correlation-based method. For each pair of

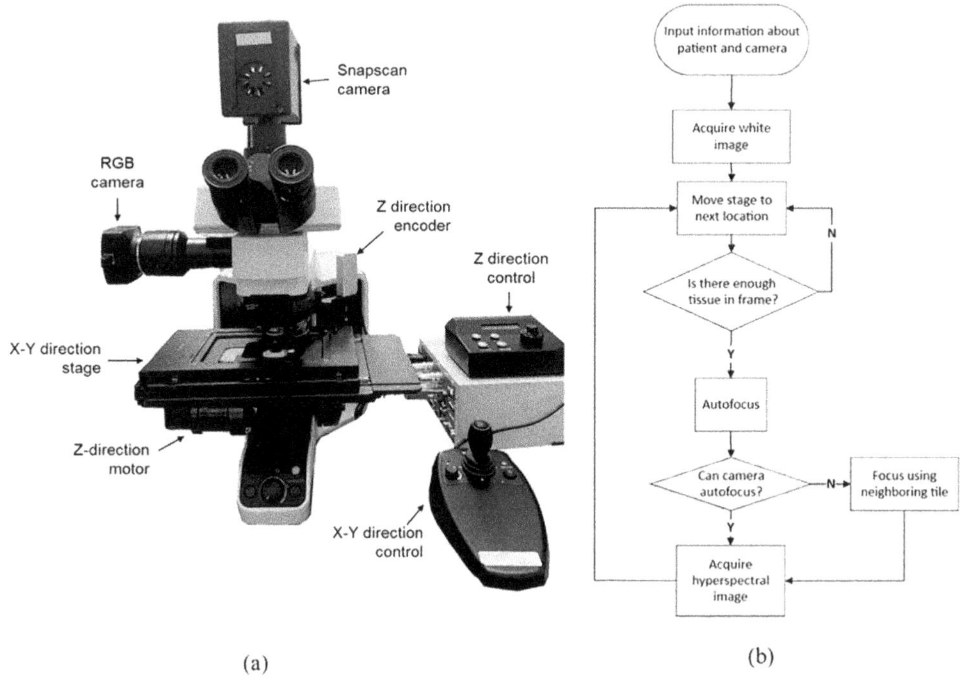

Figure 1.1. Whole-slide hyperspectral microscope system by Tran *et al.* (a) Customized, automatic hyperspectral imaging microscopic system. (b) The flowchart for the whole-slide hyperspectral image acquisition [26].

adjacent hypercubes, a 2D Hamming window and the 2D Fourier transform were applied to the spectral band with the highest contrast in each hypercube; then, the cross-power spectrum of the images was obtained by taking the complex conjugates of the Fourier transform. Finally, by calculating the maximum value in the normalized cross-correlation, the translation between two images was obtained. Figure 1.1 shows the photo of the system and its workflow.

Furthermore, a terapixel hyperspectral whole-slide imaging system based on slit-array detection and projection was developed by Liao *et al* [44]. A fabricated slit-array mask was placed on the image plane of the microscope platform and relayed to a 5-magepixel camera with a $4f$ system. A wedge prism was placed at the Fourier plane for light dispersion. This system scanned the sample along one spatial dimension in a push-broom fashion and produces rapid hyperspectral data. In addition, it uses two LEDs to acquire the focus map row-by-row in the sample, which takes about 20 s per row. However, their system is highly dependable on specific optical equipment and has rigid wavelengths selection.

1.2.2 Auto focus and extended depth of field (EDOF) imaging

One of the biggest tasks in automating HSI reliably is the problem of focusing. Liao *et al* [44, 45] illuminated the sample with two green light-emitting diodes (LEDs) from two oblique angles and recovered the focus points based on 1D autocorrelational analysis, which required no axial scanning and worked for both stained and transparent samples. A rapid focus map was acquired prior to the acquisition of the hyperspectral image, which would later be used to guide the whole-slide scanning.

However, depending on the mechanism used to produce the hypercube, different wavelengths can have different optimal focal points. Determining the best focus for each single wavelength during whole-slide scanning can be extremely time-consuming. Zhang *et al* [46] tried to overcome this by proposing an algorithm that estimates the optimal focus for different wavelengths. They proposed a Laplace operator-based autofocus algorithm and calculated the focal offsets among different spectral bands by deriving the relationship of wavelength and focal length. Therefore, the focal length could be adjusted for each single wavelength with adaptive image sharpness evaluation.

In the whole-slide hyperspectral microscope system developed by Tran *et al* [26], they reply on the single frame of the snapscan camera sensor, which had integrated Fabry–Pérot filters. A 3 × 3 filter kernel based on Brenner focus measure was applied to the frames acquired at different z positions to calculate the focus score. They performed 10 searches within 100 μm range and refined out search within 10 μm of the sharpest focus value. Finally, the z position that resulted in the frame with the highest focus score would be selected as the best focus position. Specifically, because snapscan camera sensors are integrated with filters of all spectral bands, focusing for one frame takes into account all wavelengths and thus eliminates the process of focusing for various bands one by one.

Furthermore, due to the changing thickness of histological slides and the varying focal lengths of different wavelengths, various planes of best focus can exist in a single image. This can lead to certain areas of a picture acquired being in focus while others are out of focus, precluding the use of simple autofocus techniques, such as peak-search or hill-climbing algorithms, which only try to select the image with the best focus but ignore specific regions inside of each image [46]. EDOF is a technique for ensuring that an image is in focus at all points. It takes different areas from multiple images and forms a new image with the best focus. Rathgeb *et al* [25] proposed a novel extended depth of field method for mosaic hyperspectral histological images acquired with a snapshot camera. A stack of 2D mosaicked hyperspectral images of H&E-stained histologic slides were acquired at different positions along the z-axis, and each image was demosaicked into a 3D hypercube. Then, for each band in the hypercube, a Brenner focus score was calculated for the stack of a small patch size, and the best patch is taken from the stack. The patch size kept growing until not all areas in the selected patch were in focus. Finally, all saved best patches were used to output a hyperspectral histologic image that was in focus at every point.

1.2.3 Super resolution reconstruction

Despite that several techniques have been proposed to enhance the focus and image contrast of hyperspectral histological images, the large file size and time-consuming acquisition of hyperspectral images are still challenging. A whole-slide hyperspectral image acquired at a low magnification easily exceeds 100 GB and the acquisition time can be from 10 min to 1 h. In some applications such as cancer detection, a higher magnification (20 × or 40 ×) is necessary, which may put an extreme burden on data storage devices and makes it difficult to establish a comprehensive hyperspectral microscopic dataset. State-of-the-art microscopes and whole-slide scanners are integrated with autofocusing and extended focal imaging (EFI) algorithms for RGB images. Since whole-slide scanning with a color camera has become routine in the field of pathology, making use of such advantageous features with HSI potentially improves the image quality of hyperspectral images.

Hyperspectral image super-resolution reconstruction (SRR), also known as HSI pansharpening or HSI spatial resolution enhancement, is a technique that uses the spatial information from a high-resolution (high-res) panchromatic image and the color information from a low-resolution (low-res) spectral image to generate a high-resolution spectral image [12]. Dey *et al* [78] adopted a linear degradation model to super-resolve imaging mass spectrometry with hematoxylin and eosin (H&E)-stained histological images, which neglected the nonlinearity in spectral responses and resulted in slightly noisy images. Jiang *et al* [47] used the matrix factorization method to fuse high-res RGB histological images and low-resolution hyperspectral microscopic images acquired with a push-broom camera, but the method was only tested for spatial enhancement scales of 3× and 4×.

Ma *et al* [12, 48] developed an unsupervised super-resolution reconstruction network that takes the low-res HSI and high-res RGB as inputs and generates high-res as well as low-res HSI for outputs. To consider different acquisition methods of low-res hyperspectral images, five networks were trained with different super-resolution scales, i.e., 2×, 4×, 5×, 8×, and 10×. The networks share the same architecture with slight differences in the deconvolutional layer and average pooling layer. Figure 1.2 shows the architecture of a 4 × super-resolution reconstruction

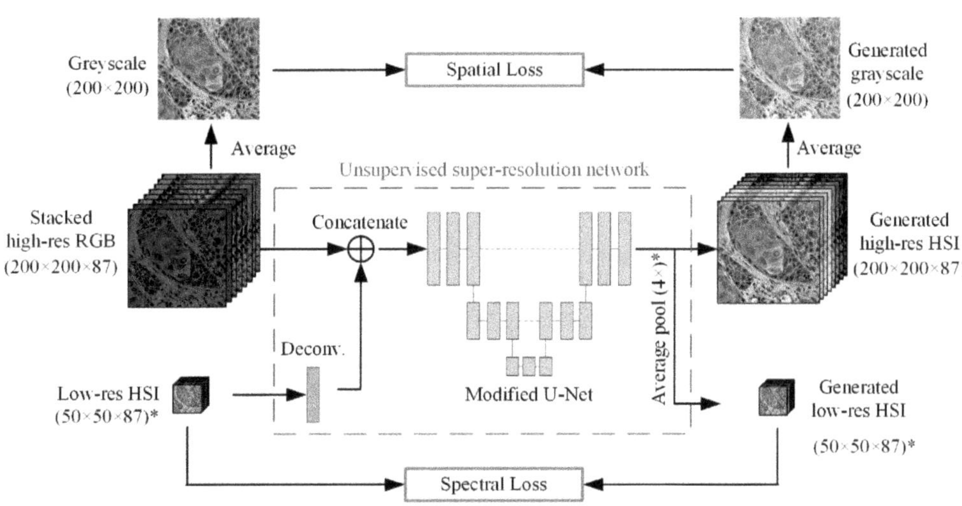

Figure 1.2. Unsupervised super-resolution reconstruction neural network by Ma *et al* [12]. * indicates the parameters that change along super-resolution scales.

network. The duplicated and stacked three channels (R, G, and B) of the input high-res RGB are concatenated with the upsampled low-res HSI input along the spectral dimension. A modified U-Net architecture took the concatenated patch as input and output a high-res HSI patch. A 4 × 4 average pooling layer was applied to the generated high-res HSI to output a low-res HSI patch with the same size as the input low-res HSI. The purpose in this work is to generate high-resolution hyperspectral images that have spatial contrast and details as clear as the high-res RGB images and spectral signatures close to the original HSI. This was fulfilled by simultaneously minimizing the spatial loss, which was the mean absolute error (MAE) between average grayscale images of input stacked high-res RGB and output high-res HSI, and the spectral loss, which was the mean squared error (MSE) between the input and output low-res HSI.

In addition, Urbina Ortega *et al* [49] proposed a relatively low computationally intensive algorithm for the spatial resolution enhancement of hyperspectral histological images. In this work, super-resolution reconstruction was achieved based on a series of different hyperspectral images of the same FOV but with sub-pixel shifts. A motion estimator computed the motion vectors for the low-res images in the sequence, and the vectors were used to shift every low-res image in a higher resolution grid. The same strategy was applied to each band using the same motion vector matrix that was calculated in the artificial single-band representation calculated via principal component analysis (PCA). Since no high-resolution RGB or grayscale image was needed in this method, the system calibration and image alignment between the high-res RGB and low-res HSI could be eliminated.

1.3 Multimodal hyperspectral microscope

Multimodal imaging involving hyperspectral imaging and another imaging modality may take advantage of both methods in a single setup. Various imaging techniques have been combined with HSI in microscopy applications, such as hyperspectral confocal microcopy for discrimination of HaCaT and melanoma cells [50] and dark-field hyperspectral imaging for nano-bio-materials detection [51]. Though not many of them are directly related to cancer study, the technology shows potential to be investigated.

1.3.1 Fluorescence imaging

Hyperspectral imaging is advantageous when used with fluorescence imaging, for its capability of resolving light signals of different wavelengths while obtaining spatial information. One important application of HSI in the medical field is to extract the spectral signature of the recorded fluorescence signal to improve the accuracy of disease detection or differentiation [5]. On the one hand, HSI can be used to differentiate multiple distinct yet spectrally overlaid emissions via spectral decomposition. On the other hand, it can be used to compute the quantitative estimates of fluorophore concentration through the processing of the recorded signal, so it can increase the system sensitivity to the fluorophore, enhance the contrast of fluorescence image, and improve the accuracy of disease detection or tissue differentiation. Meanwhile, integrating fluorescence imaging and HSI into one microscope system is fairly simple by switching the regular broadband light source to a narrow band excitation light source.

Liu *et al* [31] employed hyperspectral microscopy to image DAPI-stained hepatic carcinoma samples and analyzed the difference of fluorescent spectral characteristics between the hepatic carcinoma cells and normal hepatic cells. With a support vector machine (SVM) classifier, they achieved 99.3% sensitivity and 99.1% specificity in differentiating two types of cells, proving HSI effective. In addition to exogenous fluorescence, HSI is also useful with detection of endogenous fluorescence signals, which are beneficial for diagnostic purposes. An excitation-scanning hyperspectral imaging microscope was utilized to detect autofluorescence of colon sections to differentiate neoplastic lesions [40]. The hyperspectral microscope worked in a spectral-scanning fashion but replaced the tunable filter in front of the monochrome camera with a thin-film tunable filter array after the Xe arc lamp light source. By exciting the sample with light of different wavelengths, 39 spectral bands within the 360–550 nm range were acquired, from which the spectral signatures of neoplastic and normal colon tissues were extracted. Linear spectral unmixing was then used to estimate relative abundance of autofluorescence molecules including elastin, NADH, FAD, collagen, and PPIX, which further facilitated the analysis of colon neoplasia.

1.3.2 Polarized hyperspectral microscope

Polarized light imaging is an effective optical imaging technique to explore the structure and morphology of biological tissues through obtaining their polarization characteristics [52]. It can acquire the 2D spatial polarization information of the tissue, which reflects various physical properties of the tissue, including surface texture, surface roughness, and surface morphology information [53–57]. Polarized hyperspectral imaging (PHSI) is a combination of polarization measurement, spectral analysis, and space imaging technology. It can obtain the polarization, spectral and morphological information of the object simultaneously [58–60], and thus provides more image information for digital pathology compared to RGB histological images.

Zhou *et al* developed a dual-modality optical imaging microscope by combining hyperspectral imaging and polarized light imaging. They reported the use of the PHSI microscope for distinguishing head and neck squamous cell carcinoma (SCC) from normal tissue on H&E-stained slides based on the spectra of Stokes vector [17, 24, 28, 61]. The core components of the imaging system include an upright optical microscope with an integrated halogen light source, two linear polarizers, two liquid crystal variable retarders (LCVRs), and a customized snapscan hyperspectral camera. The LCVRs and polarizers are for polarized light imaging. The transmissive axis of Polarizer 1 was set at 45 degrees, while the transmissive axis of Polarizer 2 was at 0 degrees. The fast axis of LCVR 1 was set at 0 degree, and that of LCVR 2 at 45 degrees. The snapscan hyperspectral camera had a wavelength range of 470–750 nm with 97 spectral bands as well as an image resolution of 1200×1200 pixels.

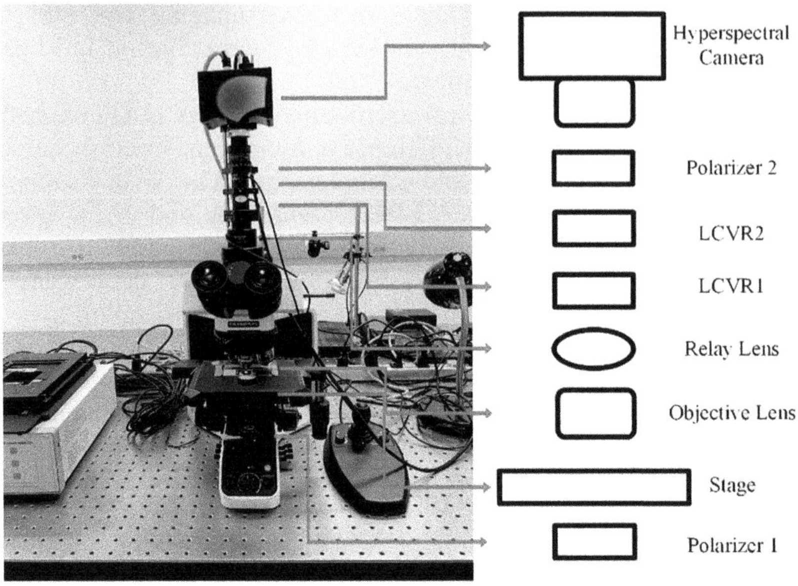

Figure 1.3. Polarized hyperspectral imaging microscope (reproduced from [17]).

The polarized light imaging components and hyperspectral imaging components worked together to acquire images in the visible-infrared wavelength range. With the LCVRs set to different retardance values, the system acquires four element images, namely I_h, I_v, I_{45}, and I_{rc}, which were used to calculate the full Stokes vector (S0, S1, S2, and S3) afterwards. The spectral signatures of four Stokes vector components show very different shapes and may help differentiate various cellular components. The customized microscope is easier to be incorporated into the standard pathological analysis process to work with the existing conventional optical microscope. Figure 1.3. demonstrates the setup of the imaging system with transmissive axis orientations of the polarizers and the fast axis orientations of LCVRs.

1.4 Applications of HSI in histological cancer detection

Hyperspectral microscopy has been actively investigated for cancer detection in recent years, including head and neck cance (HNC) [13, 16], gastrointestinal cancer [62], brain tumor [6], breast cancer [8], pulmonary cancer [63], pancreatic cancer [21], skin cancer [79], and blood cancer [37]. Here, we discuss several major types of cancer that hyperspectral microscopy has been mostly investigated in the recent decade.

1.4.1 Head and neck cancer

HNC is the sixth most common cancer worldwide, and histologic slides of head and neck cancer tissues are important for its histopathological analysis and diagnosis [80]. Utilization of HSI for head and neck histological imaging may help facilitate cancer detection as HSI provides extra spectral information. Maktabi *et al* [64] acquired hyperspectral images of histological specimens from 95 patients and employed a multi-layer perceptron to differentiate squamous epithelium cells, esophageal adenocarcinoma (EAC) cells, and tumor stroma cells using their spectral signatures. They achieved an accuracy of 78% for EAC and stroma as well as 80% for squamous epithelium, indicating the usefulness of spectral features in hyperspectral data.

HNC can be diverse due to the anatomical diversity of this region. In the oral cavity and upper aerodigestive tract, approximately 90% of cancers are SCC [14]. Cancer can occur in multiple organs including the nasopharynx, oral cavity, oropharynx, nasal cavity, paranasal sinuses, hypopharynx, larynx, and trachea [13]. Ou–Yang *et al* combined transmission and fluorescence based HSI using a push-broom system with hundreds of visible near infrared spectral bands for detection of oral SCC in 34 patient samples. The cell nuclei were identified in the basal-cell layer manually and a five-fold method combined spectral and morphological features to yield good performance on the tested patients [65]. Ma *et al* customized a dual-modal microscope system, which included a snapscan hyperspectral camera and a high-quality color camera. The microscope was used to image head and neck SCC histologic slides obtained from larynx, hypopharynx, buccal mucosa, and floor of mouth from 20 patients. They first proposed a PCA-based automatic image segmentation method to extract image patches of nuclei from hyperspectral histological images, then investigated both an SVM classifier and a convolutional neural network (CNN) for the differentiation of cancerous and normal SCC nuclei. Comparison among the classifications using only spatial information (RGB patches and CNN), only spectral information (spectral signatures and SVM), and spatial-spectral information (hyperspectral patch and CNN) was carried out, in order to evaluate the usefulness of morphological and spectral features in hyperspectral images. The results indicate that both features contribute to the differentiation of nuclei; morphological features have a dominant effect, but spectral features provide significant improvement [10, 13]. Then, they further evaluated hyperspectral microscopy in whole-slide cancer detection [11, 12]. Whole-slide hyperspectral histological images of 32 slides from 16 different patients were acquired using an automated dual-modal hyperspectral microscope, and an Inception-based neural network was implemented to carry out patch-based cancer detection in those images. In addition, they used hyperspectral super-resolution reconstruction to fuse HSI and RGB and generate high-resolution hyperspectral images with a better image quality. By comparing the image classification results using RGB, original HSI, and generated HSI, they proved that the spectral information in HSI helps with differentiation, and the generated HSI even further improved the performance. Moreover, Zhou *et al* [17, 28, 61] developed the polarized hyperspectral imaging microscope system and used it for observation and detection of SCC in histologic slides. They first employed four machine learning classifiers, i.e., SVM, random forest, Gaussian naïve Bayes, and logistic regression, to classify spectral signatures extracted from four Stokes vectors of SCC and normal tissues. The results show that SVM got the best classification performance and S3 outperformed other Stokes vectors. Then, they implemented a ResNet50 network for the classification of PHSI-synthesized RGB patches of cancerous and normal tissues and compared the results of four Stokes vectors. Results show that S3 and S0 are more effective than S1 and S2, with S3 achieving the best accuracy. Lately, they found that PHSI is beneficial to visualize collagen in SCC slides, which is one of the most structural components of the tumor microenvironment. The dense collagen and sparse collagen accumulated around tumor cells could be visualized with high contrast in Stokes vector images S1, S2, and S3, while not being clearly seen in regular non-polarized images.

The thyroid gland rests in front of the trachea in the neck, and masses can often be visually observed by the patient. To assess if a thyroid mass is benign or malignant, a fine needle aspiration (FNA) biopsy is performed and microscopically investigated, and HSI may be able to increase diagnostic ability. Thyroid cancer biopsies were studied by Hahn *et al* [66] using 100 cases of papillary thyroid carcinoma (PTC) and benign goiter (BG), developing a classifier to segment hyperspectral images and classify each region as background, PTC, or BG with successful results. Additionally, the experiments were performed with a different number of training cases, from 10 to 40 cases, without observing significant improvements in the classification results. However, the authors concluded that nuclear features offer improvement over nuclear and cytoplasmic regions when developing a classifier. In addition to biopsy samples, Tran *et al* [15, 16, 26] carried out automatic cancer detection in H&E-stained whole-slide thyroid cancer slides. They acquired a database of whole-slide hyperspectral and RGB histological images from 33 follicular thyroid carcinoma patients. VGG-19 neural networks were trained for cancer detection using RGB images, histological images, and HSI-synthesized RGB images, respectively. The network trained with hyperspectral data achieved an area under the receiver operator characteristic curve (AUC-ROC) of 0.966, outperforming both RGB and HSI-synthesized RGB. Then, they expanded the database to 49 whole-slide images. With their proposed hyperspectral data augmentation methods and a video transformer, they achieved an F-1 score of 99.1% and an accuracy of 89.64% using hyperspectral images. Finally, He *et al* [67] incorporated Muller matrix polarization HSI to distinguish papillary thyroid carcinoma tissues in unstained histological sections.

1.4.2 Breast cancer

Several approaches have been proposed in the literature for breast cancer identification in histological slides using HSI. Boucheron *et al* [68] performed a benign versus malignant nuclei classification using HSI, and compared the results with the ones obtained using three different synthetic RGB images generated from the hyperspectral images. The authors did not find a significant boost on the classification using HSI compared to conventional RGB image processing. Nevertheless, Qi *et al* [69] also explored the utility of HSI for histological breast cancer diagnosis, finding an improvement in HSI data exploitation compared to RGB. Although the instrumentation of both approaches was similar, there were some differences in the experimental procedures, especially in the type of staining, the magnification, and the image analysis approaches. While Boucheron *et al* used H&E-stained samples acquired with 40 × magnifications, Qi *et al* employed hematoxylin-only specimens acquired with 10× magnification. Even if the contradictory conclusions can be caused by the differences in magnification or stain, the image analysis frameworks present several differences. Both studies used supervised classifier approaches, but while Boucheron *et al* used the raw spectral bands of the multispectral image as features for classification, Qi *et al* used the features, extracted from the multispectral image, that were supposed to maximize the underlying differences between normal and tumor tissue samples. In another study by Ortega *et al* [8], a push-broom hyperspectral microscope was used to acquire 112 hyperspectral images of H&E-stained breast cancer slides from two patients. With the help of pathologist annotation, they extracted hyperspectral patches of cells and built a 2D-CNN to differentiate tumor and normal cells. Despite the small number of patients, their results show that HSI could bring an 8% improvement in classification accuracy compared to RGB.

Beyond the discrimination between normal and tumor tissue, more specific approaches have been recently proposed to identify ductal carcinoma *in situ* (DCIS) or mitotic cells within breast histological slides. In one approach, Khouj *et al* [70] proposed the detection of DCIS with HSI using two types of specimen preparations of breast biopsies: unstained and H&E-stained. Using as inputs some pixels manually annotated by pathologists, a semi-supervised k-means approach was applied to both types of images, suggesting a good discrimination between normal and tumor regions even in unstained samples. Additionally, mitotic cells counting is an important indicator in breast cancer grading. Ludovis *et al* [71] proposed a contest for detecting mitotic cells within H&E-stained breast cancer specimens. In this contest, three types of datasets were released: two of them composed of conventional RGB images, and a single dataset composed of MS images. In this challenge, the detection of mitotic cells was suggested to be superior to conventional imaging approaches.

1.4.3 Gastrointestinal cancer

Gastrointestinal cancer is a broad concept including all cancers in the digestive tract organs, and it is another field where hyperspectral microscopy has been actively investigated. Colorectal cancer was one of the most prominent applications. Many preliminary works have been done using HSI/MSI to discrimination between benign adenoma and malignant carcinoma tissues within H&E-stained colon histological slides since a decade ago [14]. In recent years, studies focused more on the refined methods for colon cancer detection, such as the use of texture features or CNNs. However, most studies employed MSI instead of HSI [14].

Other than colorectal cancer, HSI has shown promise in hepatic cancer detection. Wang and Li evaluated the ability of microscopic HSI to early detect bile duct carcinoma within H&E-stained rat liver samples [36]. In this research, the authors were able to quantitatively measure the tumor areas in the biopsies at different time points through the analysis of the hyperspectral data with a feature extraction method based on the morphological watershed algorithm followed by SVM classification. Chen *et al* [32] used an LCTF-based hyperspectral microscope to obtain the spatial-spectral data of H&E-stained hepatic carcinoma tissue slides, and employed an SVM classifier to differentiate the transmission spectra of cancerous and normal nuclei, which achieved 99% sensitivity and 98% specificity. Liu *et al* [31] also employed an LCTF-based system and trained an SVM model, but their classifier was used to different cells based on fluorescent spectral characteristics of DAPI-stained slides. Finally, Huang *et al* [72] used a CNN for the diagnosis of hepatobiliary tumors and got an accuracy of 85%–90%.

Three studies have been done on gastric cancer detection using hyperspectral microscopy. First, Zhu *et al* [34] divided the transmission spectra of normal and cancerous nuclei into three zones, where the spectra showed different trends. By calculating the Euclidean distance between normal and cancerous spectra, they claimed that using part of the spectra could achieve better differentiation than using the entire spectra. Then, Hu *et al* [73] proposed four deep learning classifiers using the spectral-only, spatial-spectral after dimension reduction, and full spatial-spectral features, respectively. The results show that the network based on full spatial-spectral patches has the best performance with an accuracy of 97.57%. In addition, Liu *et al* [62] used a shallow residual network for gastric cancer detection in hyperspectral images of H&E-stained slides and achieved a 91.44% accuracy, which was 13.87% higher than that of the color images.

Similarly, Ishikawa *et al* [21] compared the cancer detection performance using hyperspectral and RGB image for pancreatic tumor, and they found a 14% improvement using HSI. In this work, they developed a whole-slide scanning microscope as well as a sophisticated HSI processing pipeline, which involved construction of HDR images, band reduction, estimation of dye amount, re-estimation of absorbance, and classification of nuclei pixels. Moreover, Notarstefano *et al* [74] employed Fourier transform infrared hyperspectral imaging (FTIR-HSI) to analyze biomedical compositions (lipids, proteins, and phosphates and carbohydrates) in normal, dysplasia, pancreatic neuroendocrine tumor (PNET) and pancreatic ductal adenocarcinoma (PDAC) tissue samples.

1.4.4 Blood cancer

White blood cells, also called leukocytes, are hematopoietic cells of the immune system that are involved in protecting the body against both infectious diseases and foreign materials. The abnormal development and uncontrolled proliferation of these cells can lead to devastating blood cancers, also known as leukemia. Their timely recognition in the peripheral blood is critical to diagnosis and treatment [27]. Microscopic examination is one of the most common methods for leukemia diagnosis. In the past decade, HSI has been investigated for leukemia cell identification in several studies. Li *et al* [38] used an AOTF-based molecular hyperspectral imaging microscope to observe blood smears. They proposed an automated algorithm to identify the cytoplasm and the nucleus from leukocyte cells using both spatial features and spectral signatures. Wang *et al* [37] combined spectral and spatial features and used a marker-based learning vector quantization (MLVQ) neural network to to identify lymphoblasts from lymphocytes in hyperspectral images, which yielded 92.9% accuracy. Panda *et al* [75] used Euclidean distance and Mahalanobis distance methods to detect chronic myeloid leukemia neutrophils from hyperspectral images. Moreover, Zhou *et al* [27] used PHSI to enhance the visualization of white blood cells in leukemia blood smears. Based on their polarized imaging microscope setup, both RGB and hyperspectral images were acquired, and Stokes vectors were calculated. Based on the Stokes vectors, three polarization metrics, namely degree of polarization (DOP), degree of linear polarization (DOLP), and degree of circular polarization (DOCP) were obtained. It was found that the derived polarization metrics could improve the visualization of surface structures (protein patterns) of lymphocytes and enable subclassification of lymphocyte subpopulations.

1.5 Conclusion and discussion

In this chapter, we discussed the most relevant aspects of hyperspectral imaging for the analysis of histopathological specimens, specifically in cancer studies. The chapter focused on four major categories: the mechanism of HSI in microscopy, the hardware and software fulfillment of whole-slide hyperspectral imaging, the multi-modality microscopy involving HSI, and the recent applications of hyperspectral microscopy in cancer research.

First, we explained how different types of HSI devices were incorporated into microscope systems. Although there are four major types of HSI systems, spectral-scanning and push-broom remain the dominant types in most existing works due to their high resolution and large availability. Nevertheless, the newly developed spatial-spectral scanning snapscan hyperspectral cameras as well as the scope-free snapshot microscopy systems are very promising and may replace the conventional microscopic imaging setups in the future.

Whole-slide scanning of the histological slides and the quality of digitized whole-slide image are critical for digital pathology. Implementing hyperspectral whole-slide imaging with precise scanning and autofocusing is necessary for HSI to be integrated into routine pathology workflow. The current obstacles mainly lie in the following facts: hyperspectral image files are large, the speed of scanning-based HSI acquisition is slow, and autofocus algorithms are needed to ensure good focus for all wavelength bands. Although a few automated whole-slide hyperspectral microscopes have been developed, they are not widely employed due to the above-mentioned reasons. Super-resolution reconstruction and extended depth of field of hyperspectral histological images are promising solutions. Future works should investigate using these techniques with snapshot-based microscopy system to boost the speed and image quality of hyperspectral histological images.

As for multi-modality imaging, HSI has been combined with various imaging modalities, such as confocal microscopy, dark-field microscopy, fluorescence imaging, and polarized light imaging, whereas the last two were mostly used in cancer studies. On the one hand, HSI has been proved useful for detecting both endogenous and exogenous fluorescence signals. Especially, HSI might show great advantage if combined with the novel type of rapid slide-free histology method [76, 77]. On the other hand, a series of studies have been done on the development and utilization of a polarized hyperspectral imaging microscope system, which brings enhanced visualization of molecular compositions in histology slides. Further work needs to be done on the automation of the system, as it takes more acquisition time than normal HSI.

Finally, we reviewed the applications of HSI in cancer studies in the recent decade. Head and neck cancer, gastrointestinal cancer, and breast cancer are the three major types that HSI has been investigated on. Other than those, several studies employed HSI to analyze white blood cells in leukemia blood smears. Earlier studies tend to reply more on the transmission spectra extracted from hyperspectral images. With the development of more advanced artificial intelligence (AI) algorithms, different types of deep neural networks have been used in more recent works to exploit the rich spatial-spectral features. However, in addition to simply training the deep learning networks to automatically learn the features, research should be done to gain perspectives about the relationship between the spectral features and biomarkers. Further and deeper understanding of the hyperspectral histological images will benefit the development of AI tools specifically for medical HSI and possibly promote the future utilization of HSI in histopathology.

In conclusion, HSI is a beneficial tool for histopathological cancer research and has become an popular research topic. With future refinement of hyperspectral microscopy systems and image processing algorithms, HSI may be actively utilized in routine histopathology workflow to facilitate cancer diagnosis.

Bibliography

[1] Madabhushi A and Lee G 2016 Image analysis and machine learning in digital pathology: challenges and opportunities *Med. Image Anal.* **33** 170–5

[2] Nam S, Chong Y, Jung C K, Kwak T-Y, Lee J Y, Park J, Rho M J and Go H 2020 Introduction to digital pathology and computer-aided pathology *J. Pathol. Transl Med. JPTM* **54** 125–34

[3] Lu G and Fei B 2014 Medical hyperspectral imaging: a review *J. Biomed. Opt.* **19** 010901

[4] Fei B 2019 *Data Handling in Science and Technology* ed J M Amigo (Amsterdam: Elsevier) pp 523–65

[5] Litjens G, Bandi P, Bejnordi B E, Geessink O, Balkenhol M, Bult P, Halilovic A, Hermsen M, van de Loo R, Vogels R, Manson Q F, Stathonikos N, Baidoshvili A, van Diest P, Wauters C, van Dijk M and van der Laak J 2018 1399 H&E-stained sentinel lymph node sections of breast cancer patients: the CAMELYON dataset *GigaScience* **7** giy065

[6] Spanhol F A, Oliveira L S, Petitjean C and Heutte L 2016 A dataset for breast cancer histopathological image classification *IEEE Trans. Biomed. Eng.* **63** 1455–62

[7] Ortega S, Fabelo H, Halicek M, Camacho R, Plaza M D I L, Callicó G M and Fei B 2020 Hyperspectral superpixel-wise glioblastoma tumor detection in histological samples *Appl. Sci.* **10** 4448

[8] Ortega S, Halicek M, Fabelo H, Guerra R, Lopez C, Lejeune M, Godtliebsen F, Callico G and Fei B 2020 Hyperspectral imaging and deep learning for the detection of breast cancer

cells in digitized histological images *Proc. SPIE 11320, Medical Imaging 2020: Digital Pathology, 113200V* vol 11320 (SPIE) 113200V

[9] Ortega S, Halicek M, Fabelo H, Camacho R, Plaza M D I L, Godtliebsen F, Callicó M, Fei G and B 2020 Hyperspectral imaging for the detection of glioblastoma tumor cells in H&E slides using convolutional neural networks *Sensors* **20** 1911

[10] Ma L, Halicek M, Zhou X, Dormer J and Fei B 2020 Hyperspectral microscopic imaging for automatic detection of head and neck squamous cell carcinoma using histologic image and machine learning *Proc. SPIE 11320, Medical Imaging 2020: Digital Pathology* vol 11320 (SPIE) 113200W

[11] Ma L, Zhou X, Little J, Chen A, Myers L, Sumer B and Fei B 2021 Hyperspectral microscopic imaging for the detection of head and neck squamous cell carcinoma on histologic slides *Proc. SPIE 11603, Medical Imaging 2021: Digital Pathology* vol 11603 (SPIE) 116030P

[12] Ma L, Rathgeb A, Mubarak H, Tran M and Fei B 2022 Unsupervised super-resolution reconstruction of hyperspectral histology images for whole-slide imaging *J. Biomed. Opt.* **27** 056502

[13] Ma L, Little J, Chen A, Myers L, Sumer B and Fei B 2022 Automatic detection of head and neck squamous cell carcinoma on histologic slides using hyperspectral microscopic imaging *J. Biomed. Opt.* **27** 046501

[14] Ortega S, Halicek M, Fabelo H, Callico G M and Fei B 2020 Hyperspectral and multispectral imaging in digital and computational pathology: a systematic review [invited] *Biomed. Opt. Express.* **11** 3195–233

[15] Tran M H, Gomez O and Fei B 2023 A video transformer network for thyroid cancer detection on hyperspectral histologic images *Proc. SPIE 12471, Medical Imaging 2023: Digital and Computational Pathology* vol 12471 (SPIE) 1247107

[16] Tran M H, Ma L, Litter J, Chen A and Fei B 2022 Thyroid carcinoma detection on whole histologic slides using hyperspectral imaging and deep learning *Proc. SPIE 12039, Medical Imaging 2022: Digital and Computational Pathology* vol 12039 (SPIE) 120390H

[17] Zhou X, Ma L, Brown W, Little J, Chen A, Myers L, Sumer B and Fei B 2021 Automatic detection of head and neck squamous cell carcinoma on pathologic slides using polarized hyperspectral imaging and machine learning *Proc. SPIE 11603, Medical Imaging 2021: Digital Pathology* vol 11603 (SPIE) 116030Q

[18] Fereidouni F *et al* 2019 Dual-mode emission and transmission microscopy for virtual histochemistry using hematoxylin- and eosin-stained tissue sections *Biomed. Opt. Express.* **10** 6516–30

[19] Ortega S, Guerra R, Díaz M, Fabelo H, López S, Callicó G M and Sarmiento R 2019 Hyperspectral push-broom microscope development and characterization *IEEE Access* **7** 122473–91

[20] Halicek M, Fabelo H, Ortega S, Callico G M and Fei B 2019 In-vivo and ex-vivo tissue analysis through hyperspectral imaging techniques: revealing the invisible features of cancer *Cancers* **11** 756

[21] Ishikawa M, Okamoto C, Shinoda K, Komagata H, Iwamoto C, Ohuchida K, Hashizume M, Shimizu A and Kobayashi N 2019 Detection of pancreatic tumor cell nuclei via a hyperspectral analysis of pathological slides based on stain spectra *Biomed. Opt. Express* **10** 4568–88

[22] Takara Y, Manago N, Saito H, Mabuchi Y, Kondoh A, Fujimori T, Ando F, Suzuki M and Kuze H 2012 Remote sensing applications with NH hyperspectral portable video camera

Proc. SPIE 8527, Multispectral, Hyperspectral, and Ultraspectral Remote Sensing Technology, Techniques and Applications IV vol 8527 (SPIE) 85271G
[23] Pichette J, Charle W and Lambrechts A 2017 Fast and compact internal scanning CMOS-based hyperspectral camera: the Snapscan *Proc. SPIE 10110, Photonic Instrumentation Engineering IV* vol 10110 (SPIE) 1011014
[24] Zhou X, Ma L, Halicek M, Dormer J and Fei B 2020 Development of a polarized hyperspectral microscope for cardiac fiber orientation imaging *Proc. SPIE 11215, Diagnostic and Therapeutic Applications of Light in Cardiology 2020* vol 11213 (SPIE) 112150V
[25] Rathgeb A, Ma L, Tran M and Fei B 2023 Extended depth of field imaging for mosaic hyperspectral images *Proc. SPIE 12471, Medical Imaging 2023: Digital and Computational Pathology* vol 12471 (SPIE) 1247109
[26] Tran M H, Gomez O and Fei B 2023 An automatic whole-slide hyperspectral imaging microscope *Proc. SPIE 12391, Label-free Biomedical Imaging and Sensing (LBIS) 2023* vol 12391 (SPIE) 1239106
[27] Zhou X, Mubarak H, Ma L, Palsgrove D, Ortega S, Callicó G M, Medina E, Brimhall B, Whitted M and Fei B 2023 Polarized hyperspectral microscopic imaging for white blood cells on Wright-stained blood smear slides *Proc. SPIE 12382, Polarized Light and Optical Angular Momentum for Biomedical Diagnostics 2023* vol 12382 (SPIE) 1238207
[28] Zhou X, Mubarak H, Ma L, Palsgrove D, Summer B and Fei B 2023 Polarized hyperspectral microscopic imaging for collagen visualization on pathologic slides of head and neck squamous cell carcinoma *Proc. SPIE 12382, Polarized Light and Optical Angular Momentum for Biomedical Diagnostics 2023* vol 12382 (SPIE) 1238204
[29] Quintana L, Ortega S, Leon R, Fabelo H, Callico G M, Lopez C, Lejeune M and Bosch R 2021 Instrumentation evaluation for hyperspectral microscopy targeting enhanced medical histology In *2021 XXXVI Conf. on Design of Circuits and Integrated Systems (DCIS)* pp 1–6
[30] Tran M H and Fei B 2023 Compact and ultracompact spectral imagers: technology and applications in biomedical imaging *J. Biomed. Opt.* **28** 040901
[31] Liu K, Lin S, Zhu S, Chen Y, Yin H, Li Z and Chen Z 2021 Hyperspectral microscopy combined with DAPI staining for the identification of hepatic carcinoma cells *Biomed. Opt. Express* **12** 173–80
[32] Chen Y, Zhu S, Fu S, Li Z, Huang F, Yin H and Chen Z 2020 Classification of hyperspectral images for detection of hepatic carcinoma cells based on spectral–spatial features of nucleus *J. Innov. Opt. Health Sci.* **13** 2050002
[33] Huang Q, Li W, Zhang B, Li Q, Tao R and Lovell N H 2019 Blood cell classification based on hyperspectral imaging with modulated Gabor and CNN *IEEE J. Biomed. Health Inform.* **24** 160–70
[34] Zhu S, Su K, Liu Y, Yin H, Li Z, Huang F, Chen Z, Chen W, Zhang G and Chen Y 2015 Identification of cancerous gastric cells based on common features extracted from hyperspectral microscopic images *Biomed. Opt. Express* **6** 1135–45
[35] Wang Q, Sun L, Wang Y, Zhou M, Hu M, Chen J, Wen Y and Li Q 2020 Identification of melanoma from hyperspectral pathology image using 3D convolutional networks *IEEE Trans. Med. Imaging* **40** 218–27
[36] Wang J and Li Q 2018 Quantitative analysis of liver tumors at different stages using microscopic hyperspectral imaging technology *J. Biomed. Opt.* **23** 106002

[37] Wang Q, Wang J, Zhou M, Li Q and Wang Y 2017 Spectral-spatial feature-based neural network method for acute lymphoblastic leukemia cell identification via microscopic hyperspectral imaging technology *Biomed. Opt. Express* **8** 3017–28
[38] Li Q, Wang Y, Liu H, He X, Xu D, Wang J and Guo F 2014 Leukocyte cells identification and quantitative morphometry based on molecular hyperspectral imaging technology *Comput. Med. Imaging Graph.* **38** 171–8
[39] Leavesley S J, Griswold J R, Deal J, McAlister K, Mayes S, Browning C, Parker M, Mayes S G and Rich T C 2019 Hyperspectral imaging fluorescence excitation scanning (HIFEX) microscopy for live cell imaging *Three-Dimensional and Multidimensional Microscopy: Image Acquisition and Processing XXVI* (SPIE) pp 92–8
[40] Deal J, Mayes S, Browning C, Hill S, Rider P, Boudreaux C, Rich T C and Leavesley S J 2018 Identifying molecular contributors to autofluorescence of neoplastic and normal colon sections using excitation-scanning hyperspectral imaging *J. Biomed. Opt.* **24** 021207
[41] Yu C, Yang J, Song N, Sun C, Wang M and Feng S 2021 Microlens array snapshot hyperspectral microscopy system for the biomedical domain *Appl. Opt.* **60** 1896–902
[42] Hedde P N, Cinco R, Malacrida L, Kamaid A and Gratton E 2021 Phasor-based hyperspectral snapshot microscopy allows fast imaging of live, three-dimensional tissues for biomedical applications *Commun. Biol.* **4** 1–11
[43] Enfield K S, Martin S D, Marshall E A, Kung S H, Gallagher P, Milne K, Chen Z, Nelson B H, Lam S and English J C 2019 Hyperspectral cell sociology reveals spatial tumor-immune cell interactions associated with lung cancer recurrence *J. Immunother. Cancer* **7** 13
[44] Liao J, Jiang S, Zhang Z, Guo K, Bian Z, Jiang Y, Zhong J and Zheng G 2018 Terapixel hyperspectral whole-slide imaging via slit-array detection and projection *J. Biomed. Opt.* **23** 066503
[45] Liao J, Jiang Y, Bian Z, Mahrou B, Nambiar A, Magsam A W, Guo K, Wang S, Cho Y K and Zheng G 2017 Rapid focus map surveying for whole slide imaging with continuous sample motion *Opt. Lett.* **42** 3379–82
[46] Zhang Q, Wang Y, Li Q, Tao X, Zhou X, Zhang Y and Liu G 2022 An autofocus algorithm considering wavelength changes for large scale microscopic hyperspectral pathological imaging system *J. Biophotonics* **15** e202100366
[47] Jiang Z, Yu Z, Yu Y, Huang Z, Ren Q and Li C 2019 Spatial resolution enhancement for pushbroom-based microscopic hyperspectral imaging *Appl. Opt.* **58** 850–62
[48] Ma L, Rathgeb A, Tran M and Fei B 2022 Unsupervised super resolution network for hyperspectral histologic imaging *Proc. SPIE 12039, Medical Imaging 2022: Digital and Computational Pathology* vol 12039 (SPIE) 120390P
[49] Urbina Ortega C, Quevedo Gutiérrez E, Quintana L, Ortega S, Fabelo H, Santos Falcón L and Marrero Callico G 2023 Towards real-time hyperspectral multi-image super-resolution reconstruction applied to histological samples *Sensors* **23** 1863
[50] Bertani F R, Botti E, Ferrari L, Mussi V, Costanzo A, D'Alessandro M, Cilloco F and Selci S 2016 Label-free and non-invasive discrimination of HaCaT and melanoma cells in a co-culture model by hyperspectral confocal reflectance microscopy *J. Biophotonics* **9** 619–25
[51] Mehta N, Sahu S P, Shaik S, Devireddy R and Gartia M R 2021 Dark-field hyperspectral imaging for label free detection of nano-bio-materials *Wiley Interdiscip. Rev. Nanomed. Nanobiotechnol.* **13** e1661
[52] Tuchin V 2016 Polarized light interaction with tissues *J. Biomed. Opt.* **21** 071114

[53] Anderson R R 1991 Polarized light examination and photography of the skin *Arch. Dermatol.* **127** 1000–5

[54] Pierangelo A *et al* 2013 Polarimetric imaging of uterine cervix: a case study *Opt. Express* **21** 14120–30

[55] Raković M J, Kattawar G W, Mehrűbeoğlu M, Cameron B D, Wang L V, Rastegar S and Coté G L 1999 Light backscattering polarization patterns from turbid media: theory and experiment *Appl. Opt.* **38** 3399–408

[56] Liu B, Yao Y, Liu R, Ma H and Ma L 2019 Mueller polarimetric imaging for characterizing the collagen microstructures of breast cancer tissues in different genotypes *Opt. Commun.* **433** 60–7

[57] Chang J, He H, Wang Y, Huang Y, Li X, He C, Liao R, Zeng N, Liu S and Ma H 2016 Division of focal plane polarimeter-based 3 × 4 Mueller matrix microscope: a potential tool for quick diagnosis of human carcinoma tissues *J. Biomed. Opt.* **21** 56002

[58] Dong Y, Qi J, He H, He C, Liu S, Wu J, Elson D S and Ma H 2017 Quantitatively characterizing the microstructural features of breast ductal carcinoma tissues in different progression stages by Mueller matrix microscope *Biomed. Opt. Express* **8** 3643–55

[59] Vasefi F, MacKinnon N, Saager R B, Durkin A J, Chave R, Lindsley E H and Farkas D L 2014 Polarization-sensitive hyperspectral imaging *in vivo*: a multimode dermoscope for skin analysis *Sci. Rep.* **4** 4924

[60] Wang Z, Zheng W, Hsu C-Y S and Huang Z 2016 Polarization-resolved hyperspectral stimulated Raman scattering microscopy for label-free biomolecular imaging of the tooth *Appl. Phys. Lett.* **108** 033701

[61] Zhou X, Ma L, Mubarak H, Little J, Chen A, Myers L, Sumer B and Fei B 2022 Automatic detection of head and neck squamous cell carcinoma on pathologic slides using polarized hyperspectral imaging and deep learning *Proc. SPIE 12039, Medical Imaging 2022: Digital and Computational Pathology* vol 12039 (SPIE) 120390G

[62] Liu S, Wang Q, Zhang G, Du J, Hu B and Zhang Z 2020 Using hyperspectral imaging automatic classification of gastric cancer grading with a shallow residual network *Anal. Methods* **12** 3844–53

[63] Zhang Q, Wang Y, Qiu S, Chen J, Sun L and Li Q 2021 3D-PulCNN: pulmonary cancer classification from hyperspectral images using convolution combination unit based CNN *J. Biophotonics* **14** e202100142

[64] Maktabi M, Wichmann Y, Köhler H, Ahle H, Lorenz D, Bange M, Braun S, Gockel I, Chalopin C and Thieme R 2022 Tumor cell identification and classification in esophageal adenocarcinoma specimens by hyperspectral imaging *Sci. Rep.* **12** 1–14

[65] Ou-Yang M, Hsieh Y-F and Lee C-C 2015 Biopsy diagnosis of oral carcinoma by the combination of morphological and spectral methods based on embedded relay lens microscopic hyperspectral imaging system *J. Med. Biol. Eng.* **35** 437–47

[66] Hahn L D, Hoyt C, Rimm D L and Theoharis C 2013 Spatial spectral imaging as an adjunct to the Bethesda classification of thyroid fine-needle aspiration specimens *Cancer Cytopathol.* **121** 162–7

[67] He C, He H, Chang J, Dong Y, Liu S, Zeng N, He Y and Ma H 2015 Characterizing microstructures of cancerous tissues using multispectral transformed Mueller matrix polarization parameters *Biomed. Opt. Express* **6** 2934–45

[68] Boucheron L E, Bi Z, Harvey N R, Manjunath B S and Rimm D L 2007 Utility of multispectral imaging for nuclear classification of routine clinical histopathology imagery *BMC Cell Biol.* **8** S8
[69] Qi X, Xing F, Foran D and Yang L 2011 Comparative performance analysis of stained histopathology specimens using RGB and multispectral imaging *Proc. SPIE 7963, Medical Imaging 2011: Computer-Aided Diagnosis* vol 7963 (SPIE) 79633B
[70] Khouj Y, Dawson J, Coad J and Vona-Davis L 2018 Hyperspectral imaging and K-means classification for histologic evaluation of ductal carcinoma *in situ Front. Oncol.* **8** 17
[71] Ludovic R, Daniel R, Nicolas L, Maria K, Humayun I, Jacques K, Frédérique C, Catherine G, Gilles L N and Metin N G 2013 Mitosis detection in breast cancer histological images An ICPR 2012 contest *J. Pathol. Informatics* **4** 8
[72] Huang S, Luo J, Pu K and Wu M 2022 Diagnosis system of microscopic hyperspectral image of hepatobiliary tumors based on convolutional neural network *Comput. Intel. Neurosci.* **2022** 794844
[73] Hu B, Du J, Zhang Z and Wang Q 2019 Tumor tissue classification based on micro-hyperspectral technology and deep learning *Biomed. Opt. Express* **10** 6370–89
[74] Notarstefano V, Sabbatini S, Conti C, Pisani M, Astolfi P, Pro C, Rubini C, Vaccari L and Giorgini E 2020 Investigation of human pancreatic cancer tissues by Fourier Transform Infrared hyperspectral imaging *J. Biophotonics* **13** e201960071
[75] Panda A, Pachori R B and Sinnappah-Kang N D 2021 Classification of chronic myeloid leukemia neutrophils by hyperspectral imaging using Euclidean and Mahalanobis distances *Biomed. Signal Process. Control.* **70** 103025
[76] Fereidouni F *et al* 2017 Microscopy with ultraviolet surface excitation for rapid slide-free histology *Nat. Biomed. Eng.* **1** 957–66
[77] Fereidouni F, Morningstar T, Abraham T and Levenson R 2022 FIBI (Fluorescence Imitating Brightfield Imaging) for slide-free rapid histopathology *Biophotonics Congress: Biomedical Optics 2022 (Translational, Microscopy, OCT, OTS, BRAIN)* (Fort Lauderdale, Florida: Optica Publishing Group) p MW3A.2
[78] Dey N, Li S, Bermond K, Heintzmann R, Curcio C A, Ach T and Gerig G 2019 Multi-modal image fusion for multispectral super-resolution in microscopy *Proc. SPIE 10949, Medical Imaging 2019: Image Processing* 109490D
[79] Liu L, Qi M, Li Y, Liu Y, Liu X, Zhang Z and Qu J 2022 Staging of skin cancer based on hyperspectral microscopic imaging and machine learning *Biosensors* **12** 790
[80] Ma L, Little J V, Chen A Y, Myers L L, Sumer B D and Fei B 2022 Automatic detection of head and neck squamous cell carcinoma on histologic slides using hyperspectral microscopic imaging *J. Biomed. Opt.* **27** 046501

IOP Publishing

Spectroscopic Techniques for Cancer Diagnostics

Inbarasan Muniraj and Bryan Hennelly

Chapter 2

Advancing oral cancer detection through hyperspectral imaging and deep learning techniques

Valluri Ayyappa, Aala Suresh, Mukkara Prasanna Kumar and Sunil Chinnadurai

Cancer is a particularly dangerous disease, often leading to high mortality rates due to late-stage detection. Among the various types of cancer, oral cancer stands out as a significant threat, playing a major role in the high number of cancer-related deaths. Oral cancer, which affects the tissues of the mouth and throat, is frequently undiagnosed in its early stages, making timely intervention difficult. Despite advancements in medical science, the lack of early diagnostic tools remains a critical challenge, contributing to the significant death toll associated with this disease. To address this, advanced imaging technologies, such as hyperspectral imaging (HSI), have emerged as powerful tools for non-invasive detection. HSI captures detailed spectral information across a wide range of wavelengths, allowing for the precise differentiation between cancerous and healthy tissues. When combined with deep learning (DL) algorithms, HSI enhances the accuracy and efficiency of oral cancer diagnosis, enabling early detection and better treatment outcomes. This chapter explores various imaging techniques and DL methods that are being developed and applied to improve the detection and diagnosis of oral cancer. It also discusses the importance of diverse and comprehensive datasets in training these models. To overcome the challenge of dataset availability in oral cancer detection, we created a synthetic dataset using HSI that includes spectral signatures for both cancerous and normal tissues. This dataset is essential for developing accurate diagnostic models, as it enables the generation of realistic images through a bilinear mixing model and the extraction of key spectral signatures using vertex component analysis (VCA) and abundances using non-negative least squares (NNLS) and calculated the performance metrics are spectral angle distance (SAD) and root mean square error (RMSE). This process enhances model precision, supporting early detection efforts and demonstrating the potential of advanced imaging and AI technologies in

doi:10.1088/978-0-7503-5949-8ch2

revolutionizing cancer diagnosis. The integration of HSI with AI-driven analysis offers a promising approach to overcoming the challenges of early detection, potentially reducing the mortality associated with oral cancer.

2.1 Introduction

Cancer starts when genetic mutations cause cells to grow uncontrollably. Different types of cancer, like carcinomas and sarcomas, originate from various tissues in the body. Detecting cancer early is crucial for better treatment outcomes. New imaging techniques and DL algorithms help spot cancer more accurately and quickly. These advancements improve diagnosis and treatment, offering better chances for recovery.

2.1.1 Cancer

Cancer is a complex group of diseases characterized by the uncontrolled growth and spread of abnormal cells, which can invade surrounding tissues and metastasize to distant body parts. The genetic mutations responsible for these processes disrupt the normal regulatory mechanisms of cell division and death, leading to tumor formation. The different types of cancer include carcinomas, sarcomas, leukemias, lymphomas, melanomas, and germ cell tumors, each originating from distinct cell types and tissues. This highlights the genetic foundations of various cancers, explaining how different mutations in epithelial, connective, and hematopoietic tissues result in specific cancer types, such as carcinomas and leukemias. The chapter emphasizes the shared molecular mechanisms underlying these diverse diseases, despite their varied origins, making it a valuable reference for understanding the complexity of cancer [1].

The different types of cancers are:

- Carcinomas: cancers originating from epithelial cells, including adenocarcinoma (from glandular tissues), squamous cell carcinoma (SCC) (from squamous epithelium), and basal cell carcinoma (from the skin's basal layer).
- Sarcomas: cancers arising in connective tissues like bones, muscles, and fat, such as osteosarcoma (bone cancer), liposarcoma (fat tissue cancer), and chondrosarcoma (cartilage cancer).
- Leukemias: blood cancers characterized by the overproduction of abnormal white blood cells in the bone marrow and blood without forming solid tumors.
- Lymphomas: cancers of the lymphatic system, including Hodgkin lymphoma (with Reed–Sternberg cells) and non-Hodgkin lymphoma (a diverse group of lymphatic cancers).
- Melanomas: aggressive skin cancers originating from melanocytes, the pigment-producing cells in the skin.
- Germ cell tumors: cancers originating from reproductive cells, typically in the ovaries or testes, such as testicular cancer and ovarian germ cell tumors.

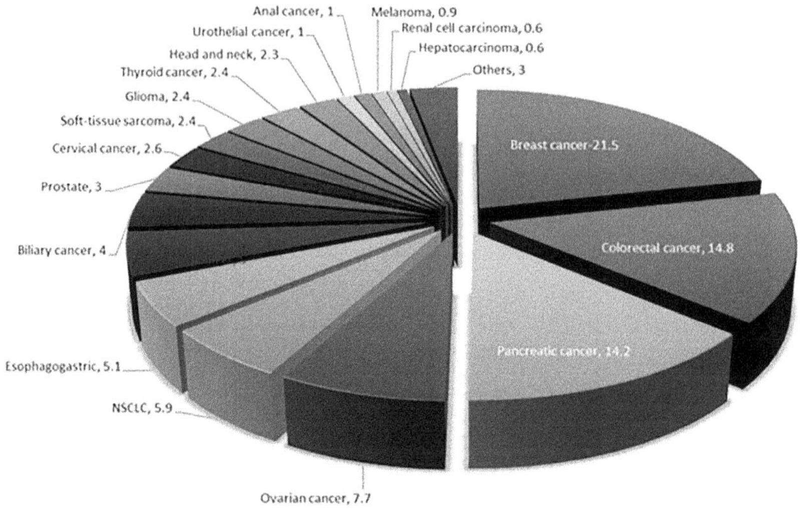

Figure 2.1. Different types of cancers with their percentages.

The different types of cancers according to their respective percentages are illustrated in the figure 2.1. Breast cancer accounts for the largest proportion, comprising 21.5% of cases. Colorectal cancer follows at 14.8%, with pancreatic cancer at 14.2%. Ovarian cancer makes up 7.7% of cases, while NSCLC (non-small cell lung cancer) and esophagogastric cancer contribute 5.9% and 5.1%, respectively. Other notable types include biliary cancer (4%), prostate cancer (3%), and cervical cancer (2.6%). Smaller percentages are observed for cancers such as glioma, thyroid, and melanoma, each representing less than 3% of the total cases. The chart highlights the relative prevalence of different cancers, with breast, colorectal, and pancreatic cancers being the most common [2].

The four stages of cancer progression, illustrated in figure 2.2, begin with the early stage, where a small tumor is present without any spread to lymph nodes or surrounding tissues. As cancer advances to the localized stage, the tumor grows larger and may spread to nearby lymph nodes, indicating a more confined spread. In the regional spread stage, the cancer further progresses, affecting surrounding tissues and spreading to distant lymph nodes, showing a more advanced state. Finally, in the distant spread stage, the cancer reaches its most severe form, spreading to distant organs or tissues, marking it advanced or metastatic. This progression highlights the increasing severity and spread of cancer as it advances through these stages.

2.1.2 Oral cancer

Oral cancer refers to malignancies that occur in the tissues of the mouth or throat, including the lips, tongue, cheeks, gums, floor of the mouth, hard and soft palates, and the pharynx (throat). Most oral cancers are SCC, which originate in the thin,

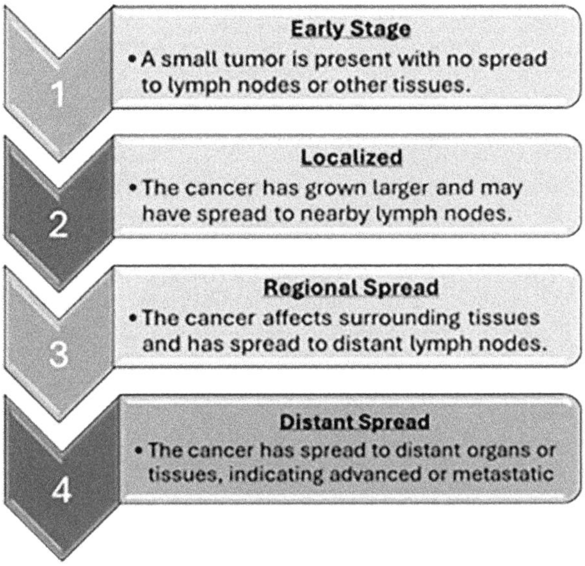

Figure 2.2. Stages of cancer.

flat cells that line the mouth and throat. Oral cancers can also manifest in the salivary glands as adenocarcinomas or mucoepidermoid carcinomas, although these are less common. Verrucous carcinoma is a slow-growing variant of SCC, while oral melanomas are rare but aggressive cancers that arise from pigment-producing cells. Lymphomas can also occur in the oral cavity, typically in the tonsils or base of the tongue. Each type of oral cancer presents unique challenges in diagnosis and treatment.

Risk factors for oral cancer are the various elements or conditions that increase an individual's likelihood of developing cancer in the mouth or surrounding areas, such as the lips, tongue, cheeks, and throat, as seen in figure 2.3. These factors can be lifestyle-related, such as tobacco use and excessive alcohol consumption, or biological, like age and genetic predisposition. Environmental exposures, poor oral hygiene, and certain infections also contribute to the risk. Understanding these risk factors is crucial for preventing, detecting, and effectively treating oral cancer [3].

- **Tobacco smoking:** A major risk factor for oral carcinogenesis involving cigarettes, cigars, pipes, and chewing tobacco.
- **Alcohol consumption:** Excessive alcohol use significantly increases oral cancer risk, particularly when combined with tobacco.
- **Betel quid use:** Commonly used in some cultures, betel quid is strongly associated with increased oral cancer risk.
- **Diet and nutrition:** Poor dietary habits, especially low intake of fruits and vegetables, contribute to a higher risk of oral cancer.
- **Aging:** The likelihood of developing oral cancer increases with age, particularly in individuals over 50 years.

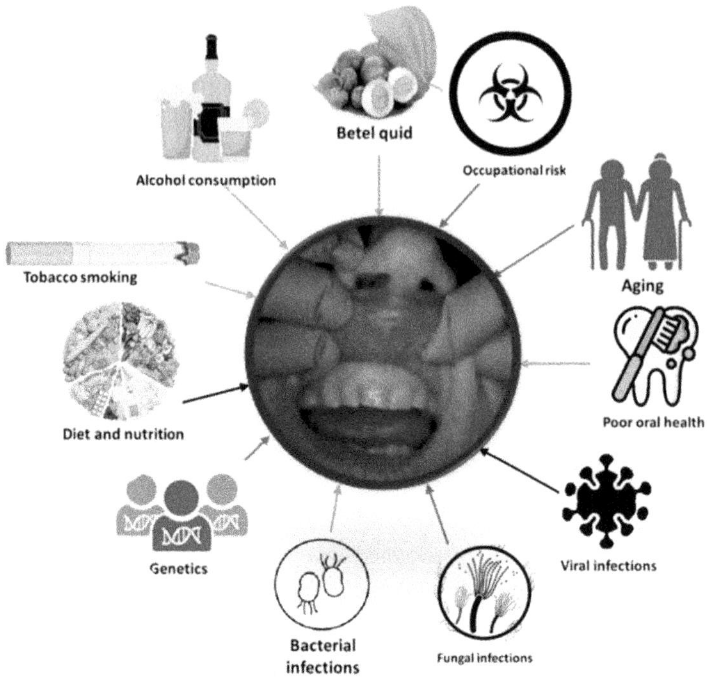

Figure 2.3. Risk factors of oral cancer. Reproduced from [4]. CC BY 4.0.

- **Genetics:** A family history of cancer enhances susceptibility to oral carcinogenesis.
- **Poor oral health:** Chronic irritation and poor dental hygiene are contributing factors to oral cancer.
- **Occupational risk:** Certain work environments may expose individuals to carcinogenic substances, increasing oral cancer risk.
- **Viral, fungal, and bacterial infections:** Infections, including HPV, significantly contribute to the development of oral cancer.

Symptoms of oral cancer can be subtle in the early stages but progressively worse if left untreated. Recognizing these signs early is crucial for timely diagnosis and treatment. The following symptoms are common indicators of oral cancer:

- **Persistent mouth sores:** Ulcers or sores in the mouth that do not heal within two weeks.
- **Lumps or thickened areas:** Unexplained lumps, bumps, or thickened areas in the mouth or throat.
- **Red or white patches:** Patches inside the mouth that are red, white, or a combination of both.
- **Unexplained bleeding:** Bleeding in the mouth without an obvious cause.

- **Numbness or pain:** Numbness, tenderness, or pain in any area of the face, mouth, or neck.
- **Difficulty swallowing:** Trouble with swallowing, chewing, or moving the jaw or tongue.
- **Changes in voice:** Hoarseness, chronic sore throat, or changes in voice.
- **Ear pain:** Persistent earache without hearing loss.
- **Loose teeth:** Teeth becoming loose for no apparent reason.
- **Weight loss:** Unexplained weight loss can be a sign of advanced oral cancer.

2.1.3 Clinical management and detection methods of oral cancer

The clinical management of oral cancer involves examining its effects, determining the stage, and planning appropriate treatment. Diagnosis includes a clinical examination, biopsy, and imaging to assess the presence and extent of cancer. Treatment typically involves surgery, radiation, and/or chemotherapy based on the cancer's stage. Prognosis varies, with earlier stages generally having a better outlook compared to more advanced stages. Each one is explained in detail below.

Diagnosis of oral cancer involves a combination of clinical examination, biopsy, and imaging techniques to detect and assess the extent of the disease. Traditional methods such as visual inspection, palpation, and biopsy remain the gold standard, while imaging techniques like computed tomography scans, MRIs, and PET scans provide valuable information on the spread of the disease. Studies like those by Kaur *et al* (2021) highlight the development of point-of-care devices that improve survival rates by enabling early-stage diagnosis [5]. Additionally, other research emphasizes the role of light-based technologies and fluorescence imaging in detecting early oral cancer lesions, offering a non-invasive alternative to traditional biopsy methods [6]. These advancements and conventional methods provide a comprehensive approach to oral cancer diagnosis.

Treatment for oral cancer varies based on the tumor's stage and location, with options including surgery, radiation therapy, chemotherapy, and newer approaches like targeted therapy and immunotherapy. Surgery remains the primary treatment for resectable tumors, often combined with radiation or chemotherapy to enhance outcomes. Recent research has explored advanced techniques, such as nanomedical drug delivery systems, which improve the selectivity and efficacy of chemotherapeutic agents, reducing toxicity to healthy tissues [7]. The Cochrane review by Worthington *et al* (2023) evaluates surgical interventions and supports elective neck dissection for better survival rates in patients with clinically negative neck nodes [8]. Additionally, Shah *et al* (2023) discuss the challenges associated with chemotherapy and radiotherapy, including their adverse effects and economic burden, highlighting the need for improved management strategies [9]. These studies underscore the complexity of oral cancer treatment and the continuous evolution of therapeutic approaches to enhance patient outcomes.

Prognosis of oral cancer is influenced by several key factors, including the stage of the disease at diagnosis, tumor size, lymph node involvement, and response to treatment. Early-stage oral cancers generally have a more favorable prognosis compared to advanced stages, where the presence of metastasis and poor differentiation significantly worsen outcomes. For instance, a study by Boonpoapichart *et al* (2021) identifies critical prognostic factors in oral tongue SCC, highlighting that advanced tumor, node and mestastais stage, poor histologic grade, and large tumor size are associated with lower survival rates [10]. Another study by Mes *et al* (2017) demonstrates that integrating gene expression profiles with clinical variables can significantly enhance survival prediction, particularly in early-stage oral SCC, which could prevent overtreatment in many cases [11]. These studies underscore the importance of a comprehensive approach in assessing prognosis, combining clinical staging with molecular and histopathological factors to tailor treatments.

Oral cancer detection involves various methods designed to identify abnormalities in the oral cavity, ranging from visual inspections to advanced imaging techniques. Each method has its own strengths and limitations, influencing its effectiveness in diagnosing and staging the disease. Early detection is crucial for improving outcomes, but challenges such as false positives, invasive procedures, and the need for specialized equipment can impact the diagnostic process. The following methods provide a comprehensive approach to detecting oral cancer, each with its specific role and considerations, and each method is explained in detail below.

1. **Visual examination:** Dentists and healthcare providers typically begin with a thorough visual inspection of the oral cavity, looking for any abnormalities such as sores, lumps, or discolored patches. Limitations: early-stage oral cancer can be difficult to distinguish from benign conditions, leading to potential delays in diagnosis. Visual exams rely heavily on the clinician's experience and may miss subtle or hidden lesions [12].
2. **Palpation:** This involves physically feeling the tissues in the mouth and neck for lumps or thickened areas that may indicate cancer. Limitations: palpation may not detect deep or early-stage tumors, and it is less effective in identifying cancers that do not present as palpable masses [12].
3. **Toluidine blue staining:** A dye that selectively stains abnormal tissues is applied to the mouth. Areas that retain the dye may indicate cancerous or precancerous lesions. Limitations: while useful, toluidine blue can produce false positives, staining normal tissues, leading to unnecessary anxiety or biopsies [5].
4. **Brush biopsy (OralCDx):** A brush is used to collect cells from a suspicious area for microscopic examination. Limitations: brush biopsy is non-invasive but may not be as definitive as a surgical biopsy. It is also less reliable for diagnosing deep or invasive cancers [12].
5. **Biopsy:** The gold standard for diagnosing oral cancer involves taking a tissue sample from the suspicious area and examining it histologically. Limitations: while highly accurate, biopsies are invasive, may cause discomfort, and

require expertise to interpret. There is also a risk of missing the cancer if the biopsy sample does not include the malignant area [5].

6. **Imaging tests (CT, MRI, PET scans):** Used to determine the extent of the cancer and whether it has spread to other areas. Limitations: imaging can be expensive and is usually not part of initial screenings. These methods are typically used after a diagnosis to stage the cancer, rather than for early detection [12].
7. **Fluorescence imaging:** This method uses special lights to detect changes in the tissues that are not visible under normal lighting, identifying abnormal areas for further investigation. Limitations: fluorescence imaging can be influenced by normal factors, leading to false positives. It also requires specific equipment and expertise, limiting its availability in standard clinical settings [5].
8. **Salivary diagnostics:** Experimental approaches involve analysing saliva for biomarkers that indicate the presence of oral cancer. Limitations: these methods are still in the research stage and are not widely available. They also face challenges in differentiating cancer-specific markers from those caused by other oral conditions [12].

2.1.4 Hyperspectral imaging

HSI is an advanced imaging technique that captures data across a broad spectrum of light, far beyond the capabilities of the human eye and conventional cameras. Unlike traditional imaging, which typically relies on three primary colors (red, green, and blue), HSI gathers information across hundreds of narrow wavelength bands. This capability allows for the creation of a detailed spectral signature for each pixel in an image, enabling precise identification and analysis of materials based on their unique spectral properties. Originally developed for remote sensing and space exploration, HSI has now expanded into various fields, including agriculture, environmental monitoring, and industrial quality control. The technique offers significant advantages, such as providing detailed and accurate spectral information, being non-invasive and non-destructive, and exhibiting high sensitivity to subtle differences in materials. Furthermore, HSIs can be integrated with real-time analysis systems, making them particularly valuable for applications that require immediate decision-making. Recent studies have demonstrated its effectiveness in diverse areas, such as non-invasive blood oxygen saturation assessment in medical diagnostics [13], monitoring agricultural conditions like nutrient deficiencies and pest infestations [14], and forensic science for analysing complex crime scene materials [15].

1. **Hyperspectral imaging in cancer detection:** In medical imaging, HSI has emerged as a powerful tool for cancer detection and diagnosis. Its ability to capture detailed spectral data from biological tissues allows for the differentiation of healthy, precancerous, and cancerous tissues based on their unique spectral signatures. This capability is particularly valuable in

oncology, where early detection of cancer can significantly improve patient outcomes. HSI's non-invasive nature means that it can be used repeatedly without causing harm to the patient, making it ideal for monitoring disease progression or response to treatment. Furthermore, the high sensitivity of HSI enables it to detect even subtle changes in tissue composition, which might be indicative of early-stage cancer. Compared to traditional imaging techniques like X-rays or MRIs, HSI offers the advantage of providing more specific information about the biochemical and molecular composition of tissues, potentially leading to earlier and more accurate diagnoses [13, 16].

2. **Hyperspectral imaging in oral cancer:** When applied to oral cancer, HSI offers several significant advantages over traditional detection methods. HSI can capture and analyse the light reflected from oral tissues across a wide range of wavelengths, creating detailed spectral signatures that can distinguish between healthy, precancerous, and cancerous tissues. This level of detail is often beyond the capabilities of other methods, such as visual examination, palpation, or even standard imaging techniques. Unlike these traditional methods, which may miss subtle or hidden lesions, HSI can detect early-stage cancer by identifying minute changes in tissue composition that are not visible to the naked eye.

   Figure 2.4 is an example of hyperspectral oral cancer, which has a spatial resolution of 512 × 512 pixels and contains 204 spectral bands. These bands correspond to different wavelengths of light, which allows the analysis of the tissue's biochemical and structural properties at a microscopic level. This detailed data is crucial for distinguishing between healthy tissue and

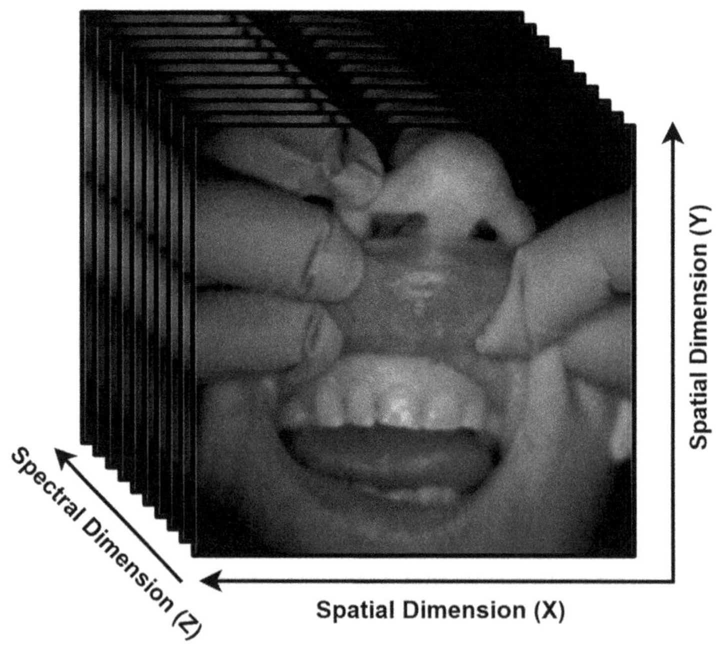

Figure 2.4. Hyperspectral image of oral cancer. Reproduced from [4]. CC BY 4.0.

cancerous tissue, which have different spectral signatures. Moreover, HSI is non-invasive, unlike biopsies, which require tissue removal and can be uncomfortable for the patient. This makes HSI an excellent tool for routine screenings and early detection, potentially reducing the need for invasive procedures. Additionally, HSI can reduce the likelihood of false positives compared to methods like toluidine blue staining, which can stain normal tissues. By offering a more accurate and less invasive means of detecting oral cancer, HSI could play a crucial role in improving early diagnosis and patient outcomes [5, 12].

2.1.5 Artificial intelligence in medical imaging

The role of DL and machine learning (ML) in cancer detection is revolutionizing oral cancer detection by significantly enhancing diagnostic accuracy and efficiency compared to traditional methods. Traditional techniques, such as visual examination, palpation, and biopsy, can be subjective, invasive, and less precise, potentially missing early-stage lesions or leading to false positives. In contrast, ML and DL analyse large datasets and complex medical images with high precision. ML algorithms are adept at identifying patterns in patient data and predicting cancer risk, while DL models, particularly convolutional neural networks (CNNs), excel at processing histopathological and hyperspectral images, detecting and classifying lesions that might be invisible to the naked eye.

Recent advancements underscore the effectiveness of integrating ML and DL with HSI and other non-invasive techniques. For instance, combining DL with hyperspectral imaging allows for a detailed analysis of tissue spectral signatures, greatly improving early cancer detection without the need for invasive procedures [5]. Additionally, ML algorithms facilitate personalized risk prediction and automated image analysis, further enhancing the accuracy and efficiency of cancer screenings. These technologies collectively offer a more precise, efficient, and less invasive approach to oral cancer detection, addressing the limitations of traditional methods and significantly improving overall patient outcomes [12].

2.2 Hyperspectral imaging in oral cancer detection

HSI is an advanced technique that captures detailed spectral information from each pixel, enabling precise material identification and analysis beyond traditional imaging methods. It offers significant advantages, such as non-invasive and highly accurate tissue characterization, which is especially valuable in medical diagnostics like oral cancer detection. HSI's capabilities are enhanced by modern hyperspectral cameras, which are tailored for specific applications with high spectral and spatial resolution, making them indispensable tools for early and accurate diagnosis.

2.2.1 Principles of hyperspectral imaging

HSI is an advanced imaging technique that captures and analyzes a broad spectrum of light from each pixel in an image, providing detailed information far beyond what is visible to the human eye or conventional RGB cameras. Unlike standard imaging, which captures data in just three color bands (red, green, and blue), HSI records data across hundreds of narrow and contiguous wavelength bands, spanning the visible, near-infrared, and sometimes even thermal infrared regions. Each pixel in a hyperspectral image contains a complete spectrum of light, resulting in a 'data cube' where the x and y dimensions represent spatial information, and the z dimension represents spectral information. This rich spectral data allows for precise material identification and analysis based on unique spectral signatures, making HSI a powerful tool for various applications, including remote sensing, environmental monitoring, and medical imaging [16].

The spectral range and resolution of HSI systems are critical factors that influence their performance and suitability for different applications. Spectral range refers to the wavelengths that the hyperspectral sensor can capture, which can vary from visible light (400–700 nm) to extended wavelengths such as near-infrared (700–2500 nm) and even thermal infrared (above 2500 nm). The choice of spectral range depends on the application and the specific features of the materials being studied. Spectral resolution, on the other hand, refers to the ability of the imaging system to distinguish between closely spaced wavelengths. High spectral resolution is crucial for applications requiring detailed spectral analysis, such as detecting subtle changes in tissue composition in medical imaging, where precise differentiation between materials based on their spectral features is essential [13].

Advances in HSI technology have led to significant improvements in both spectral range and resolution, enhancing its capabilities and expanding its applications. Modern hyperspectral sensors can achieve high spectral resolution with narrow wavelength bands, allowing for the detection of fine spectral features and the analysis of complex materials. This is particularly beneficial in fields such as medical diagnostics, where accurate identification of tissue types and early detection of abnormalities are crucial. Innovations in sensor design, data processing algorithms, and integration with other technologies like ML and artificial intelligence have further enhanced the ability of HSI systems to provide detailed and actionable information. These advancements have solidified HSI as a valuable tool in diverse areas, including agriculture, environmental monitoring, and healthcare, where precise material characterization and analysis are essential [17].

2.2.2 Advantages of HSI over traditional imaging

HSI significantly enhances tissue characterization compared to traditional imaging techniques by capturing and analysing detailed spectral data from each pixel. Traditional imaging methods, such as color photographs or standard digital imaging, typically use only three primary color channels (red, green, and blue) to create an image. This limited color information restricts the ability to differentiate between tissues with similar appearances but distinct biochemical compositions. In contrast, HSI acquires data across hundreds of narrow and contiguous wavelength bands, creating a comprehensive spectral profile for each pixel. This allows for precise identification and differentiation of various tissue types based on their unique spectral signatures, such as differences in protein, lipid, and water content. For instance, while traditional imaging might struggle to distinguish between benign and malignant lesions based on visual appearance alone, HSI can detect subtle biochemical changes indicative of cancerous tissue, thus improving diagnostic accuracy and early detection [17]. This advanced capability leads to better-informed treatment decisions and potentially better patient outcomes.

The non-invasive nature of HSI offers a significant advantage over traditional diagnostic techniques, especially for routine screenings and monitoring. Traditional methods, such as biopsies, endoscopies, and imaging modalities like x-rays or MRIs, often involve physical interaction with the patient's body, which can be uncomfortable and carry risks such as infection, bleeding, or adverse reactions. Biopsies, for example, require the extraction of tissue samples for analysis, which can be invasive, distressing, and potentially lead to complications. In contrast, HSI provides a completely non-invasive approach by capturing spectral data from the surface of the tissue through light reflection or absorption without direct physical contact. This approach not only reduces patient discomfort but also avoids the risks associated with invasive procedures, eliminating the need for recovery time. Furthermore, HSI allows for repeated examinations over time to monitor disease progression or treatment response without additional discomfort or risk, making it particularly suitable for applications like routine oral cancer screenings [5]. The combination of safety, comfort, and efficiency underscores HSI's advantages over more invasive diagnostic methods, enhancing early detection and patient management.

2.2.3 Hyperspectral camera technology

Hyperspectral camera technology is vital in oral cancer detection, with several types of cameras suited to different applications. Push-broom cameras offer high spatial resolution by scanning scenes line by line, while snapshot cameras capture entire scenes instantly, making them ideal for quick medical imaging. The key technical specifications for oral cancer detection include a spectral range within the visible and near-infrared wavelengths (400–1000 nm) to detect tissue composition, high spectral resolution (5–10 nm) for distinguishing subtle tissue differences, and adequate spatial resolution (0.1–1 mm) for detailed imaging. High frame rates, sufficient field of view, and high sensitivity with low noise are also critical to ensure accurate and efficient cancer detection. These specifications help optimize HSI for early and non-invasive oral cancer diagnosis. The below table 2.1, has the specifications of HSI cameras.

2.3 Datasets for oral cancer detection

HSI for oral cancer captures detailed spectral information across various wavelengths to detect and analyze tissue types non-invasively. Datasets in HSI research are categorized into animal, human, artificial, *in vivo*, and *ex vivo* types. Animal datasets aid in preclinical studies, human datasets are crucial for real-world applications, and artificial datasets simulate conditions for model refinement. *In vivo* imaging is performed on living organisms, while *ex vivo* imaging involves high-resolution analysis of removed tissues. Synthetic hyperspectral images

Table 2.1. Specifications of different HSI cameras for oral cancer detection

HSI camera	Model	Company	Spectral range	Spectral resolution	Spatial resolution
Push-broom	Pika L	Resonon	400–1000 nm (VNIR)	2.1 nm	Up to 1500 pixels across the line
Push-broom	FX10	Specim	400–1000 nm	5 nm	1024 pixels across the line
Snapshot	Hyper-Cam	Telops	400–1000 nm (VNIR)	2 nm	Up to 640 × 480 pixels
Snapshot	OCI-F	BaySpec	400–1000 nm (VNIR)	4.5 nm	900 × 500 pixels
Whiskbroom	AisaFENIX	Specim	380–2500 nm (VNIR)	3.5 nm	1024 pixels across the line
Imaging Spectrometer	HySpex VNIR-1800	Norsk Elektro Optikk (NEO)	400–1000 nm (VNIR)	3.5 nm	1800 pixels across the line

generated using models like the bilinear mixing model (BMM), mimic real-world conditions to enhance diagnostic tool accuracy.

2.3.1 Sources of oral cancer dataset

HSI is an advanced imaging technique that captures detailed spectral information across different wavelengths, allowing for the non-invasive detection and analysis of various tissue types. In the field of oral cancer research, HSI plays a crucial role in identifying cancerous tissues, monitoring disease progression, and guiding surgical interventions. Datasets used in HSI research are vital for developing and validating these imaging techniques.

These datasets can be categorized based on their origin (animal or human), the nature of the data (artificial or real), and the environment in which the imaging occurs (*in vivo* or *ex vivo*). The following figure 2.5 categorizes these datasets, illustrating the various types of data sources used in oral cancer imaging with HSI.

1. **Animal versus human:**
    - **Animal:** Animal datasets are derived from non-human subjects, such as mice or rats, often used in preclinical studies. These datasets are invaluable for studying the progression of oral cancer and testing responses to treatments in a controlled environment. For instance, HSI can be used to monitor tumor growth in mice, providing insights that are crucial before transitioning to human trials. ML models trained on these datasets can help in identifying spectral signatures unique to cancerous tissues in animal models, which can later be adapted for human studies.

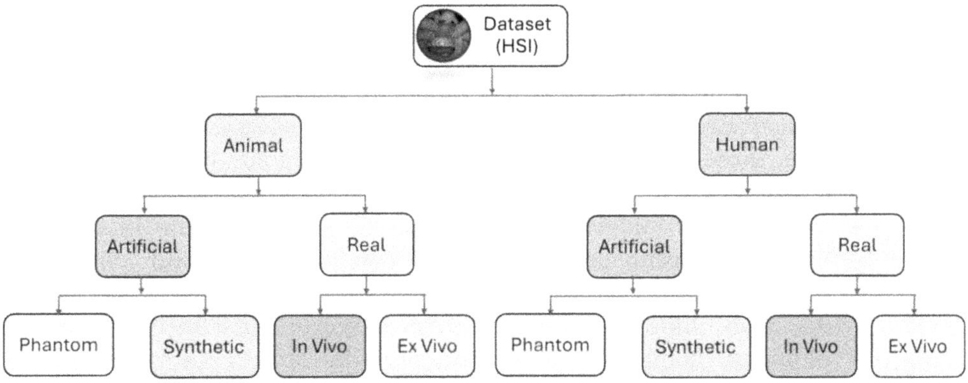

Figure 2.5. Sources of oral cancer datasets for HSI applications. Reproduced from [4]. CC BY 4.0.

- **Human:** Human datasets are obtained from real patients, offering insights into oral cancer within the actual physiological environment of humans. These datasets are critical for developing diagnostic tools, treatment strategies, and validating findings from animal models. For example, hyperspectral images taken during clinical procedures can be used to distinguish between malignant and benign tissues in real time, with ML models trained on such datasets enhancing diagnostic accuracy.

2. **Artificial versus real:**
    - **Artificial:** Artificial datasets are synthetically generated, often through computational simulations or models, to supplement real data. These datasets are particularly useful when real data is limited or difficult to obtain. For instance, synthetic hyperspectral data can be created to simulate different stages of oral cancer, helping in the development and testing of ML models before they are applied to real-world data.
    - **Real:** Real datasets are acquired directly from experiments or clinical procedures involving actual subjects, whether they are animal models or human patients. This type of data reflects true physiological conditions, making it essential for accurate diagnosis and treatment planning. In oral cancer research, real hyperspectral images captured during surgery or biopsy can be used to train DL models to detect and classify cancerous tissues with high precision.
3. **Phantom versus synthetic:**
    - **Phantom:** Phantom datasets involve artificial models that mimic the optical properties of biological tissues. In oral cancer HSI, phantoms are used to calibrate imaging systems and validate algorithms in a controlled environment. For example, phantoms might simulate the spectral characteristics of oral mucosa, allowing researchers to test the accuracy of HSI systems in detecting cancerous tissues under controlled conditions.
    - **Synthetic:** Synthetic datasets are computer-generated and designed to replicate the statistical properties of real data, although they may not

necessarily mimic physical tissue characteristics. These datasets are used to train ML models, test hypotheses, and explore various scenarios in oral cancer detection. For instance, synthetic hyperspectral images can be used to augment training datasets, improving the robustness of ML models in different imaging conditions.

4. ***In vivo* versus *ex vivo*:**
   - ***In vivo*:** This imaging refers to capturing hyperspectral images from living organisms during clinical procedures. For oral cancer, this involves imaging the oral cavity in real time during surgery or diagnosis, allowing for the study of cancerous tissues in their natural biological context. This method provides critical information about factors like blood flow and tissue oxygenation, which are essential for real-time decision-making in clinical settings.
   - ***Ex vivo*:** This imaging involves capturing images from tissues that have been removed from the organism, such as during a biopsy. This method allows for high-resolution imaging in a controlled lab environment, aiding in the detailed pathological analysis of oral cancer tissues. *Ex vivo* datasets are often used to train ML models to distinguish between cancerous and normal tissues with greater accuracy, which can then be applied to *in vivo* imaging.

2.3.2 Hyperspectral synthetic dataset for oral cancer

A hyperspectral synthetic dataset is a collection of computer-generated images that replicate real-world hyperspectral data. These images feature numerous narrow spectral bands, offering detailed information about the materials or objects in each pixel. Researchers use synthetic datasets to simulate various conditions and tissue types, allowing them to test and improve algorithms for detecting differences between cancerous and normal tissues. This helps validate models and methods without the need for real hyperspectral images. Such datasets are especially valuable in fields like remote sensing, medical imaging, and material analysis. Below, we have created a synthetic dataset specifically for distinguishing between cancerous and normal tissues in oral cancer.

2.3.2.1 Importance of synthetic datasets in hyperspectral imaging for oral cancer detection

The necessity of creating synthetic datasets for HSI in oral cancer detection stems from the inherent challenges associated with obtaining real-world data. HSI is a powerful tool that captures extensive spectral information across different wavelengths, allowing for precise differentiation between healthy and diseased tissues. However, acquiring real-world datasets for oral cancer is difficult due to several factors, including privacy concerns, the invasive nature of data collection, ethical considerations, and the requirement for accurate ground-truth labeling by medical experts. These challenges lead to a scarcity of real-world data, limiting the ability to develop, train, and validate robust diagnostic models using ML and DL techniques.

To address the challenges of obtaining real-world data for oral cancer detection, synthetic datasets are crucial. These datasets are created using known spectral signatures of both cancerous and healthy tissues to generate detailed hyperspectral images that resemble real biological tissues. By using synthetic data, researchers can simulate different scenarios and variations in tissue, allowing them to train algorithms in a controlled setting. This helps make up for the lack of real-world data and improves the reliability and effectiveness of diagnostic models. As a result, these models become better at handling the diversity and complexity of real clinical cases, advancing non-invasive cancer detection.

2.3.2.2 Introduction of synthetic dataset

This study aims to create a synthetic HSI dataset to enhance the differentiation between cancerous and normal tissues, thereby improving medical imaging techniques. We start by smoothing the spectral data to clarify the tissue signatures and generate abundance maps showing tissue distribution. A bilinear mixing model is then used to create a realistic synthetic image that simulates how different tissues interact in real scenarios. After generating this synthetic HSI image, the unmixing process is applied to analyze each pixel's composition in detail. VCA identifies the key spectral signatures of the tissues, while NNLS estimates the proportion of each tissue type within each pixel. This step is crucial for accurately mapping the spatial distribution of cancerous and normal tissues. The effectiveness of our approach is evaluated using performance metrics: SAD measures how closely our spectral signatures match the actual ones, and RMSE assesses the precision of our abundance maps.

2.3.2.3 Creation of synthetic dataset

The creation of a synthetic hyperspectral image dataset for distinguishing cancerous and normal tissues begins by smoothing spectral data using a Savitzky–Golay filter. Spectral signatures for each tissue type are defined, and abundance maps are generated to show the distribution of these tissues. A synthetic image is then produced using a bilinear mixing model that combines linear mixtures and nonlinear interactions of the tissue spectra, as shown in figure 2.6. This approach creates a realistic HSI that mimics actual tissue appearance in medical imaging. The resulting data can be used to improve imaging algorithms and techniques for medical diagnostics.

1. **Selection of endmember:** The spectral signatures are the endmembers of cancerous and normal tissues are taken from online. An endmember represents the pure spectral signature of a material or tissue type. In this case, two endmembers are selected, which are the spectral signature (endmember) of normal tissue (ENT) and the spectral signature (endmember) of cancerous tissue (ECT). These endmembers are crucial for generating synthetic hyperspectral images.
2. **Preprocessing (filtering)** The preprocessing typically involves filtering the spectral data to remove unwanted spikes, noise, and enhancing the quality of the spectral signatures. It ensures that the data is clean and suitable for further analysis and modeling, which is essential for accurately generating

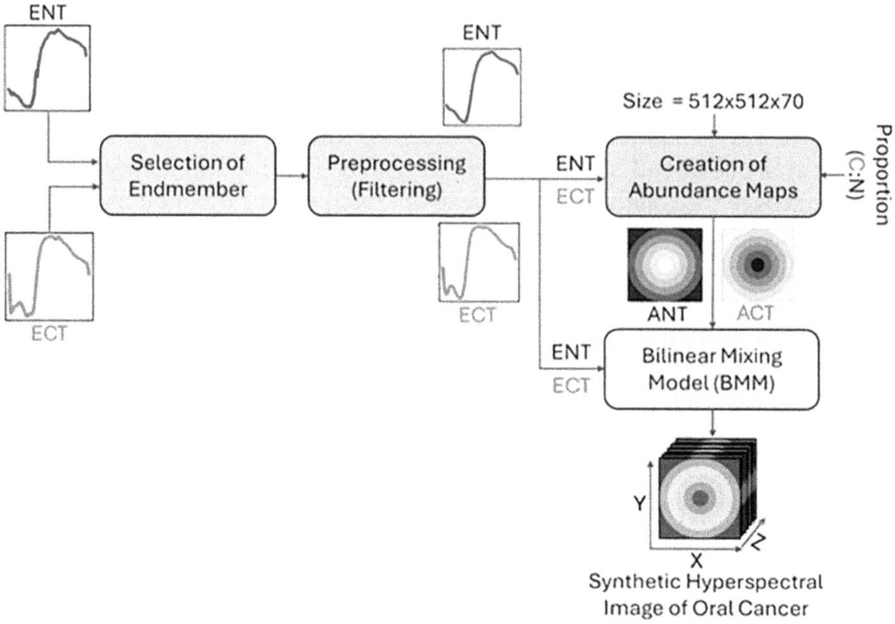

Figure 2.6. Creating a synthetic hyperspectral Iimage dataset for oral cancer.

synthetic images. Here, the Savitzky–Golay filter we are using is a digital filter used to smooth a set of data points, reducing noise while preserving the shape and features of the data's signal.

$$y_i' = \sum_{j=-m}^{m} c_j y_{i+j} \tag{2.1}$$

where:

- y_i': The smoothed value at the ith data point.
- y_{i+j}: The original data points within the window centered at y_i.
- c_j: The filter coefficients determined by the polynomial fit, which dictate the weight of each data point in the window. These coefficients are derived based on the chosen polynomial order and window size.
- m: Half the window size, such that the total number of data points considered in the smoothing process is $2m + 1$.

In the context of the normal and cancerous spectral signatures from HSI data, this filter is applied to improve the quality of the spectral data by smoothing out fluctuations that are considered noise while retaining important spectral features, which are crucial for differentiating between cancerous and normal tissues. The filtered endmembers are called true cancerous and true normal tissues. The spectral signature ECT is shown in figure 2.7, which has 70 spectral bands, each representing a specific wavelength of light. The curve on the graph indicates how much light the cancerous tissue reflects at each wavelength.

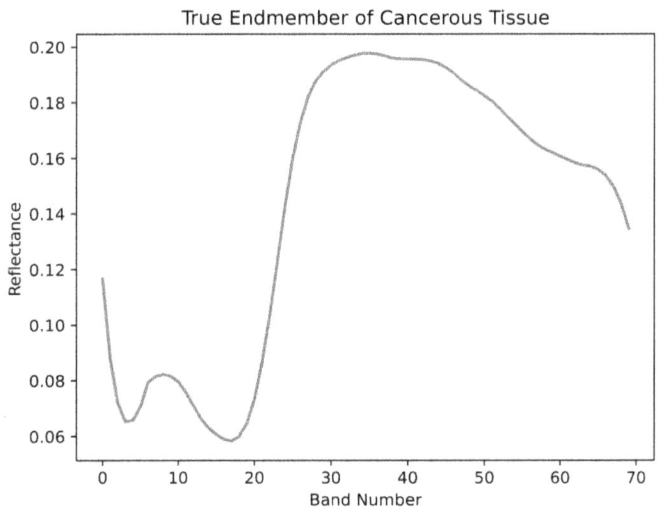

Figure 2.7. True ECT.

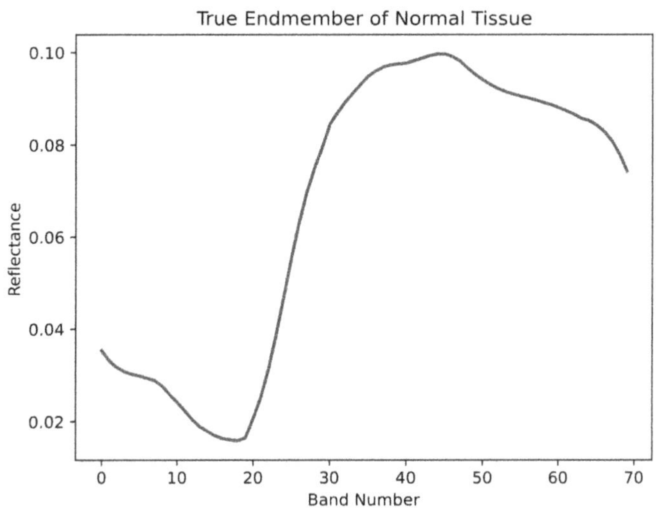

Figure 2.8. True ENT.

This information helps in identifying cancerous areas. The spectral signature ENT is figure 2.8, which has 70 spectral bands, each representing a specific wavelength of light. The shape of the graph and reflectance values on the y-axis indicate how much light the normal tissue reflects at each wavelength means bands, represented on the x-axis.

3. **Creating the abundance maps:** Abundance maps represent the proportion of different materials (in this case, cancerous and normal tissues) present in each pixel of the hyperspectral images. It initializes a blank abundance map of size is 512, 512, 2 for a 512 × 512 image with two classes (cancer and normal). Concentric circular regions are created within the abundance map based on

their distance from the centre. The abundance values are set according to the distance from the centre depends upon the type of tissue which are shown below figures as true abundance maps for cancerous tissue and normal tissue. Cancer abundance values decrease as the distance increases, and the normal abundance is set as the complement.

The formula below calculates the distance from the center point (i, j) to any other point (i', j') for generating abundance maps:

$$\text{Distance} = \sqrt{(i - i')^2 + (j - j')^2} \tag{2.2}$$

These abundance maps are matrices with a size of 512 × 512. For a pixel located at (x, y), the abundance values are represented as $a_N(x, y)$ for normal tissue and $a_C(x, y)$ for cancerous tissue, where:

$$a_N(x, y) + a_C(x, y) = 1 \tag{2.3}$$

This equation ensures that the sum of the abundances for all endmembers at any given pixel equals 1, reflecting the full representation of the pixel by these tissue types.

The abundance map of cancerous tissue (ACT) is a vital visual tool in synthetic hyperspectral image analysis, with dimensions of 512 × 512 pixels. Each pixel corresponds to a specific location within the tissue sample, where the map accurately represents the concentration of cancerous tissue using various shades of red—darker shades signify higher concentrations, while lighter shades indicate lower concentrations. The map displays concentric circles that figure 2.9 illustrates: the actual spread of cancerous cells: the innermost circle represents 100% cancerous tissue, followed by rings with 80%, 60%, 40%, and 20% cancerous tissue, progressively transitioning to the outermost region, which is completely normal. This gradient pattern is essential for understanding the real distribution and clustering of cancerous tissues. The map is derived from analysing data across 70 spectral bands, each capturing distinct wavelengths, and processing this information to obtain an accurate abundance value for each pixel. This detailed representation allows for a precise visual assessment of cancer distribution, assisting in identifying areas that may require more aggressive treatment and enhancing medical decision-making.

The abundance map of normal tissue (ANT) is an essential visual tool in synthetic oral cancer hyperspectral image analysis, with dimensions of 512 × 512 pixels. Each pixel corresponds to a specific location within the tissue sample, accurately representing the concentration of normal tissue. Using various shades of blue darker shades indicate higher concentrations, while lighter shades denote lower concentrations. The map features concentric circles that figure 2.10 illustrates: the innermost circle represents 0% normal tissue, and subsequent rings show progressively increasing concentrations of

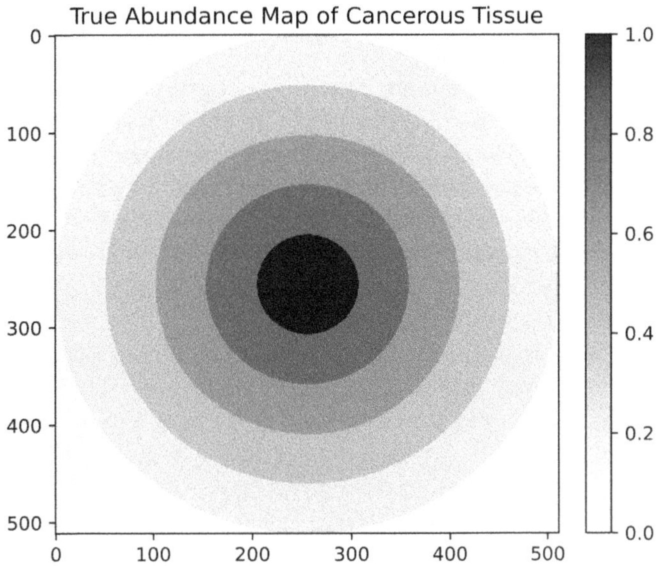

Figure 2.9. True ACT.

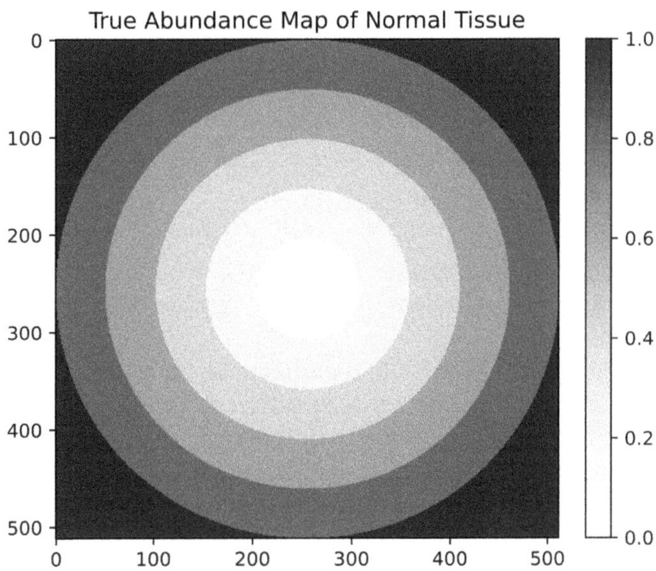

Figure 2.10. True ANT.

normal tissue are 20%, 40%, 60%, and 100%. This gradient pattern is crucial for understanding the distribution and prevalence of normal tissue. The map is generated by analysing data across 70 spectral bands, capturing distinct wavelengths, and processing this information to compute accurate abundance values for each pixel. This detailed visualization supports precise assessments of tissue distribution, aiding in better diagnostic and treatment planning decisions.

4. **Synthetic hyperspectral image:** The image spatial dimensions are 512 × 512, the range of wavelengths from 450 nm to 900 nm, with 70 bands, was generated using a BMM. This model combines linear mixing with nonlinear interactions between the different tissue types to simulate realistic tissue spectra. This model combines the cancerous and normal spectral signatures to form a hyperspectral image with their abundance maps. The BMM combines the ENT and ECT with their respective ANT and ACT to generate the synthetic hyperspectral image.

   The BMM is used to generate the synthetic hyperspectral image with both linear and nonlinear mixing of spectral signatures. The BMM formula, as given below, shows that for each pixel (i, j) in the hyperspectral image, the spectral signature $S_{ij}(\lambda)$ at each wavelength λ is given by:

$$S_{ij}(\lambda) = \sum_{l=1}^{L} A_{ij}^{(l)} \cdot E^{(l)}(\lambda) + \sum_{l=1}^{L} \sum_{m=l+1}^{L} A_{ij}^{(l)} \cdot A_{ij}^{(m)} \cdot (E^{(l)}(\lambda) \circ E^{(m)}(\lambda)) \tag{2.4}$$

   where:

   - L is the number of endmembers; in this case, $L = 2$ for cancerous and normal tissues.
   - $\boldsymbol{A}_{ij}^{(l)}$ is the abundance of endmember l at pixel (i, j).
   - $\boldsymbol{E}^{(l)}(\lambda)$ is the spectral signature (reflectance) of endmember l at wavelength λ.
   - The first term, $\sum_{l=1}^{L} \boldsymbol{A}_{ij}^{(l)} \cdot \boldsymbol{E}^{(l)}(\lambda)$, represents the linear mixing of the endmembers based on their abundances.
   - The second term, $\sum_{l=1}^{L} \sum_{m=l+1}^{L} \boldsymbol{A}_{ij}^{(l)} \cdot \boldsymbol{A}_{ij}^{(m)} \cdot (\boldsymbol{E}^{(l)}(\lambda) \circ \boldsymbol{E}^{(m)}(\lambda))$, represents the nonlinear interactions between the different endmembers.
   - '$\circ$' represents the Hadamard product between two spectral signatures or endmembers.
   - m is the index of the second endmember in a pair used to calculate the nonlinear interactions between different endmembers.

The model accounts for interactions between different materials or tissue types, providing a more realistic representation of how these elements mix in the real world. This model outputs a synthetic hyperspectral image with dimensions 512 × 512 × 70, where X and Y are spatial dimensions (512 × 512 pixels), and Z represents the spectral dimensions (70 spectral bands). The final created synthetic hyperspectral image for oral cancer as shown below, figure 2.11.

The 36th band of oral cancer synthetic hyperspectral image is indicated in figure 2.12, in which the dark red regions (from center) indicate the higher abundance of the cancerous tissue and lower abundance of the normal tissue signature, which means that cancerous tissue is gradually decreasing towards the edge of the image; the dark blue regions (near edge part of image) indicate higher abundance of the normal tissue signature and lower

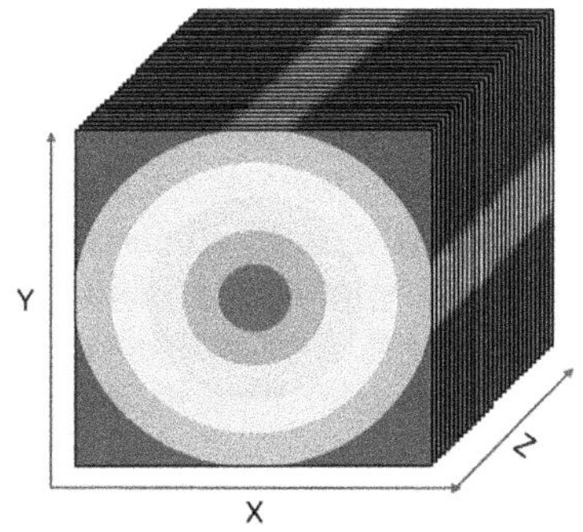

Figure 2.11. Synthetic hyperspectral image.

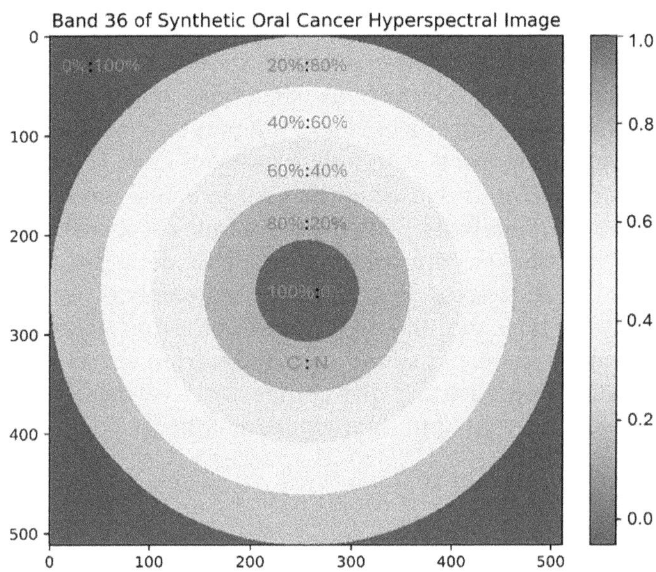

Figure 2.12. 36th band of oral cancer synthetic hyperspectral image.

abundance of the cancerous tissue signature, which means that the normal tissue is increasing towards the edge part of image from center.

The synthetic hyperspectral image effectively simulates the varying presence of cancerous and normal tissues across the image, which is crucial for training ML models to accurately differentiate between these two. In this figure the C is represented as spreading percentages cancerous tissue, which is decreasing from 100% at the center to 0% at the edge of the image, and N represents percentagesof normal tissue, which is decreasing from 100% at edge of the image to 0% at the center.

2.3.2.4 Unmixing of synthetic hyperspectral oral cancer

In HSI, unmixing is the process of decomposing each pixel into a combination of pure spectral signatures, known as endmembers, to determine their proportion (abundance) within that pixel. The study starts with a synthetic hyperspectral image of oral cancer, created using a BMM with dimensions 512 × 512 pixels and 70 spectral bands. The VCA is then applied to identify the most distinct spectral signatures (endmembers) in the image. Following this, the NNLS unmixing model estimates the spatial abundance of each identified endmember across the image. Finally, performance metrics, including SAD for endmembers and RMSE for abundance, are calculated to assess the accuracy of the unmixing process. This systematic approach provides valuable insights into the spectral and spatial distribution of different tissue types in the synthetic oral cancer HSI.

1. **Synthetic hyperspectral image:** The synthetic hyperspectral image of oral cancer is a detailed image with dimensions of 512 × 512 pixels and 70 spectral bands, created to mimic the spectral properties of cancerous tissues, which is shown in figure 2.13. It uses a bilinear mixture model to combine different light interactions, simulating how various tissue types might appear in a real-world scenario. This image serves as the starting point for analysing and identifying different tissue components within the cancerous area. It is essential for testing and improving methods that could be used in actual medical imaging.
2. **Vertex component analysis:** VCA is a technique used to identify pure spectral signatures, known as endmembers, from HSI data. In the context of oral cancer, the VCA process assumes two endmembers, each representing a different tissue type: normal tissue and cancerous tissue. The goal is to extract the most distinct spectral signatures from the HSI data, which can then be used to characterize the composition of the tissue. The equation below is used for estimating the two endmembers.

$$E = \{E^{(1)}, E^{(2)}, \ldots, E^{(L)}\} \tag{2.5}$$

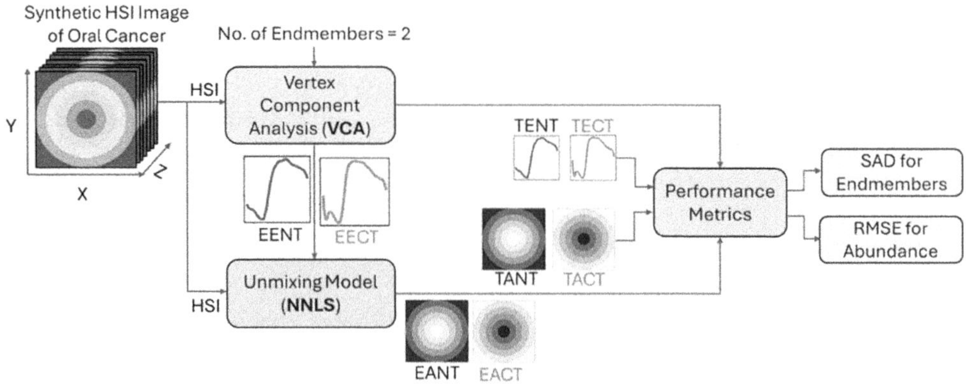

Figure 2.13. NNLS-based unmixing on synthetic hyperspectral image of oral cancer.

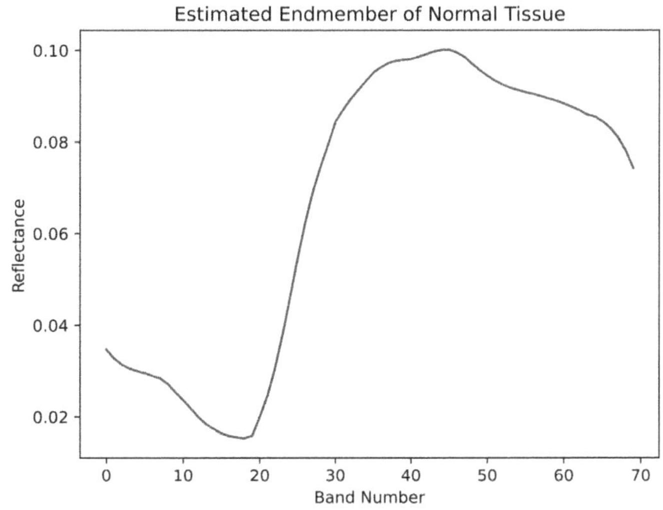

Figure 2.14. EENT.

where $E^{(L)}$ represents the number of extracted endmembers, in this case, EENT (estimated endmember of normal tissue) and EECT (estimated endmember of cancerous tissue).

The EENT, represented by the blue curve, is shown in figure 2.14. The graph plots reflectance against band number, highlighting how normal tissue reflects light across different spectral bands. The reflectance gradually increases from around band 10, peaks near band 40, and slightly decreases towards the higher bands. This curve serves as a reference for identifying regions in the HSI data that correspond to normal tissue.

The EECT, represented by the red curve, is shown in figure 2.15. It plots the reflectance against band number, but with higher reflectance values overall. The curve for cancerous tissue shows a sharp increase in reflectance around band 20, followed by a peak near band 40, and then a gradual decline. This distinct spectral profile helps in differentiating cancerous tissue from normal tissue in the hyperspectral image. Together, these endmember profiles provide essential information for the subsequent unmixing process, which aims to map the spatial distribution of these tissue types within the image.

3. **Non-negative least squares:** The unmixing model is a key step in hyperspectral image analysis, used to estimate how much of each identified endmember is present in every pixel of the image. After identifying the pure spectral signatures, or endmembers, through VCA, the NNLS model calculates the abundance of each endmember across the entire image. This process is crucial for mapping the spatial distribution of different tissue types within the HSI data.

$$\min_{A_{ij}} \left| S_{ij} - \sum_{l=1}^{L} A_{ij}^{(l)} \cdot E^{(l)} \right|^2 \quad \text{subject to} \quad A_{ij}^{(l)} \geqslant 0 \tag{2.6}$$

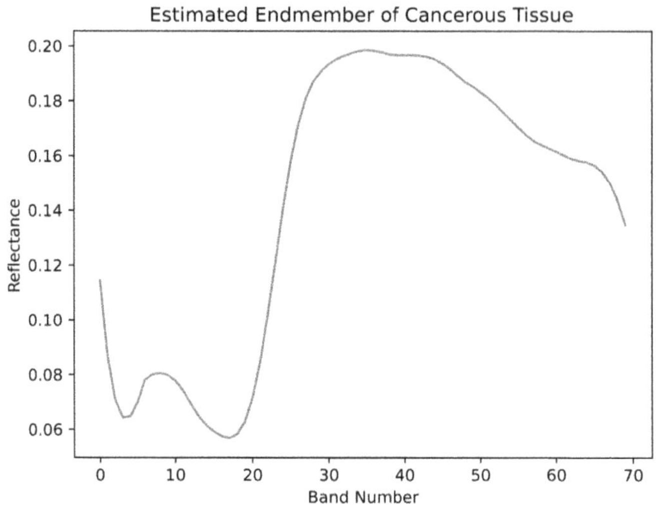

Figure 2.15. EECT.

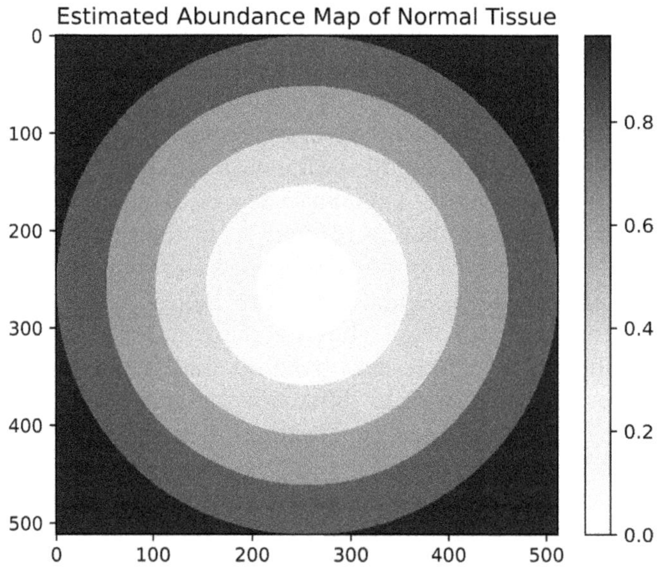

Figure 2.16. EANT.

Where,

- $\boldsymbol{A}_{ij}^{(l)}$ represents the estimated abundances for each endmember.
- $\boldsymbol{S}_{ij}$ is the observed pixel spectrum.
- $\boldsymbol{E}^{(l)}$ is the estimated endmember of the type of tissue.

The solution provides abundance maps EANT and EACT, which are explained and shown in figures 2.16 and 2.17.

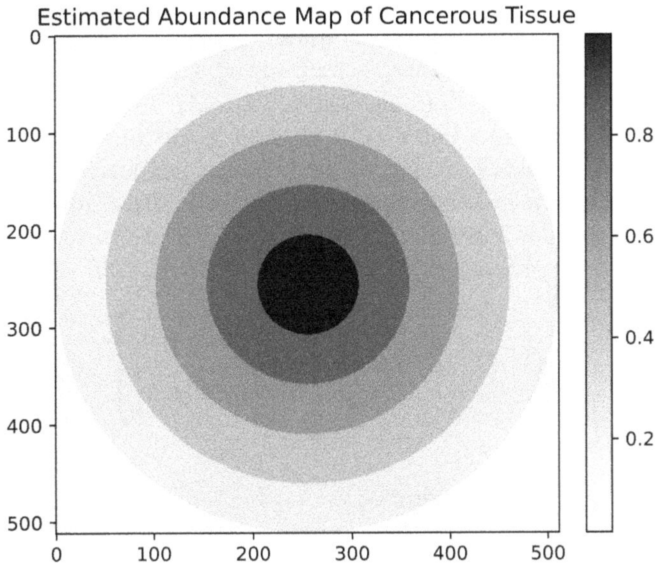

Figure 2.17. EACT.

The EANT, derived from a synthetic hyperspectral image with dimensions of 512 × 512 pixels, visually represents the concentration of normal tissue using shades of blue. Darker shades indicate higher concentrations, while lighter shades represent lower concentrations, forming concentric circles. The innermost circle shows 0% normal tissue, with increasing concentrations of 20%, 40%, 60%, and up to 100% as you move outward. This gradient pattern helps in understanding the distribution of normal tissues, aiding in precise diagnostic and treatment planning.

The EACT, derived from a synthetic hyperspectral image with dimensions of 512 × 512 pixels, visually represents the concentration of cancerous tissue using shades of red. Darker shades indicate higher concentrations, while lighter shades represent lower concentrations, forming concentric circles. The innermost circle shows 100% cancerous tissue, with decreasing concentrations of 80%, 60%, 40%, and down to 20% as you move outward, eventually reaching normal areas at the edges. This gradient pattern helps in understanding the distribution and clustering of cancerous tissues, aiding in precise diagnostic and treatment planning.

4. **Performance metrics:** The performance metrics are the SAD for endmembers and RMSE for abundances, and are crucial for evaluating spectral unmixing. SAD measures the accuracy of spectral signatures, while RMSE assesses the precision of abundance estimates. These metrics collectively determine the reliability of unmixing results and impact critical analyses and decision-making processes.

SAD is a metric used to measure how accurately the model has identified the spectral signatures of tissues in oral cancer imaging. It calculates the angle between the estimated and actual spectral profiles of different tissue types, with each dimension representing a specific wavelength. A smaller SAD value indicates that the model closely matches the true spectral signature of the tissue, meaning it accurately distinguishes between normal and cancerous tissues. A larger SAD value suggests a potential error in identifying these tissue characteristics, which is critical for accurate diagnosis and treatment planning.

$$\mathrm{SAD}(\boldsymbol{E}^{(l)}, \widehat{\boldsymbol{E}^{(l)}}) = \arccos\left(\frac{\boldsymbol{E}^{(l)} \cdot \widehat{\boldsymbol{E}^{(l)}}}{\left|\boldsymbol{E}^{(l)}\right|\left|\widehat{\boldsymbol{E}^{(l)}}\right|}\right) \tag{2.7}$$

where:

- $\boldsymbol{E}^{(l)}$ is the true endmember.
- $\widehat{\boldsymbol{E}^{(l)}}$ is the estimated endmember.

RMSE quantifies the error in estimated abundance maps from the spectral unmixing process. It measures the difference between actual abundance values (from ground truth or reference data) and those estimated by the unmixing model. RMSE is calculated as the square root of the average squared differences between these values. A lower RMSE indicates accurate abundance estimation, reflecting a well-represented spatial distribution of materials, while a higher RMSE points to potential inaccuracies in the mapping.

$$\mathrm{RMSE}(A_{\text{true}}, A_{\text{estimated}}) = \sqrt{\frac{1}{N}\sum_{i=1}^{N}(A_{\text{true},i} - A_{\text{estimated},i})^2} \tag{2.8}$$

where:

- A_{true} is the true abundance map (TANT for normal, TACT for cancerous).
- $A_{\text{estimated}}$ is the estimated abundance map (EANT for normal, EACT for cancerous).

The final performance metrics for unmixing on the synthetic hyperspectral image of oral cancer show the SAD values are 0.0080 for cancerous tissue and 0.0052 for normal tissue, reflecting effective identification of spectral signatures. RMSE of 0.0229 for cancerous tissue and 0.0247 for normal tissue, indicating good accuracy in abundance estimation. These metrics demonstrate that the unmixing process was successful in accurately mapping the distribution of cancerous and normal tissues, as shown in table 2.2.

Table 2.2. Performance metrics.

S.No	Metrics	Normal tissue	Cancerous tissue
1	SAD	0.0052	0.0080
2	RMSE	0.0247	0.0229

2.4 Deep learning for hyperspectral image analysis

DL is a specialized subset of ML that utilizes artificial neural networks composed of multiple layers to model and understand complex patterns within data. These multilayered structures emulate the functioning of the human brain by allowing data to be processed through interconnected nodes, enabling the model to learn hierarchical representations from raw inputs automatically. Unlike traditional ML techniques that often rely on manual feature extraction, DL algorithms can autonomously discern intricate features and relationships within large datasets. This capability has led to significant advancements across various domains, including computer vision, natural language processing, and speech recognition, where DL models have achieved superior performance and accuracy [18]. The proliferation of DL has been supported by the availability of extensive datasets, powerful computational resources, and sophisticated optimization algorithms such as stochastic gradient descent (SGD) and adaptive moment estimation (Adam), which effectively minimize errors during the training process [19].

2.4.1 Data preprocessing and feature extraction

In the context of oral cancer detection using HSI, the initial step involves meticulous preprocessing of the captured spectral data to enhance its quality and suitability for analysis. This preprocessing encompasses techniques such as noise reduction to eliminate irrelevant signal disturbances, normalization to standardize data scales, and dimensionality reduction to manage the vast amount of spectral information efficiently. Methods like principal component analysis (PCA) and minimum noise fraction (MNF) are commonly employed to condense the data while preserving critical spectral characteristics essential for accurate diagnosis [20]. Subsequently, DL models, particularly CNNs, are utilized to automatically extract and learn meaningful features from the pre-processed hyperspectral images. These models adeptly identify distinctive spectral patterns that differentiate healthy, precancerous, and cancerous oral tissues based on their unique biochemical compositions, thereby facilitating precise and reliable cancer detection [21].

2.4.2 Model training and validation

Train the DL models for effective hyperspectral oral cancer detection necessitates the use of comprehensive and well-annotated datasets where different tissue types are accurately labeled. Given the high-dimensional nature of hyperspectral data, large and diverse datasets are essential to ensure robust learning and generalization. Techniques such as transfer learning can be employed to leverage pre-trained models, adapting them to specific oral cancer detection tasks with improved efficiency [22]. Throughout the training process, validation methods like cross-validation are utilized to monitor model performance and prevent overfitting, ensuring that the models maintain high accuracy when applied to new, unseen data. Evaluation metrics including accuracy, sensitivity, specificity, and the area under the receiver operating characteristic (ROC) curve are used to assess and refine the models' diagnostic capabilities comprehensively [23].

2.4.3 Classification and segmentation

After feature extraction and model training, advanced DL architectures are applied for the classification and segmentation of hyperspectral images to accurately identify and localize cancerous tissues within the oral cavity. Models such as CNNs, 3D CNNs, and U-Net networks are trained to classify different tissue regions by analyzing their spectral signatures comprehensively. These networks effectively discern patterns associated with various stages of oral cancer, enabling differentiation between normal, dysplastic, and malignant tissues with high precision [24]. Segmentation models like U-Net further enhance diagnostic capabilities by precisely outlining areas of concern, providing clear visual maps that assist clinicians in identifying regions that may require further examination or intervention [25]. This detailed segmentation is critical for planning effective treatment strategies and improving patient outcomes.

2.4.4 Real-time analysis

Once adequately trained and validated, DL models can be integrated into real-time analysis systems to provide immediate and actionable insights during oral examinations and surgical procedures. These models can rapidly process incoming hyperspectral data to detect and highlight suspicious tissue areas, thereby assisting clinicians in making swift and informed diagnostic and treatment decisions [26]. The incorporation of these systems into clinical workflows enhances the accuracy and efficiency of oral cancer detection, reducing the reliance on time-consuming and invasive diagnostic methods. Additionally, these models can be integrated into comprehensive clinical decision support systems, providing healthcare professionals with detailed analyses and recommendations based on spectral data, which supports personalized treatment planning and improves overall patient care [27].

2.4.5 Oral cancer detection framework using deep learning models

Once adequately trained and validated, DL models can be integrated into real-time analysis systems to provide immediate and actionable insights during oral examinations and surgical procedures, as shown in figure 2.18. These models can rapidly process incoming hyperspectral data to detect and highlight suspicious tissue areas, thereby assisting clinicians in making swift and informed diagnostic and treatment decisions [26]. The incorporation of these systems into clinical workflows enhances the accuracy and efficiency of oral cancer.

1. **Data collection:** The process begins with the collection of HSI data, which includes both cancerous and normal oral tissue samples. This dataset forms the foundation for further analysis.
2. **Oral (cancer and normal) dataset:** The collected HSI images are organized into a dataset that categorizes images into cancerous and normal groups. This categorization is crucial for training the DL model.

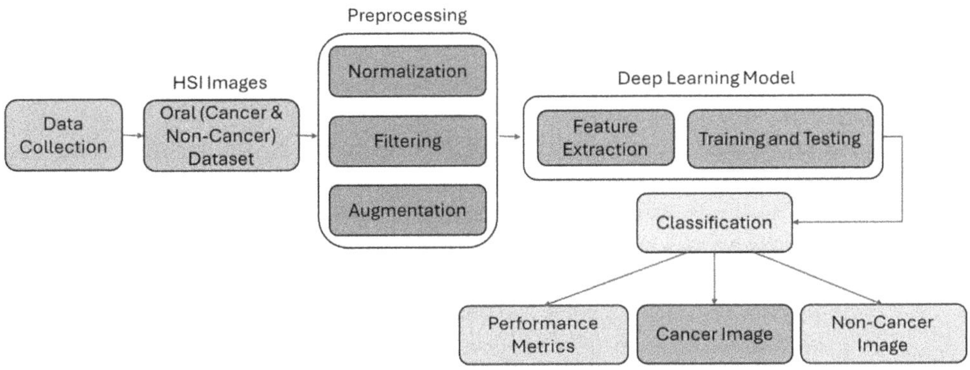

Figure 2.18. Block diagram of oral cancer detection using DL.

3. **Preprocessing: normalization:** The HSI images are standardized to ensure consistent intensity values across the dataset. This step reduces variability due to lighting conditions or other external factors.

   Filtering: Noise is removed from the images using various filtering techniques to enhance the clarity of the relevant features within the tissue samples.

   Augmentation: The dataset is artificially expanded by applying transformations like rotation, scaling, or flipping to the images. This step helps prevent overfitting and improves the model's robustness.
4. **Deep learning model: feature extraction:** The DL model automatically identifies and extracts significant features from the pre-processed images that are indicative of cancerous or normal tissues.

   Training and testing: The dataset is split into training and testing subsets. The model is trained on the training data to learn the patterns associated with cancer, and then tested on the test data to evaluate its performance as per the applications which are classification, unmixing, segmentation.
5. **Classification:** After training, the model classifies new HSI images into either cancerous or normal categories. This classification is based on the features identified during the training phase.
6. **Performance metrics:** The performance of the DL model is evaluated using various metrics such as accuracy, precision, recall, and F1-score. These metrics help in assessing how well the model can distinguish between cancerous and normal images.
7. **Cancer image or non-cancer image:** The final output of the model categorizes each image into either 'Cancer Image' or 'Non-Cancer Image,' providing a clear indication of the presence or absence of oral cancer in the tissue sample.

2.4.6 CNN-based classification of cancerous and normal oral tissues using hyperspectral imaging

In the context of oral cancer, the dataset used for this CNN model consists of HSIs that capture detailed spectral information of oral tissues. Each image has a spatial resolution of 512 × 512 pixels and contains 204 spectral bands. These bands correspond to different wavelengths of light, which allows the model to analyse the tissue's biochemical and structural properties at a microscopic level. This detailed data is crucial for distinguishing between healthy tissue and cancerous tissue, which have different spectral signatures.

1. **Input layer:** The input layer of the CNN takes the hyperspectral image stack as input, with each image representing a different spectral band of the oral tissue. This layer feeds the rich spectral data into the network, where each band is treated as a separate channel (like color channels in standard images). This enables the model to process and analyze the complex information contained in the HSI, crucial for detecting subtle signs of oral cancer.
2. **Convolution layer-1:** In the first convolutional layer (Conv-1), several filters are applied to the input image stack. These filters scan across the image to detect basic features like edges, textures, or simple patterns within the oral tissue. Each filter creates a feature map that highlights specific aspects of the tissue, such as the structure of cells or the presence of abnormalities, which are important in distinguishing cancerous tissues from healthy ones.
3. **Max pooling layer:** Following Conv-1, a max pooling layer is applied to reduce the spatial dimensions of the feature maps. This layer selects the most prominent features from small regions of the image, which helps to focus on the most significant patterns. By reducing the size of the feature maps, this layer makes the network more efficient and better at generalizing, which is important for accurately identifying cancerous tissues across different patients.
4. **Convolution layer-2:** The second convolutional layer (Conv-2) takes the pooled feature maps and applies more complex filters. These filters detect higher-level features by combining the basic patterns identified in Conv-1. This layer is crucial for recognizing more detailed structures in the oral tissue, such as irregularities in cell arrangement or tissue texture, which may indicate the presence of cancer.
5. **Convolution layer-3:** The third convolutional layer (Conv-3) further refines the features detected in the previous layers. At this stage, the network can identify even more complex patterns, such as specific molecular signatures or structural anomalies that are unique to cancerous tissues. This layer plays a key role in capturing the subtle differences between cancerous and normal tissues that may not be visible in conventional imaging.
6. **Max pooling layer:** Another max pooling layer is applied after Conv-3 to further reduce the size of the feature maps. This step simplifies the data and makes the model more efficient, helping it focus on the most critical features while avoiding overfitting. By concentrating on the most significant information, this layer improves the model's ability to correctly classify tissues as cancerous or normal.
7. **Fully connected layer:** The fully connected layers take the flattened feature maps from the final convolutional layer and combine them into a single vector. These layers function like a traditional neural network, where each neuron is connected to every input. They synthesize all the extracted

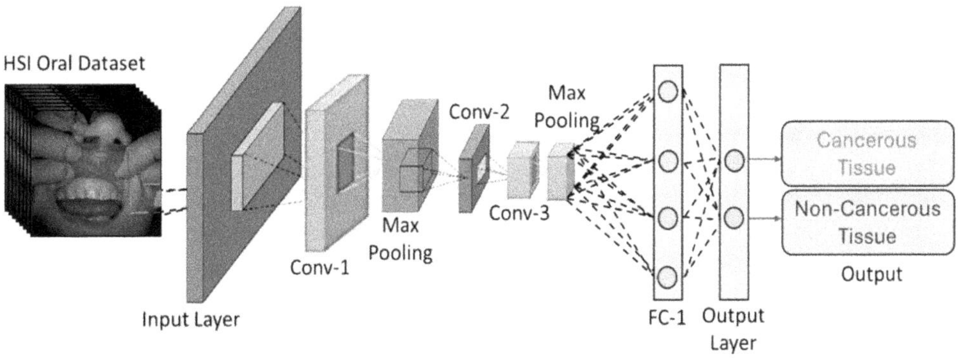

Figure 2.19. CNN architecture for classifying cancerous and normal oral tissues using hyperspectral imaging. Reproduced from [4]. CC BY 4.0.

features to make a final decision, determining the likelihood that a given tissue sample is cancerous based on the patterns learned from the HSI data.

8. **Output layer:** The output layer consists of two nodes, representing the classes of cancerous and normal tissue. This layer uses the features processed by the fully connected layers to predict the probability of each class. The model then assigns the tissue to the class with the higher probability, effectively labeling the tissue as either cancerous or normal.
9. **Cancerous tissue:** Cancerous tissue in the oral cavity refers to regions where cells have become malignant. These tissues exhibit distinct spectral signatures due to changes in their biochemical composition and structure, which are captured by the HSI and recognized by the CNN. If the network identifies these features, it classifies the tissue as cancerous, indicating the presence of oral cancer.
10. **Normal tissue:** Normal tissue represents healthy, normal tissue in the oral cavity that does not show signs of malignancy. The CNN identifies these tissues by recognizing the spectral characteristics that are typical of healthy cells. If the network finds that the features of the tissue match those of normal tissue, it classifies the sample accordingly, indicating that the tissue is free from cancer.

The CNN architecture illustrated in figure 2.19 is specifically designed to process high-dimensional HSI data, enabling accurate early detection and diagnosis of oral cancer by distinguishing cancerous tissues from normal ones based on their spectral and spatial signatures.

2.4.7 Current research on oral cancer using deep learning algorithms

Research on oral cancer, focusing on the application of various DL algorithms, is explained below. These studies aim to improve the accuracy and efficiency of detection and classification. Additionally, the contributions of different authors who have published significant papers on oral cancer are also explained below.

The study uses a dataset of oral images, including both healthy and diseased conditions such as thrush, lichen, hairy tongue, and leukoplakia. A pre-trained DenseNet169 model, fine-tuned with transfer learning and enhanced through data augmentation, was used for classification. The DenseNet model showed outstanding performance with 94.08% accuracy, 94.16% precision, 94.7% recall, and 94.7% F1-score. In contrast, the LeNet model underperformed with an F1-score of 63.01% and an accuracy of 64.02%. The study highlights that DL, particularly the DenseNet model, has strong potential for oral cancer detection, though further tuning is necessary for real-world application [28].

The authors propose a method using three feature extraction techniques Zernike Moment, wavelet features, and the histogram of directed gradients optimized by fuzzy particle swarm optimization (FPSO). These features are then classified using the faster region-based CNN (Faster RCNN). The study aims to assess the method's efficiency by evaluating overall accuracy is 98.8%, contributing to early oral cancer detection [29].

The diagnostic approach for oral cancer detection using the EfficientNet DL architecture highlights the importance of early diagnosis, which can be improved by combining DL with feature extraction and transfer learning. The proposed model uses pre-trained weights to enhance accuracy and speed in image processing, demonstrating the potential of advanced technology to improve oral cancer diagnostics and patient outcomes [30].

The cutting-edge approach for detecting and classifying oral cancer using HSI focused on the maxillofacial region. Oral and neck cancer is prevalent, particularly among socio-economically disadvantaged populations. The study proposes a fusion of deep Boltzmann machine (DBM) and support vector machine (SVM) for the classification of cancerous and normal tissues in hyperspectral images. This method addresses the lack of modern digital tools for early cancer detection. The proposed framework achieves a classifier accuracy of 94.75% through classifier fusion by majority voting, outperforming conventional DL techniques [31].

The processing of hyperspectral tissue data by a neural network allows the automated classification of tissue samples with increasing model accuracies. Our research deals with the classification of healthy oral fat, muscle and mucosa by using hyperspectral reflectance values and thus differs to alternative approaches built upon HSIs and CNNs. To eliminate the accuracy gap, future studies will emphasize convolutional building blocks and image data [32].

To improve the consistency and accuracy of oral SCC (OSCC) diagnosis uses the FD-Net, a novel segmentation network applied to microscopic hyperspectral images of H&E-stained pathological sections. This method aims to reduce human error and variability in traditional diagnoses by segmenting cancerous and noncancerous nuclei, first coarsely and then finely, to assist pathologists in identifying lesions. The FD-Net outperforms other segmentation networks, particularly in predicting and marking cancerous nuclei without manual intervention. As the OSCC dataset grows, FD-Net's segmentation capabilities are expected to strengthen, further reducing pathologists' workload by simplifying and automating the labeling process [33].

The novel approach for early detection of oral cancer using DL, specifically a restricted Boltzmann machine (RBM), was applied to HSI. The authors emphasize the importance of early diagnosis, which can significantly improve patient survival rates. Their enhanced RBM technique achieves a high accuracy of 95.75% in differentiating between benign and malignant tissues at early stages, demonstrating its potential to improve cancer diagnostics and patient outcomes by identifying the disease earlier than current methods [34].

The study integrates polarized hyperspectral imaging (PHSI) with DL to automatically detect head and neck SCC on H&E-stained tissue slides. The researchers used a PHSI microscope to collect Stokes vector data (S0, S1, S2, and S3) from SCC samples of 17 patients. They generated synthetic RGB images from these data, cropped them into patches, and applied a ResNet50-based CNN for classification through transfer learning. Testing across multiple patients showed that the S3 parameter achieved the highest average accuracy of 84.2%, outperforming S0. The results suggest that PHSI combined with DL could enhance the accuracy and automation of SCC detection in pathological slides [35].

The novel DL approach for early oral cancer diagnosis using a computer-assisted medical image classification system. The authors developed a partitioned deep CNN to process hyperspectral images, achieving a classification accuracy of 91.4%, with a sensitivity of 0.94 and specificity of 0.91 in distinguishing between benign and malignant tumors. This CNN outperformed traditional methods like Support SVM and Deep Belief Networks (DBN), highlighting its effectiveness in improving diagnostic accuracy and quality in oral cancer detection. The study underscores the potential of advanced imaging techniques and AI in enhancing cancer treatment outcomes [36].

The study explores the use of label-free, reflectance-based HSI and autofluorescence imaging for detecting SCC at the surgical margins of head and neck tissue specimens. Involving 293 samples from 102 patients, the research shows that HSI and autofluorescence imaging outperform traditional methods, including proflavin dye and standard RGB imaging, in accurately identifying cancer margins. Specifically, HSI achieved an AUC of 0.82 in detecting SCC up to 3 mm from the margin, while autofluorescence imaging detected HPV-positive SCC with an AUC of 0.99. These techniques demonstrated superior accuracy in both intra-patient and inter-patient settings. The findings suggest that these non-ionizing imaging modalities could significantly aid surgeons in reducing inadequate surgical margins during SCC resections, thereby improving patient outcomes [37].

The study explores HSI as a non-invasive tool for early detection of oral cancer, aiming to improve clinical outcomes by diagnosing cancers at earlier stages. Using an animal model with chemically induced tongue carcinogenesis, researchers acquired hyperspectral images of both *In vivo* and *Ex vivo* mouse tongues. They evaluated various ML algorithms, including discriminant analysis, ensemble learning, and SVM, to detect neoplasia, validating the results with pathological gold-standard maps. The findings suggest that HSI, combined with ML techniques, could be an effective non-invasive method for quantitatively detecting and delineating squamous neoplasia in oral cancers [38].

The HSI combined with DL for non-invasive detection of head and neck cancer. HSI captures high-resolution images across numerous spectral bands, offering detailed data for distinguishing between different tissue types. The researchers implemented a CNN to automatically learn and classify pixels in HSI as either tumor or normal tissue. The method was tested on a dataset of hyperspectral images from 12 tumor-bearing mice, achieving an average accuracy of 91.36%. The findings suggest that this DL approach can effectively detect head and neck tumors in animal models using HSI [39].

The study provides a systematic review of the use of machine learning techniques for diagnosing and predicting oral cancer, a highly dangerous cancer affecting areas like the lips, tongue, mouth roof, and oropharynx. Key risk factors include tobacco, alcohol, cigarettes, and HPV infection. Early detection and accurate treatment are crucial for improving survival rates. The review also discusses the limitations and concerns that clinicians face when integrating machine learning models into routine clinical practice for oral cancer diagnosis and prognosis [40].

The study focuses on developing a CNN model to accurately detect oral epithelial dysplasia (OED), a precursor to oral SCC (OSCC), in whole-slide pathology images. Given the high variability and misdiagnosis rates among experts when grading OED, the researchers aimed to create a reliable automated tool. They optimized the model using 112 annotated cases and compared two CNN architectures, DeepLabv3 + and UNet++, for their effectiveness in OED detection. DeepLabv3+ outperformed UNet++ in accuracy, precision, and segmentation, achieving a 93.3% overall accuracy and a 90.9% F1-Score on a test set. The study demonstrates the feasibility of using CNNs for detecting premalignant oral lesions, paving the way for future clinical applications [41].

The HSI, combined with DL for non-invasive, early detection of head and neck tumors, specifically laryngeal cancer. Traditional diagnosis methods rely on subjective assessments, leading to high variability. HSI offers a potential solution by identifying unique spectral signatures of cancerous tissues. However, processing HSI data is challenging due to its complexity. To address this, the researchers developed and evaluated CNNs that integrate both 2D spatial and 3D spatio-spectral convolutions within a Densenet architecture. Tested on an *in vivo* dataset of the oral cavity and oropharynx, their 3D spatio-spectral Densenet achieved an average accuracy of 81%, demonstrating that combining spatial and spectral data significantly improves cancer detection accuracy [42].

The automatic detection of medically relevant features in oral and dental hyperspectral images using advanced DL techniques, specifically Mask R-CNN for instance segmentation. The approach helps dentists identify and classify unhealthy areas without exposing patients to ionizing X-ray radiation, using spectral imaging in the visible and near-infrared ranges. The dataset includes 116 hyperspectral images from 18 patients, annotated with 38 classes in six sub-groups by dental experts. Preliminary results demonstrate the high potential and accuracy of this method for accurately classifying and segmenting different areas, potentially aiding in disease prevention [43].

Developing an advanced DL algorithm for the early detection and classification of oral cancer using hyperspectral images. The proposed system, based on a regression-based partitioned deep CNN, aims to improve the accuracy of computer-aided diagnosis by labeling regions of interest in multidimensional images. The model achieved a classification accuracy of 91.4%, with a sensitivity of 0.94 and specificity of 0.91 when distinguishing between cancerous and benign tumors. For distinguishing cancerous tumors from normal tissue, the accuracy reached 94.5% with more extensive training. Compared to traditional methods, the partitioned deep CNN demonstrated superior performance, enhancing the quality of oral cancer diagnosis [44].

The DL-based approach for the real-time identification and prediction of oral cancer aiming to improve early detection and patient outcomes. By leveraging CNNs, the researchers have developed a system that combines patient questionnaires with oral cavity images to create a more accurate and reliable prediction model. This method addresses the limitations of traditional diagnostic approaches, which often rely on subjective visual assessments by healthcare professionals, leading to potential delays in diagnosis. The proposed system is non-invasive, user-friendly, and accessible, allowing individuals to participate actively in their healthcare. It also facilitates communication with healthcare professionals, ensuring timely guidance and intervention, ultimately enhancing patient-centric care and improving the management of oral health [45].

The challenge of diagnosing oral cancer, a highly prevalent and severe malignancy, particularly in India, where it claims 130 000 lives annually. Traditional diagnostic methods, like biopsies, struggle to accurately distinguish and classify cancer cells. To improve early detection and classification, the study employs digital processing technology alongside DL algorithms. It uses three feature extraction methods wavelet features, Zernike moments, and bagged histograms of oriented gradients to identify cancer cells in the oral region. The fuzzy particle swarm optimization (FPSO) technique then selects the optimal texture features, which are classified using a CNN. The study's results show that combining Artificial Bee Colony (ABC) FPSO and CNN yields the best performance for accurately identifying oral cancer, demonstrating improved classification accuracy, precision, and recall rates [46].

This study introduces an advanced approach for improving oral cancer detection using a Deep CNN combined with an optimized Long Short-Term Memory (LSTM) technique. The process begins with preprocessing OSCC images using median filtering and CLAHE, followed by feature extraction through the Local Tetra Pattern (LTrP). The HHHLO algorithm is then used to select the optimal features, which are classified by the hybrid DCNN-LSTM model with the accuracy of 97.5% [47].

Developing a CNN model to detect oral cancer, particularly in images of lips and tongue, which are affected by factors like alcohol, tobacco, and smoking. The CNN model, named Oral Cancer Detection, is designed to classify images as either cancerous or Normal. The model was tested and demonstrated high effectiveness, achieving an accuracy of 94% with low complexity and faster processing time.

The results indicate that this CNN-based approach is both efficient and accurate in diagnosing oral cancer through image analysis [48].

Raman spectroscopy was combined with DL to detect and classify multiple types of oral cancer tissues, including tongue, gingival, and buccal SCC. The researchers collected 16 200 Raman spectra from 180 tissue samples of 90 patients and tested various deep neural network models, including AlexNet, VGGNet, ResNet50, MobileNetV2, and Transformer. ResNet50 performed the best, achieving an overall accuracy of 92.81%, precision of 92.93%, and recall of 92.86% in distinguishing cancerous from normal tissues. Based on these findings, a prototype intelligent detection system was developed using these models, potentially guiding and improving oral cancer detection and advancing clinical diagnostic tools [49].

A DL framework was developed to improve the detection of oral cancer by automating the processes of feature extraction, preprocessing, and classification. The framework utilizes Contrast-limited Adaptive Histogram Equalization (CLAHE) for enhancing image contrast, and Gray Level Co-occurrence Matrix (GLCM) for extracting texture-based features. For classification, a modified CNN was employed. When tested, the framework achieved a high accuracy of 99.13%, surpassing existing state-of-the-art methods. This demonstrates the potential of the proposed approach in enhancing early detection and improving prognosis outcomes for oral cancer [50].

DL methods for the accurate identification and classification of oral cancer: a new CANet model and a Swin Transformer-based model. CANet leverages attention mechanisms combined with location information to enhance classification, while the Swin Transformer segments images into blocks processed through multiple layers. Both models were trained the CANet, achieving superior results: an accuracy of 97.00%, sensitivity of 97.82%, specificity of 97.82%, and F1-Score of 96.61% [51].

The use of DL techniques for detecting oral cancer from histopathology images: specifically, it analyses 10 pre-trained deep CNN models using transfer learning. Among these, the VGG19 model with data augmentation achieved the highest classification accuracy of 96.26% for distinguishing between normal tissue and oral squamous cell carcinoma. To further enhance performance, the VGG19 model was integrated with a custom naïve inception block, addressing issues like vanishing gradients and high computational demands. This combined model demonstrated superior detection capabilities, showcasing its potential to improve oral cancer diagnosis [52].

The global challenge of oral cancer, the fifth most common cancer, is primarily caused by alcohol, betel nut, and tobacco use. One research method focused on developing an AI-driven model to improve early diagnosis, which is crucial for better survival outcomes. A fusion-based DL network was created to recognize oral cancer using a publicly available dataset of tongue and lip images. Data augmentation was applied to balance the dataset, and hyperparameters were optimized for higher accuracy. The proposed model achieved an overall accuracy of 94.62%, outperforming other state-of-the-art DL models, indicating its potential for early detection and classification of oral cancer in medical diagnosis systems [53].

2.5 Conclusion

The integration of HSI with DL marks a significant advancement in the early detection of oral cancer, greatly enhancing patient outcomes. HSI provides detailed spectral information that enables precise differentiation between cancerous and healthy tissues, while DL algorithms improve the accuracy and efficiency of data analysis. The non-invasive nature of HSI and its potential for real-time analysis make it an excellent tool for routine screenings and early diagnosis, potentially reducing the need for invasive procedures. However, challenges such as model robustness, data availability, and computational demands must be addressed. Future research should focus on improving model reliability, validating effectiveness through clinical trials, and developing comprehensive datasets, including synthetic ones. Overall, the combination of HSI and AI-driven analysis offers a promising approach to overcoming early detection challenges, with the potential to significantly reduce mortality rates and improve patient care.

2.6 Future scope

Generating synthetic hyperspectral datasets with varying random proportions of cancerous, normal, and different oral cancer tissue types will be crucial for evaluating DL algorithms across tasks like hyperspectral unmixing, classification, and segmentation. By incorporating a diverse range of tissues, these datasets will enhance the realism and robustness of model evaluations. The research focuses on identifying the most effective models for accurately distinguishing between various tissue types, which is vital for advancing medical imaging, particularly for detecting different stages and forms of oral cancer. Additionally, these techniques can be adapted for broader applications, such as environmental monitoring and precision agriculture, further expanding their impact across various fields.

References

[1] Bunz F 2008 The genetic basis of cancer *Principles of Cancer Genetics* (Springer) pp 1–47

[2] Réda M, Richard C, Bertaut A, Niogret J, Collot T, Fumet J D, Blanc J, Truntzer C, Desmoulins I, Ladoire S *et al* 2020 Implementation and use of whole exome sequencing for metastatic solid cancer *EBioMedicine* **51** 102624

[3] Senevirathna K, Jayasinghe Y A, Jayawickrama S M, Amarasinghe H and Jayasinghe R D 2023 Oral cancer disease among the poor: a Sri Lankan context *Oral* **3** 420–36

[4] Hyttinen J, Fält P, Jäsberg H, Kullaa A and Hauta-Kasari M 2020 Oral and dental spectral image database—ODSI-DB *Appl. Sci.* **10** 7246

[5] Kaur J, Srivastava R and Borse V 2021 Recent advances in point-of-care diagnostics for oral cancer *Biosens. Bioelectron.* **178** 112995

[6] Gupta P 2017 An update on light-based technologies and fluorescent imaging in oral cancer detection *Oncobiol. Targets* **4** 3155

[7] Liu Y and Deng H 2024 Tumor-targeting nanomedical drug delivery system and the application in oral cancer *E3S Web of Conferences* vol 553 (EDP Sciences) p 05033

[8] Worthington H V, Bulsara V M, Glenny A-M, Clarkson J E, Conway D I and Macluskey M 2023 Interventions for the treatment of oral cavity and oropharyngeal cancers: surgical treatment *Cochr. Database Syst. Rev.* **8** CD006205

[9] Shah R, Shah H, Thakkar K and Parikh N 2023 Conventional therapies of oral cancers: highlights on chemotherapeutic agents and radiotherapy, their adverse effects, and the cost burden of conventional therapies *Crit. Rev. Oncogenesis.* **28** 1–10

[10] Boonpoapichart S, Punyavong P, Jenwitheesuk K, Surakunprapha P and Winaikosol K 2021 Significant prognostic factors influencing the survival difference of oral tongue squamous cell carcinoma *Plast. Reconst. Surgery-Glob. Open* **9** e3889

[11] Mes S W, Te Beest D, Poli T, Rossi S, Scheckenbach K, Van Wieringen W N, Brink A, Bertani N, Lanfranco D, Silini E M *et al* 2017 Prognostic modeling of oral cancer by gene profiles and clinicopathological co-variables *Oncotarget* **8** 59312

[12] Chakraborty D, Natarajan C and Mukherjee A 2019 Advances in oral cancer detection *Adv. Clin. Chem.* **91** 181–200

[13] Wu J 2024 Hyperspectral imaging for non-invasive blood oxygen saturation assessment *Photodiag. Photodyn. Therapy* **45** 104003

[14] Kumar A, Bharti V, Kumar V, Meena P D and Suresh G 2017 Hyperspectral imaging applications in rapeseed and mustard farming *J. Oilseeds Res.* **34** 1–8

[15] de Cássia Mariotti K, Ortiz R S and Ferrão M F 2023 Hyperspectral imaging in forensic science: an overview of major application areas *Sci. Justice* **63** 387–95

[16] Banu K S, Lerma M, Ahmed S U and Gardea-Torresdey J L 2024 Hyperspectral microscopy-applications of hyperspectral imaging techniques in different fields of science: a review of recent advances *Appl. Spectrosc. Rev.* **59** 935–58

[17] Akewar M and Chandak M 2023 Hyperspectral imaging algorithms and applications: a review TechRxiv https://www.techrxiv.org/users/706929/articles/692094-hyperspectral-imaging-algorithms-and-applications-a-review?commit=853ecccdea95eedfb8dddf299a78d2b4a77cb7e9

[18] LeCun Y, Bengio Y and Hinton G 2015 Deep learning *Nature* **521** 436–44

[19] Kingma D P 2014 Adam: a method for stochastic optimization preprint arXiv:1412.6980.

[20] Yang X, Ye Y, Li X, Lau R Y K, Zhang X and Huang X 2018 Hyperspectral image classification with deep learning models *IEEE Trans. Geosci. Remote Sens.* **56** 5408–23

[21] Li S, Song W, Fang L, Chen Y, Ghamisi P and Benediktsson J A 2019 Deep learning for hyperspectral image classification: an overview *IEEE Trans. Geosci. Remote Sens.* **57** 6690–709

[22] Hussain M, Bird J J and Faria D R 2019 A study on cnn transfer learning for image classification *Advances in Computational Intelligence Systems: Contributions Presented at the 18th UK Workshop on Computational Intelligence, September 5-7, 2018, Nottingham, UK* (Springer) pp 191–202

[23] Sokolova M and Lapalme G 2009 A systematic analysis of performance measures for classification tasks *Inf. Process. Manage.* **45** 427–37

[24] Gao K, Liu B, Yu X, Qin J, Zhang P and Tan X 2020 Deep relation network for hyperspectral image few-shot classification *Remote Sens.* **12** 923

[25] Ronneberger O, Fischer P and Brox T 2015 U-net: convolutional networks for biomedical image segmentation *Medical Image Computing and Computer-Assisted Intervention–MICCAI 2015: 18th International Conference, Munich, Germany, October 5-9, 2015, proceedings, part III 18* (Springer) pp 234–41

[26] Guo Y, Liu Y, Oerlemans A, Lao S, Wu S and Lew M S 2016 Deep learning for visual understanding: a review *Neurocomputing* **187** 27–48

[27] Esteva A, Kuprel B, Novoa R A, Ko J, Swetter S M, Blau H M and Thrun S 2017 Dermatologist-level classification of skin cancer with deep neural networks *Nature* **542** 115–8

[28] Chavva R *et al* 2024 Oral cancer detection using deep learning *2024 Int. Conf. on Science Technology Engineering and Management (ICSTEM)* (IEEE) pp 1–6

[29] Koustubha S, Srividya C N, Leela D C and Gowda N 2024 Oral cancer detection using deep learning *Int. J. Innov. Res. Eng.* **5** 195–202

[30] Kalaivani P, Iyyanar P, Rajan C, Harshini Priya R, Janani P and Jayasudha A S 2024 Oral cancer detection using deep learning *2024 2nd Int. Conf. on Artificial Intelligence and Machine Learning Alications Theme: Healthcare and Internet of Things (AIMLA)* (IEEE) pp 1–4

[31] Jeyaraj P R, Panigrahi B K and Samuel Nadar E R 2022 Classifier feature fusion using deep learning model for non-invasive detection of oral cancer from hyperspectral image *IETE J. Res.* **68** 4031–42

[32] Daniel G E Thiem, Römer P, Gielisch M, Al-Nawas B, Schlüter M, Plaß B and Kämmerer P W 2021 Hyperspectral imaging and artificial intelligence to detect oral malignancy–part 1-automated tissue classification of oral muscle, fat and mucosa using a light-weight 6-layer deep neural network *Head Face Med.* **17** 1–9

[33] Zhang X, Li Q, Li W, Guo Y, Zhang J, Guo C, Chang K and Lovell N H 2024 Fd-net: feature distillation network for oral squamous cell carcinoma lymph node segmentation in hyperspectral imagery IEEE *J. Biomed. Health Inform.* **28** 1552–63

[34] Kiruthikaa K V and Vijay Franklin J 2021 Detection of oral cancer in hyperspectral images using restricted Boltzmann machines *Int. J. Aquat. Sci.* **12** 1760–6

[35] Zhou X, Ma L, Mubarak H K, Little J V, Chen A Y, Myers L L, Sumer B D and Fei B 2022 Automatic detection of head and neck squamous cell carcinoma on pathologic slides using polarized hyperspectral imaging and deep learning *Medical Imaging 2022: Digital and Computational Pathology* vol 12039 (SPIE) pp 91–100

[36] Rajan Jeyaraj P and Samuel Nadar E R 2019 Computer-assisted medical image classification for early diagnosis of oral cancer employing deep learning algorithm *J. Cancer Res. Clin. Oncol.* **145** 829–37

[37] Halicek M, Dormer J D, Little J V, Chen A Y, Myers L, Sumer B D and Fei B 2019 Hyperspectral imaging of head and neck squamous cell carcinoma for cancer margin detection in surgical specimens from 102 patients using deep learning *Cancers* **11** 1367

[38] Lu G, Wang D, Qin X, Muller S, Wang X, Chen A Y, Chen Z G and Fei B 2018 Detection and delineation of squamous neoplasia with hyperspectral imaging in a mouse model of tongue carcinogenesis *J. Biophoton.* **11** e201700078

[39] Ma L, Lu G, Wang D, Wang X, Chen Z G, Muller S, Chen A and Fei B 2017 Deep learning based classification for head and neck cancer detection with hyperspectral imaging in an animal model *Medical Imaging 2017: Biomedical Applications in Molecular, Structural, and Functional Imaging* vol 10137 (SPIE) pp 632–9

[40] Sulochana C and Sumathi M 2022 A systematic review on oral cancer diagnosis and prognosis using machine learning techniques *J. Algebr. Stat.* **13** 3542–50

[41] Liu Y, Bilodeau E, Pollack B and Batmanghelich K 2022 Automated detection of premalignant oral lesions on whole slide images using convolutional neural networks *Oral Oncol.* **134** 106109

[42] Bengs M, Westermann S, Gessert N, Eggert D, Gerstner A O H, Mueller N A, Betz C, Laffers W and Schlaefer A 2020 *Spatio-spectral deep learning methods for* in vivo *hyper-spectral laryngeal cancer detection Medical Imaging 2020: Computer-Aided Diagnosis* vol 11314 (SPIE) pp 369–74
[43] Boiko O, Hyttinen J, Fält P, Jäsberg H, Mirhashemi A, Kullaa A and Hauta-Kasari M 2019 Deep learning for dental hyperspectral image analysis *27th Color and Imaging Conference Final Program and Proceedings* (Society for Imaging Science & Technology)
[44] Vinay Kumar K, Palakurthy S, Balijadaddanala S H and Reddy S 2024 Early detection and diagnosis of oral cancer using deep neural network *J. Comput. Allied Intell.* **2** 22–34
[45] Pradeep Singh S M, Shariff M, Subramanyam D P, Varun M H, Shruthi K and Poornima A S 2023 Real time oral cavity detection leading to oral cancer using CNN *2023 Int. Conf. on Network, Multimedia and Information Technology (NMITCON)* (IEEE) pp 1–7
[46] Yadav R K, Ujjainkar P and Moriwal R 2023 Oral cancer detection using deep learning approach *2023 Int. Students' Conf. on Electrical, Electronics and Computer Science (SCEECS)* (IEEE) pp 1–7
[47] Subbulakshmi A and Nagarajan S 2023 A novel meta heuristic approach with optimal deeplearning neural network based oral cancer detection model *Ind. J. Sci. Technol.* **16** 4164–76
[48] Bansal S, Jadon R S and Gupta S K 2023 Lips and tongue cancer classification using deep learning neural network *2023 6th Int. Conf. on Information Systems and Computer Networks (ISCON)* (IEEE) pp 1–3
[49] Chang X, Yu M, Liu R, Jing R, Ding J, Xia J, Zhu Z, Li X, Yao Q, Zhu L *et al* 2023 Deep learning methods for oral cancer detection using Raman spectroscopy *Vib. Spectrosc.* **126** 103522
[50] Santhiya M, Sindhuja M, Jegatha R and Manikandan J 2023 An effective automated framework for oral cancer detection by enhanced convolutional neural networks *2023 12th Int. Conf. on Advanced Computing (ICoAC)* (IEEE) pp 1–7
[51] Chen R, Wang Q and Huang X 2024 Intelligent deep learning supports biomedical image detection and classification of oral cancer *Technol. Health Care* **32** 465–75
[52] Redie D K, Bilgaiyan S and Sagnika S 2023 Oral cancer detection using transfer learning-based framework from histopathology images *J. Electron. Imaging* **32** 053004
[53] Dwivedi K, Patel K, Pandey J P and Garg P 2024 An automatic robust deep learning and feature fusion-based classification method for early diagnosis of oral cancer using lip and tongue images *2024 2nd Int. Conf. on Disruptive Technologies (ICDT)* (IEEE) pp 391–5

IOP Publishing

Chapter 3

Fourier transform infrared (FTIR) spectroscopy as a tool for the diagnosis of cancer

Neha Sylvia Walter and Shalmoli Bhattacharyya

FTIR is a simple, rapid and non-invasive spectroscopic method utilized by the chemists for characterizing the structures of molecules. Recent advances have generated interest in this tool for a wide variety of applications including cancer diagnosis. There are remarkable variations in the frequencies of absorption and intensities of absorption bands in the spectra of healthy and tumour samples. The variations are due to alterations in the nucleic acid and lipids content in the diseased samples resulting in unique vibrational frequencies of key functional groups. The technique holds promise for screening and diagnosing cancer as well as for tracking the progression or regression disease following treatment. Owing to its simplicity, reproducibility, non invasiveness, small sample requirement and no sample destruction, FTIR can be established as a robust and reliable technique for early detection and diagnosis of different types of human cancer.

3.1 Introduction

Over four decades, there have been substantial advances in IRS (infrared spectroscopy). The structure of complex biomolecules is now typically determined in many research laboratories employing various techniques *viz*, mass spectrometry, x-ray diffraction, and two-dimensional nuclear magnetic resonance (NMR), Nonetheless, IRS still playing a significant role. IRS offers substantial details that cannot be obtained by other means, and is complementary to that of other methods. The ability to examine materials in all stages of matter is one of IRS's biggest advantages. If infrared spectra of material in each state are to be measured as efficiently as possible and provide the most of the information, it is imperative to comprehend the distinctions between the spectra of gases, liquids, and solids. The advancement in IRS led to the development of a new instrument called FTIR which is an analytical tool to recognize polymeric, organic, and occasionally inorganic

doi:10.1088/978-0-7503-5949-8ch3

materials. When measuring, all resolution elements are measured continuously (Fellgett's advantage). Furthermore, with every resolution element, more radiation may flow between the source and the detector. This leads to far quicker and more sensitive measurements of reflection, emission, and transmission spectra. Infrared light is scanned across the test materials using the FTIR detection technique to evaluate chemical characteristics. To detect the sample, nearly, 10 000–100 cm^{-1} of IR radiation are passed through a sample and a part of which is absorbed while others are transmitted. The sample molecules absorb the radiation and convert it into rotating and/or vibrational energy.

More precisely, in 1891, Michelson first created the two-beam interferometer which is the basic structure of FTIR. It functions by using a beamsplitter to split a beam into two directions, one beam reflected by a stationary mirror while the other by an oscillating glass. Once a difference of route is established, resulting in interference between the beams, they converge at the beamsplitter. The rotating mirror causes a change in the travel distance of second beam, resulting in a shift in the produced IR light frequency distribution. The detector signal is obtained as a time-domain interferogram which is then converted to the IR spectrum by Fourier transform [1]. FTIR is a versatile tool that may be used for a wide range of tasks, including quality control, analysing the chemical composition of microscopic particles, detecting contamination in or on material, and identifying organic molecules and particular functional groups. In failure analysis studies, FTIR can also detect uncured monomers, breakdown, or oxidation. Literature suggests that to examine the clinical samples, FTIR spectroscopy can be utilized as a non-invasive, quick, economical, non-destructive method which requires a small sample volume, nonetheless, FTIR spectroscopy has not yet taken the lead. Since FTIR can monitor the vibrational signature of clinical samples *viz*, biofluids; breast milk, tears, saliva, blood, urine, and pancreatic juice etc, cells, and tissue fluids to identify metabolic changes, it is a potential method for detecting illnesses and distinguishing between healthy and abnormal samples such as cancer cells.

Cancer refers to abnormalities of the biostructure that include unregulated cell proliferation, invasive cell growth and metastatic implantation into neighbouring tissue or to other body regions. As per the data, around 10 million deaths globally were attributed to cancer in 2020. Due to factors i.e., a high body mass index, alcohol and tobacco consumption, a diet poor in fruits and vegetables, air pollution (lung cancer), and a lack of physical exercise susceptibility to cancer increases. The most prevalent malignancies are breast, lung, colon, rectal, and prostate cancers. Thirty percent or more of cancer cases in poor and developing nations are caused by viruses, namely hepatitis and HPV (human papillomavirus) [2]. Most malignancies are initially detected by either by clinical sign and symptoms, or screening the patient by endoscopy, CT scan and x-rays which consume time and resources. Recent research has indicated the utility of an FTIR tool along with machine learning as a simple, non-invasive and reliable diagnostic technique for cancer. The following section outlines the application of FTIR spectroscopy in the early diagnosis of different human cancers.

3.2 FTIR in cancer diagnosis

Several optical techniques have been studied in detail to be developed as a diagnostic modality for different diseases including cancer. FTIR spectroscopy is one such technique capable of providing information at the molecular level about the chemical composition of the biological materials. This technique has been routinely utilized for characterizing the molecular structures by medicinal chemists. In recent years, this tool has developed as an important analytical method for a diverse range of applications. Nonetheless, the potential of this technique as a diagnostic modality for cancer has been recognized for decades [3].

FTIR spectroscopy can be employed for cancer diagnosis due to the ability of this technique to detect the structural and chemical alterations in the diseased cells and tissues in contrast to the normal on the basis of their characteristic spectral properties which can also help to identify novel disease biomarkers [4]. The structural alterations can be readily observed in IR spectra and a biomarker can be identified to highlight any tissue's pathological state [5]. Thus, this technique possesses the capability to illustrate the cell's structural alterations at the molecular level in different cancers. Alterations in structure induced by cancer results in different vibration modes of the molecules in the cells and tissues. These unique frequencies of vibration of key functional groups cause alterations in the FTIR spectra thereby helping to differentiate normal and tumour cells by their characteristic spectra. The major advantage of this FTIR spectroscopy is its simplicity, reproducibility, minimal preparation, lack of specific reagents, small sample requirement and no sample destruction. FTIR spectroscopy can not only be employed for screening, diagnosis and prognosis of cancer but also for continually assessing the response to treatment as well as monitoring the progression or regression of disease.

Specimens analysed by the technique for cancer diagnosis and management include blood, urine, saliva, tissues, sputum, bladder wash, bile and extracellular vesicles (EVs). Though blood and tissues are the most commonly used samples, recently EVs have captured focus because of their association with cancer. EVs range in size from 30 to 1000 nm and contain varied biological molecules *viz.* nucleic acids, proteins and lipids. These vesicles are secreted by different cells and are important for cellular communication thereby providing important information about the condition of cells and disease progression.

Several studies have illustrated the application of FTIR analysis (see for instance, figure 3.1) for detecting and diagnosing lung, colorectal, breast, cervix, ovaries, prostate, gastric and oral cancer, which are outlined below.

3.2.1 Lung cancer

This is one of the commonly prevalent cancer types and a major cause of mortality worldwide. The incidence of this disease has increased in recent years due to a rise in smoking and environmental pollution. The current clinical diagnostic tools for lung cancer include chest x-ray, bronchoscope and computerized tomography. Though effective, these techniques are unable to identify lung cancer at an early stage pinpointing the need to develop an efficient tool for early detection of the disease.

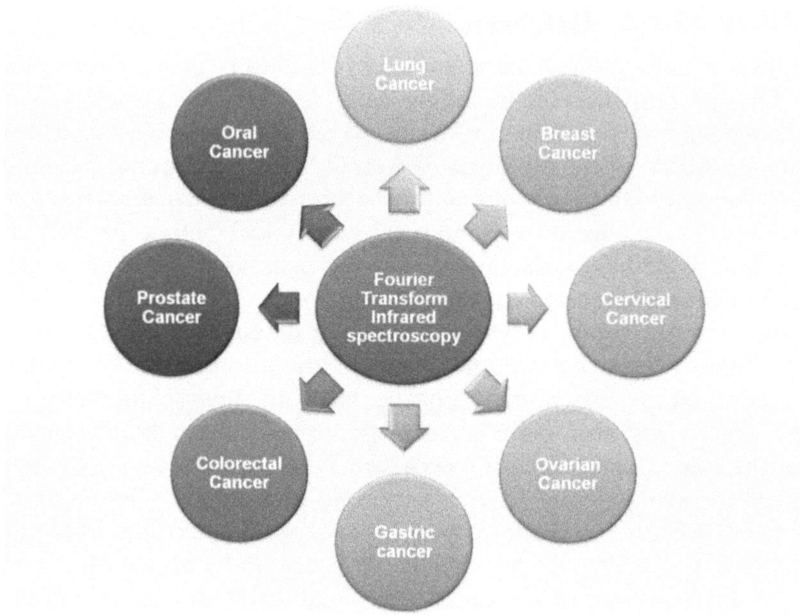

Figure 3.1. FTIR for diagnosis for different types of cancer.

Studies have evaluated FTIR spectroscopy for the diagnosis of lung cancer using sputum samples [6]. Multivariate analysis revealed five significant wavenumbers that distinguished spectra of cancer cells from the normal. These observations highlight the potential of FTIR as a low cost, highly sensitive, specific, non-invasive technique for screening sputum samples for diagnosing lung cancer.

Confocal Raman microscope and attenuated total reflectance-Fourier transform infrared microscope (ATR-FTIR) were also tested for the diagnosis of cancer wherein significant variations were evident in the spectra of malignant and normal tissues, relative to Raman shift, positions of IR peak and intensities of spectra [7]. ATR-FTIR spectroscopy also showed itself to be a promising detection method in distinguishing malignant and non-malignant lung tissues in approximately 60 samples with 96.7% sensitivity and specificity [8]. FTIR spectra of serum samples dried under vacuum on a BaF_2 window revealed differences in the secondary structure of serum proteins among lung cancer patients and healthy subjects [9]. Likewise, IRS in tissue samples from normal and lung cancer patients revealed variations in wavenumber in functional groups of the major biomolecules [10]. IRS was used in combination with PCA (principal component analysis) and HCA (hierarchical cluster analysis) to classify benign and malignant lung tissue sections the inferences of which were in agreement with histopathological studies [11]. ATR-FTIR spectroscopy was also employed along with chemometrics to effectively differentiate the serum samples of lung cancer patients and healthy individuals. This method was relatively simpler and can be developed for clinical screening and diagnosis of the disease [12].

3.2.2 Breast cancer

Due to its high frequency an early and rapid diagnosis is of utmost significance to prevent the mortality due to the disease. The available diagnostic modalities for the disease include mammography, ultrasound, magnetic resonance imaging (MRI) and punching biopsies which are highly subjective and time consuming. FTIR can be employed as a potential modality for the early diagnosis of breast cancer along with the chemometric methods, for instance HCA, PCA and to differentiate malignant and normal spectra. ATR-FTIR was able to distinguish IDC (invasive ductal carcinoma) from normal breast tissue, ductal carcinoma in situ (DCIS), and metaplastic carcinoma.

DCIS (ductal carcinoma *in situ*) can be used reliably and reproducibly without destruction of tissue samples [13]. Another study reported detection of the disease employing FTIR spectroscopy along with artificial neural networks (ANNs) or cluster analysis requiring only 1 μl of serum sample [14]. ATR-FTIR spectroscopy of serum followed by PCA and principal component regression (PCR) revealed a range of 1306–1250 cm^{-1} (corresponding to functional groups of RNA and DNA) to be significant for diagnosing breast cancer [15]. ATR-FTIR spectroscopy along with ANN was employed to identify unique IR absorption spectrum of lipid, carbohydrates, phospholipid and nucleic acid, regions to efficiently differentiate between malignant and benign breast tumours [16].

FTIR spectroscopy in conjunction with the Kennard-Stone (KS) algorithm, back propagation neural network (BPNN) model (94.2% accuracy) and support vector machine (SVM) model (92.9% accuracy) was used to differentiate normal control from ductal carcinoma *in situ* as well as invasive breast cancer in serum samples. The frequency ranges 1475–1710 cm^{-1} (corresponding to proteins) and 900–1425 cm^{-1} (corresponding to nucleic acids, lipids, sugar, proteins) exhibited best accuracy [17].

A recent study analysed plasma-derived small EVs from healthy controls and breast cancer patients by FTIR followed by PCA and identified spectroscopic lipid-to-lipid ratio I2960/I2929 as a robust marker of the disease having 100% sensitivity and specificity [18]. Moreover, a multi-modal ATR-FTIR and surface-enhanced Raman scattering (SERS) approach were uitlized to characterize the RNA biomarkers in the sera of breast cancer patients. PCA on the data followed by the application of machine learning algorithms led to the identification of key molecular fingerprints having >90% accuracy, specificity and sensitivity. The SVM model depicted the best area under the curve (AUC = 0.9979) indicative of excellent performance. These findings highlighted the FTIR as an effective and reliable tool for early identification of the disease. The technique can be developed as a potential adjunct to currently available diagnostic modalities for accurate diagnosis of breast cancer.

3.2.3 Cervical cancer

This is the second most frequent cancer affecting women after breast cancer. The conventional methods for the disease diagnosis include colposcopy and Pap smear which are observer dependant and have low sensitivity. FTIR spectroscopy can be used as a novel, sensitive tool capable of detecting biochemical alterations at a molecular level. Infrared microspectroscopy along with probabilistic neural networks showed a high (>95%) accuracy in biopsied tissue from normal and cervical cancer patients [19]. FTIR spectroscopy has been employed in conjunction with machine and deep learning algorithms (SVM model) to effectively distinguish between patients having cervical cancer and hysteromyoma from healthy individuals [20].

FTIR was used in combination with a particle swarm optimization-CNN model for early screening and discrimination between cervical cancer, hysteromyoma, cervical intraepithelial neoplasia (CIN I), CIN II, and CIN III with 87.2% accuracy [21]. ATR-FTIR spectroscopy and chemometric analysis using PCA in the 970–1150 cm^{-1} range was used for to distinguish cervical cancer cell lines (SiHa, HeLa and C33A) from primary fibroblasts with high sensitivity [22]. Another study reported analysis of squamous cell carcinoma (SCC) and normal cryopreserved samples employing FTIR microspectroscopy and an SVM classification model with >90% accuracy [23].

These findings highlight the ability of this method in the early detection of the disease.

3.2.4 Ovarian cancer

This is the most lethal gynaecological cancer primarily due to factors such as high recurrence rate, drug resistance and diagnosis at advanced stages. Being simple, non-invasive and convenient, FTIR spectroscopy offers immense potential in diagnosing ovarian cancer concomitant with identification of the characteristics of different forms of the disease, monitoring real-time cancer progression and drug resistance [24, 25]. The technique can differentiate the molecular differences between malignant and normal tissues employing a wide range of samples *viz.* blood, urine, and tissues.

ATR-FTIR of plasma, serum and urine followed by chemometric analysis illustrated considerable spectral differences in ovarian cancer patients with neo-adjuvant chemotherapy and without previous chemotherapy in a large cohort of patients. Best sensitivity (76%) and specificity (98%) for detection of ovarian cancer was achieved using the serum samples [26]. FTIR (2974 cm^{-1}, 1777 cm^{-1}) and FT-Raman spectroscopy along with PCA and machine learning algorithms illustrated high specificity, accuracy, and sensitivity in the detection of chemical alterations between platinum-sensitive and resistant ovarian cancer tissues due to increased protein, phospholipid and lipid content in the latter [27]. Thus, the technique can not only successfully distinguish normal ovarian tissue from malignant tissues based on IR spectral signatures but also identify the drug resistant cancer. The tool can therefore be used with other available tools for disease diagnosis.

3.2.5 Gastric cancer

Gastric cancer is one of the main health challenges, being the fifth most frequent cancer globally. It is one of the highly aggressive and lethal malignant tumours with a low survival rate [28]. FTIR has shown promise as a novel technique for diagnosing gastric cancer. FTIR and SVM method was employed to distinguish normal and malignant gastric cancer tissue samples with 100% sensitivity, 83.3%

specificity and 92.2% total discrimination accuracy [29]. Entropy weight local-hyperplane *k*-nearest neighbour based on frequency domain information (EWHFI) along with the adaptive weight local-hyperplane *k*-nearest neighbour (AWHK) algorithm with fine Fourier transform data in the frequency domain was found to be effective for the early gastric cancer diagnosis in endoscopic biopsy gastric tissue samples [30].

Dong *et al* employed an FTIR tool and PCA and Fisher's discriminant analysis (FDA) for diagnosis of lymph node metastasis of the disease with 95% sensitivity. Non-metastatic and metastatic LN spectra were split into two different groups by PCA with significant bands at wavenumbers 3260, 1740, 1640and 1080 cm^{-1} [31]. Recently, ATR-FTIR spectroscopy, PCA and machine learning algorithms were utilized to distinguish serum samples from patients with gastric cancer and normal individuals (3500–3000, 1700–1600, and 1090–1070 cm^{-1}) with 89.7% sensitivity and 87.2% specificity [32]. These reports indicate FTIR spectroscopy along with chemometrics as a practical and reliable tool for diagnosis and clinical screening of the disease.

3.2.6 Colorectal cancer

This ranks third among the most prevalent cancers and is the second highest cause of mortality due to cancer globally. The disease is often diagnosed at advanced stages wherein limited treatment alternatives are available. The evaluation process of the disease is quite challenging and subjective as colon carcinogenesis progresses through several overlapping stages. Currently, physical examination, imaging techniques, for instance computed tomography scans, abdominal ultrasound, magnetic resonance imaging, histopathological examination, molecular testing and colonoscopy or sigmoidoscopy, are employed for diagnosing the disease. FTIR spectroscopy has also been employed for diagnosing colorectal cancer as a fast and efficient technique for detecting biopsies of colon cancer.

Studies have demonstrated the efficiency and reliability of ATR-FTIR micro-spectroscopy along with chemometric methods to differentiate healthy colon tissues from malignant ones [33, 34]. The spectral region of 1800–900 cm^{-1} illustrated considerable variability in the FTIR spectrum of cancerous and normal colon biopsies. The specificity (100%), accuracy (93.3%) and sensitivity (88.2%) of this method fulfil the requirements of clinical diagnosis. Dong *et al* reported FTIR spectroscopy and PCA and FDA to differentiate tumour cells from normal with 96.6% sensitivity [35].

PCA-linear discriminant analysis (PCA-LDA) and FTIR spectroscopy have also been employed to identify the spectral differences between healthy colon, cancerous pre- and post-chemotherapy colon tissues as well as the surgical margin of colorectal tumour [36]. The spectral analysis highlighted the variation between the normal and cancer tissue and post-chemotherapy samples suggestive of pathophysiological interpretation as well as monitoring treatment efficacy. The study highlighted the effectiveness of the FTIR tool to define tumour margin of even single cancer cells, prior to resection procedure as it can enhance the chances of a patient's survival.

A recent study also illustrated the potential of FTIR spectroscopy and different machine learning algorithms as an alternative and reliable diagnostic method for colon cancer. The method depicted 87%–100% accuracy, 88.1%–100% sensitivity and 82.9%–100% specificity in both high wavenumber (2700–3700 cm^{-1}) and low wavenumber (1000–1760 cm^{-1}) range [37]. Moreover, Magno *et al* performed a meta-analysis on FTIR spectroscopy for detecting colorectal cancer employing blood-based samples [38]. Being simple, cost-effective, non-invasive, and due to its excellent discriminating potential, FTIR can be employed as a screening tool in asymptomatic populations as well incorporated for routine clinical diagnosis after further research.

3.2.7 Prostate cancer

This is the third most frequent cancer and a major reason of mortality in men as per the World Health Organization. The diagnostic modalities for the disease include physical examination, imaging techniques, biopsy, Gleason score and PSA (prostate specific antigen) test. FTIR microspectroscopy along with principal component-discriminant function analysis was utilized for analysis of prostate cancer tissues. The technique could effectively distinguish the signature spectra of confined and invasive prostate cancer with 83.6% sensitivity and 86.0% specificity based on the Gleason criteria [39].

EVs derived from blood samples were also employed for the detection and differentiation of the disease from normal utilizing FTIR and Raman spectroscopy. The study reported spectral signature of the EVs from cancer patients as a useful screening tool for early detection of the disease [40]. EVs from the urine of suspected prostate cancer patients were analysed by FTIR and following PCA, the method was found to differentiate prostate cancer with 59% sensitivity and 81%.specificity suggestive of the ability of this tool as a novel, non-invasive strategy for screening of prostate cancer [41]. FTIR-ATR also illustrated highest absorbance and marked variability in the spectra of sera from prostate cancer patients and normal individuals highlighting the potential of this tool for accurate and early diagnosis of this cancer [42].

3.2.8 Oral cancer

Oral cancer is an important public health concern, being the sixth most frequent cancer type globally with a 45% mortality rate. Oral cancer diagnosis is routinely done by biopsy followed by histopathological studies. FTIR spectroscopy can be utilized for diagnosing oral cancer employing varied samples *viz.* cells, tissues and body fluids. Menzies *et al* illustrated FTIR as a simple, low cost, non-invasive and reliable tool to differentiate between normal and oral, oropharyngeal and laryngeal cancer sputum at wavenumbers 1042 1550 and 1650 cm^{-1} [43]. Studies on IRS in oral cancer research and detection have been summarized in detail by Wang and Wang [44].

Exosomes isolated from whole saliva samples of healthy individuals and patients with oral cancer were evaluated utilizing ATR-FTIR spectroscopy, PCA-LDA and

SVM classification as a diagnostic modality for oral cancer [45]. The spectral signature of salivary exosomes from oral cancer patient was markedly distinct from those of healthy subjects. The method illustrated high specificity, sensitivity and accuracy. The technique was also successfully reported to differentiate serum samples of premalignant and buccal mucosa cancer patients with >90% accuracy showing promise of earlier diagnosis [46].

Another study highlighted FTIR spectral signatures (biomarker band at 1075 cm^{-1}) of saliva sample from oral and oropharyngeal cancer patients to be markedly different (90% accuracy) from that of the control on account of the biomolecular changes caused by the disease [47]. Likewise, ATR-FTIR along with machine learning could distinguish oral squamous cell carcinoma from the normal with 83.33% sensitivity, 91.66% accuracy and 100.0% specificity and precision [48].

3.3 Conclusion

At length FTIR spectroscopy holds potential as an important tool for the early detection and diagnosis of cancer as delayed diagnosis worsens treatment outcomes. As evidenced by numerous studies, the technique can differentiate normal samples from those of cancer with a high degree of accuracy, sensitivity and specificity. The major advantage of the technique is that it is a rapid, simple, non-invasive, non-destructive technique for diagnosing cancer. The characteristic spectra along with the different machine learning provide essential information about the disease origin, progression, identification chemotherapy resistant cancer and follow up of therapy on the basis of biochemical changes in the molecules. FTIR spectroscopy is emerging as a promising alternative tool for clinical diagnosis in addition to the other available diagnostic modalities in cancer.

Conflict of interest statement

The authors declare that there is no conflict of interest.

References

[1] Griffiths P R and de Haseth J A 2006 *Fourier Transform Infrared Spectrometry* (Hoboken, NJ: Wiley)

[2] WHO 2024 Cancer https://who.int/news-room/fact-sheets/detail/cancer (accessed 23 September 2024)

[3] Woernley D L 1952 Infrared absorption curves for normal and neoplastic tissues and related biological substances *Cancer Res.* **12** 516–23

[4] Le Naour F, Sandt C, Peng C, Trcera N, Chiappini F, Flank A M, Guettier C and Dumas P 2012 *In situ* chemical composition analysis of cirrhosis by combining synchrotron fourier transform infrared and synchrotron x-ray fluorescence microspectroscopies on the same tissue section *Anal. Chem.* **84** 10260–6

[5] Bunaciu A A, Fleschin Ş and Aboul-Enein H Y 2015 Cancer diagnosis by FTIR spectrophotometry *Rev. Roum. Chim.* **60** 415–26

[6] Lewis P D, Lewis K E, Ghosal R, Bayliss S, Lloyd A J, Wills J, Godfrey R, Kloer P and Mur L A 2010 Evaluation of FTIR spectroscopy as a diagnostic tool for lung cancer using sputum *BMC Cancer* **10** 640

[7] Lv J, Zhang L, Feng J, Liu Y, Wang Z, Zhao M and Shi R 2011 Optical observation of lung cancer with Attenuated Total Reflectance Fourier Transform Infrared Microscope (ATR-FTIR) and confocal raman microscope *Spectrosc. Lett.* **44** 312–7

[8] Sun X, Xu Y, Wu J, Zhang Y and Sun K 2013 Detection of lung cancer tissue by attenuated total reflection-fourier transform infrared spectroscopy-a pilot study of 60 samples *J. Surgical. Res.* **179** 33–8

[9] Wang X, Shen X, Sheng D, Chen X and Liu X 2014 FTIR spectroscopic comparison of serum from Lun-G cancer patients and healthy persons *Spectrochim. Acta A Mol. Biomol. Spectrosc.* **122** 193–7

[10] Kaznowska E, Depciuch J, Łach K, Kołodziej M, Koziorowska A, Vongsvivut J, Zawlik I, Cholewa M and Cebulski J 2018 The classification of lung cancers and their degree of malignancy by FTIR, PCA-LDA analysis, and a physics-based computational model *Talanta* **186** 337–45

[11] Bangaoil R, Santillan A, Angeles L M, Abanilla L, Lim A Jr, Ramos M C, Fellizar A, Guevarra L Jr and Albano P M 2020 ATR-FTIR spectroscopy as adjunct method to the microscopic examination of hematoxylin and eosin-stained tissues in diagnosing lung cancer *PLoS One* **15** e0233626

[12] Yang X, Ou Q, Qian K, Yang J, Bai Z, Yang W, Shi Y and Liu G 2021 Diagnosis of lung cancer by ATR-FTIR spectroscopy and chemometrics *Front. Oncol.* **11** 753791

[13] Rehman S, Movasaghi Z, Darr J A and Rehman I U 2010 Fourier transform infrared spectroscopic analysis of breast cancer tissues; Identifying differences between normal breast, invasive ductal carcinoma, and ductal carcinoma *in situ* of the breast *Appl. Spectrosc. Rev.* **45** 355–68

[14] Backhaus J, Mueller R, Formanski N, Szlama N, Meerpohl H G, Eidt M and Bugert P 2010 Diagnosis of breast cancer with infrared spectroscopy from serum samples *Vib. Spectrosc.* **52** 173–7

[15] Sitnikova V E, Kotkova M A, Nosenko T N, Kotkova T N, Martynova D M and Uspenskaya M V 2020 Breast cancer detection by ATR-FTIR spectroscopy of blood serum and multivariate data-analysis *Talanta* **214** 120857

[16] Tomas R C *et al* 2022 Detection of breast cancer by ATR-FTIR spectroscopy using artificial neural networks *PLoS One* **17** e0262489

[17] Du Y, Xie F, Yin L, Yang Y, Yang H, Wu G and Wang S 2022 Breast cancer early detection by using Fourier-transform infrared spectroscopy combined with different classification algorithms *Spectrochim. Acta A Mol. Biomol. Spectrosc.* **283** 121715

[18] Mishra A, Zehra S, Bharti P K, Mathur S R, Ranjan P, Batra A, Inampudi K K, Modi G P, Nikolajeff F and Kumar S 2024 Spectroscopic insight into breast cancer: profiling small extracellular vesicles lipids via infrared spectroscopy for diagnostic precision *Sci. Rep.* **14** 9347

[19] Podshyvalov A, Sahu R K, Mark S, Kantarovich K, Guterman H, Goldstein J, Jagannathan R, Argov S and Mordechai S 2005 Distinction of cervical cancer biopsies by use of infrared microspectroscopy and probabilistic neural networks *Appl. Opt.* **44** 3725–34

[20] Xue Y, Zheng X, Wu G and Wang J 2023 Rapid diagnosis of cervical cancer based on serum FTIR spectroscopy and support vector machines *Lasers Med. Sci.* **38** 276

[21] Ma Y, Liang F, Zhu M, Chen C, Chen C and Lv X 2022 FT-IR combined with PSO-CNN algorithm for rapid screening of cervical tumors *Photodiagnosis Photodyn. Ther.* **39** 103023
[22] Cañas R Z, Moran O Z, Flores M E J, Ruiz V V, Leyva J R, Macuil R D and Gayou V L 2023 Characterization and differentiation of cervical cancer cell lines using ATR-FTIR spectroscopy and multivariate data analysis *Biomed. Signal Process. Control.* **86** 105169
[23] Félix M M, Tavares M V, Santos I P, Batista de Carvalho A L M, Batista de Carvalho L A E and Marques M P M 2024 Cervical squamous cell carcinoma diagnosis by FTIR micro-spectroscopy *Molecules* **29** 922
[24] Li L *et al* 2018 Characterization of ovarian cancer cells and tissues by Fourier transform infrared spectroscopy *J. Ovarian Res.* **11** 64
[25] Li L, Wu J, Yang L, Wang H, Xu Y and Shen K 2021 Fourier transform infrared spectroscopy: an innovative method for the diagnosis of ovarian cancer *Cancer Manag. Res.* **13**
[26] Giamougiannis P, Morais C L M, Rodriguez B, Wood N J, Martin-Hirsch P L and Martin F L 2021 Detection of ovarian cancer (± neo-adjuvant chemotherapy effects) via ATR-FTIR spectroscopy: comparative analysis of blood and urine biofluids in a large patient cohort *Anal. Bioanal Chem.* **413** 5095–107
[27] Kluz-Barłowska M, Kluz T, Paja W, Pancerz K, Łączyńska-Madera M, Miziak P, Cebulski J and Depciuch J 2024 FT-Raman and FTIR spectroscopy as a tools showing marker of platinum-resistant phenomena in women suffering from ovarian cancer *Sci. Rep.* **14** 11025
[28] Ilic M and Ilic I 2022 Epidemiology of stomach cancer *World J. Gastroenterol.* **28** 1187–203
[29] Li Q, Wang W, Ling X and Wu J G 2013 Detection of gastric cancer with Fourier transform infrared spectroscopy and support vector machine classification *BioMed. Res. Int.* **2013** 942427
[30] Li Q, Zhao R, Shi S and Li W 2019 Diagnosis of gastric endoscopic biopsies using attenuated total reflectance (ATR) Fourier transform infrared (FT-IR) spectroscopy with entropy weight local-hyperplane *k*-nearest neighbor based on frequency domain information (EWHFI) *Ana. Lett.* **52** 1914–25
[31] Dong L, Duan X, Bin L, Wang J, Gao Q, Sun X and Xu Y 2022 Evaluation of Fourier transform infrared (FTIR) spectroscopy with multivariate analysis as a novel diagnostic tool for lymph node metastasis in gastric cancer *Spectrochim. Acta A Mol. Biomol. Spectrosc.* **289** 122209
[32] Pang N, Yang W, Yang G, Yang C, Tong K, Yu R and Jiang F 2024 The utilization of blood serum ATR-FTIR spectroscopy for the identification of gastric cancer *Discov. Oncol.* **15** 350
[33] Khanmohammadi M, Garmarudi A B, Ghasemi K, Jaliseh H K and Kaviani A 2009 Diagnosis of colon cancer by attenuated total reflectance-fourier transform infrared micro-spectroscopy and soft independent modeling of class analogy *Med. Oncol.* **26** 292–7
[34] Khanmohammadi M, Bagheri Garmarudi A, Samani S, Ghasemi K and Ashuri A 2011 Application of linear discriminant analysis and attenuated total reflectance Fourier transform infrared microspectroscopy for diagnosis of colon cancer *Pathol. Oncol. Res.* **17** 435–41
[35] Dong L *et al* 2014 Evaluation of FTIR spectroscopy as diagnostic tool for colorectal cancer using spectral analysis *Spectrochim. Acta A Mol. Biomol. Spectrosc.* **122** 288–94
[36] Kaznowska E, Depciuch J, Szmuc K and Cebulski J 2017 Use of FTIR spectroscopy and PCA LDC analysis to identify cancerous lesions within the human colon *J. Pharm. Biomed. Anal.* **134** 259–68

[37] Maria L, Gallo C, Capozzi V and Giuseppe Perna G 2023 Discrimination of healthy and cancerous colon cells based on FTIR spectroscopy and machine learning algorithms *Appl. Sci.* **13** 10325

[38] Magno G M, Lotilla G E, Ambrosio E R, Nagera F L, Grino M I, Castro M R, Millan J A, Manzano J A, Tiongco R E and Albano P M 2024 Blood-based FTIR spectroscopy as a minimally invasive diagnostic method for colorectal cancer: a meta-analysis *Asian Pac. J. Cancer Prev.* **25** 1487–95

[39] Baker M J, Gazi E, Brown M D, Shanks J H, Clarke N W and Gardner P 2009 Investigating FTIR based histopathology for the diagnosis of prostate cancer *J. Biophotonics* **2** 104–13

[40] Krafft C, Wilhelm K, Eremin A, Nestel S, von Bubnoff N, Schultze-Seemann W, Popp J and Nazarenko I 2017 A specific spectral signature of serum and plasma-derived extracellular vesicles for cancer screening *Nanomed* **13** 835–41

[41] Yap X L, Wood B, Ong T A, Lim J, Goh B H and Lee W L 2021 Detection of prostate cancer via IR spectroscopic analysis of urinary extracellular vesicles: a pilot study *Membranes (Basel)* **11** 591

[42] Harjan A H, Kadhim S A and Almayahi B A 2022 Prostate cancer serum spectra as indicators of early diagnosis using FTIR-ATR Fourier Transform Infrared Spectroscopy *J. Pharma. Negat. Results.* **13** 829–35

[43] Menzies G E, Fox H R, Marnane C, Pope L, Prabhu V, Winter S, Derrick A V and Lewis P D 2014 Fourier transform infrared for noninvasive optical diagnosis of oral, oropharyngeal, and laryngeal cancer *Transl. Res.* **163** 19–26

[44] Wang R and Wang Y 2021 Fourier transform infrared spectroscopy in oral cancer diagnosis *Int. J. Mol. Sci.* **22** 1206

[45] Zlotogorski-Hurvitz A, Dekel B Z, Malonek D, Yahalom R and Vered M 2019 FTIR-based spectrum of salivary exosomes coupled with computational-aided discriminating analysis in the diagnosis of oral cancer *J. Cancer Res. Clin. Oncol.* **145** 685–94

[46] Duckworth E, Hole A, Deshmukh A, Chaturvedi P, Chilakapati M K, Mora B and Roy D 2022 Improving vibrational spectroscopy prospects in frontline clinical diagnosis: Fourier transform infrared on buccal mucosa cancer *Anal. Chem.* **94** 13642–6

[47] Falamas A, Faur C I, Ciupe S, Chirila M, Rotaru H, Hedesiu M and Cinta Pinzaru S 2021 Rapid and noninvasive diagnosis of oral and oropharyngeal cancer based on micro-Raman and FT-IR spectra of saliva *Spectrochim. Acta A Mol. Biomol. Spectrosc.* **252** 119477

[48] Shree P, Aggarwal Y, Kumar M, Majhee L, Singh N N, Prakash O, Chandra A, Mahuli S A, Shamsi S and Rai A 2024 Saliva based diagnostic prediction of oral squamous cell carcinoma using FTIR spectroscopy *Indian J. Otolaryngol. Head Neck Surg.* **76** 2282–9

IOP Publishing

Spectroscopic Techniques for Cancer Diagnostics

Inbarasan Muniraj and Bryan Hennelly

Chapter 4

Advancing trustworthy virtual staining in histopathology using infrared spectroscopic imaging

Kianoush Falahkheirkhah, Jihun Oh and Rohit Bhargava

Microscopic imaging of biological materials relies on staining to visualize morphology; subsequently, a human examines the morphology to manually recognize patterns of staining indicative of disease. Virtual staining (VS), on the other hand, offers a transformative approach to translating label-free modalities into realistic stained images. This approach has become even more powerful through the use of advanced deep learning (DL) methods, potentially optimizing the speed and affordability of histopathological evaluations by eliminating staining and need for extensive manual examinations. Here we first review the state of the art in spectroscopic analyses and provide an overview of the approach. We then introduce the basic tenets of VS. Despite its apparent success, a significant and persistent challenge with this technology is the occurrence of hallucinations—unreal content that can introduce errors in cancer diagnosis and treatment. To ensure the reliability of VS, it is essential to understand and disclose potential uncertainties, helping clinicians and pathologists avoiding errors rooted in hallucinations. This work presents a preliminary exploration into methods for quantifying uncertainty in VS and introduces an efficient approach for estimating it during inference. Ultimately, this study underscores the importance and potential of trustworthy VS, bridging the divide between algorithmic development and clinical application.

4.1 Introduction

Need in histopathology: The practice of pathology is essential to many diagnostic and research tasks in varied diseases such as cancer. However, it remains highly labor-intensive, involving significant effort at each stage from tissue preparation to diagnostic interpretation. Ordinarily, thin tissue sections are stained and analysed under bright-field microscopy by skilled pathologists. Complex cases often require

doi:10.1088/978-0-7503-5949-8ch4

multiple rounds of staining along with detailed immunohistochemistry (IHC) analyses to reach a conclusive diagnosis. While microscopic assessment by a pathologist is the gold standard, current assessment methods have concordance issues [1–4], do not involve the tumor microenvironment [5–10] and incorporate little knowledge of molecular expression [11–13]. Recent efforts have aimed to prescribe individualized treatments by including patient clinical data, histologic characteristics of the biopsy and molecular biomarkers of the tumor [14]; however, the search for useful new technologies to improve pathology is an active area. In addition to the need for more information or improvements in current processes, time is often of the essence in diagnoses.

The current diagnostic choices are between the long wait times (several days) for gold standard formalin fixed paraffin embedded (FFPE) sections or the 'real-time' ($<$1 h) results with the workflow complexities and high resource needs for rapid, intraoperative frozen section (FS) pathology [15]. As a result, intraoperative pathology is only practiced in highly skilled and infrastructure-rich settings. Pathologists resist frozen section pathology because reviewing poor quality sections can have significant clinical impact on diagnosis and an incorrect evaluation of the FS can lead to inappropriate or incorrect surgery. Interpretation is challenging due to staining inconsistency, artifacts and the need for an experienced pathologist. Modern technologies that enable a rapid assessment of tissue that is compatible with clinical workflow, can produce archival-quality images in minutes using artificial intelligence (AI), and helping interpret diagnostic regions can be very helpful. If validated, these advances can provide improved diagnoses, reduce re-operation rates, improve outcomes, and reduce costs.

A new contrast in microscopy by spectroscopic imaging: To address these needs, we first examine optical microscopy and its limitations. Originally microscopy was 'label-free' [16] but bright-field optical microscopy offers little native contrast. Hence, tissue staining prior to microscopy is the standard practice for the last 125 + years. An additional source of contrast has now become accessible that can be label-free but provide significantly more contrast than (a few) dyes. The chemically specific mechanisms of mid-infrared (IR) absorption and Raman scattering [17, 18] have emerged in microscopy formats over the last two decades and present an opportunity for pathology. The examination of tissue with IR spectroscopy predates the discovery of the Raman effect and has been a long-standing area of investigation. While bulk IR spectroscopy has been used to examine biological materials since around the same time as staining became popular [19], spectra could only be acquired from microscopic regions around 1949 [20]. Unfortunately, the signal-to-noise ratio (SNR) of the data were too low and scanning of large tissues to examine them in the manner of optical microscopy was not possible. Larger areas could be mapped with the coupling of interferometers and IR microscopes in the 1980s, leading to the availability of Fourier transform IR (FT-IR) mapping [21]. However, the ability to measure a typical biomedical sample like a typical pathology specimen was limited by both the low throughput (and SNR) of the microscopes as well as the slow scanning to build up low-resolution ($\sim$50 μm pixels sizes) maps of small areas ($\sim$ 1 mm × 1 mm). The next advance was the incorporation of array detectors for IR imaging [22], providing high speed and enabling measurements with sufficient SNR to be useful. These advances provided impetus for many proof of concept studies by numerous groups across the world. Despite progress, typical commercially-available FT-IR imaging systems' performance [23] made it too slow for routine pathology ($\sim$1 day/sample). Techniques like high-definition Fourier transform infrared (FT-IR) [24–26] spectroscopy offer hyperspectral resolution, though this often comes at the cost of throughput, with slower acquisition times and substantial data redundancy posing challenges in clinical settings. The emergence of quantum cascade lasers (QCLs) [27, 28] provided orders of magnitude higher intensity and allowed new designs of IR microscopes that provide both rapid and high-fidelity imaging [29–32]. QCL systems [27, 30, 33–36] can also provide rapid, targeted spectral imaging that preserves essential biochemical information without redundant data, making it more suitable for clinical applications.

By harnessing the unique vibrational spectral fingerprints of biomolecules—including proteins, lipids, nucleic acids, and collagen—IR imaging quantifies their distribution and concentration at each pixel, capturing intricate spatial morphology. Several example studies are available for the application of IR imaging to pathology [23, 38–45]. Herein, molecular composition encoded in the optical spectral profile at every pixel is interpreted via AI algorithms, providing a previously inaccessible molecular contrast for pathology [23]. IR spectral contrast is the strongest optical molecular signal. IR spectra have been used to describe optical molecular signatures [46] of health and disease [40, 47] and offers a powerful signal as it arises from fundamental vibrational mode absorption. IR imaging capabilities and their comparison with other imaging techniques for pathology has been recently discussed [37]. Complementary to traditional pathology (figure 4.1), IR imaging can provide 'stainless' images, use machine learning (ML) to provide diagnostic information in easy to interpret, color-coded images, provide information that may otherwise need extensive staining and examination (e.g. tumor infiltrating lymphocytes), and generate new information (e.g. collagen quality of the stroma) that is commonly not sought in today's pathology or may not even be possible to obtain with current methods. Some studies have even correlated observed biochemical physiology to cancer driving mutations [31, 48].

Infrared-based tissue segmentation: Advancements in QCL-based IR imaging are revolutionizing the field of pathology, particularly in applications where real-time assessment is essential. One such critical setting is the intraoperative frozen lab, where rapid and accurate diagnostic evaluations are crucial for guiding surgical decisions [49, 50]. Traditional methods, such as formalin fixation and H&E staining, although reliable, require significant time for sample preparation and staining, often exceeding several hours. By contrast, IR imaging offers a transformative approach, enabling chemical and structural assessments of fresh tissue samples without the need for stains, significantly accelerating the diagnostic workflow. IR imaging's real-time capabilities are enabled by its ability to acquire and analyze spatial-spectral data at unprecedented speeds. When combined with cryostat-prepared fresh frozen tissue, this technology facilitates near-instantaneous imaging and diagnosis. Cryostat microtomes allow the preparation of thin tissue sections in a matter of

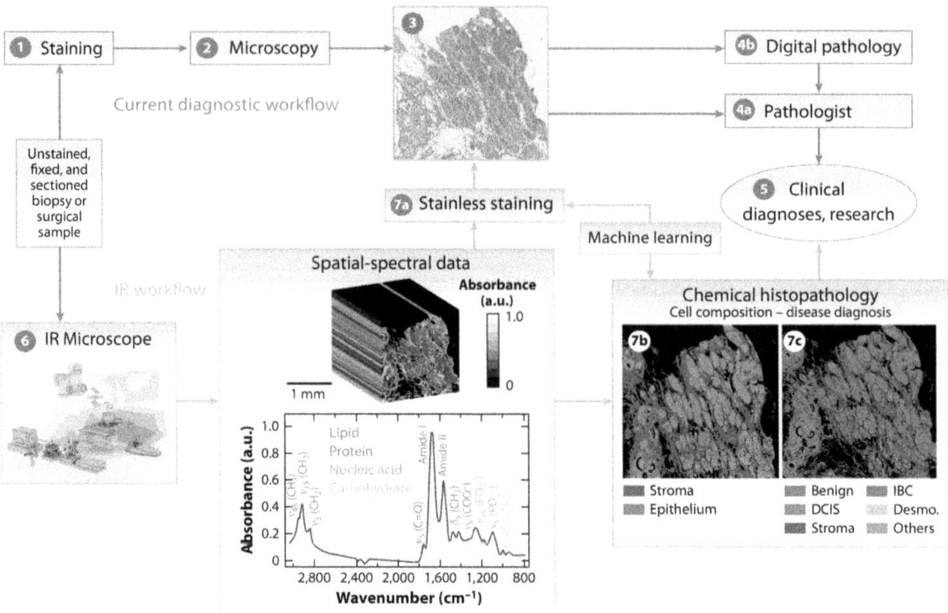

Figure 4.1. Concept of all-digital pathology by IR imaging. Current pathology workflow (blue boxes) starts from slide samples and proceeds via staining, ML to segment tissue into cell types and disease (histopathology) or use stainless staining to provide stain-equivalent images. Reproduced with permission from a prior study [37] CC BY 4.0.

minutes, providing a direct pathway from surgical excision to imaging. This rapid workflow aligns perfectly with the clinical demands of intraoperative diagnostics, where surgeons rely on timely information to make critical decisions. In this context, QCL-IR imaging stands out for its ability to preserve the chemical and structural integrity of fresh tissue, enabling high-resolution imaging and advanced data analysis within a timeframe of less than an hour. Unlike conventional histopathological methods, IR imaging does not rely on staining or subjective human interpretation. Instead, it employs ML algorithms to analyze the spectral-spatial data and make automated, objective assignments of disease states. For example, in our recent study [36], using annotations from experts (figures 4.2(a) and 4.2(b)), a U-Net [51] DL model (figure 4.2(c)) was trained to segment fresh frozen prostate tissues into three key histological classes: benign epithelium, malignant epithelium, and non-epithelial stroma. Importantly, IR imaging demonstrated clear differentiation between these histological classes as can be seen in figures 4.2(d–f), providing results that were consistent with parallel H&E-stained sections (figures 4.2(g) and 4.2(h)). This capability is particularly valuable in complex tissue architectures, where traditional methods may face challenges in accurately identifying the boundaries between benign and malignant regions. By offering rapid and precise segmentation, IR imaging supports more informed decision-making during surgical procedures. Beyond its immediate clinical applications, the use of IR imaging in frozen labs has broader implications for the field of pathology. The label-free nature of the technique preserves

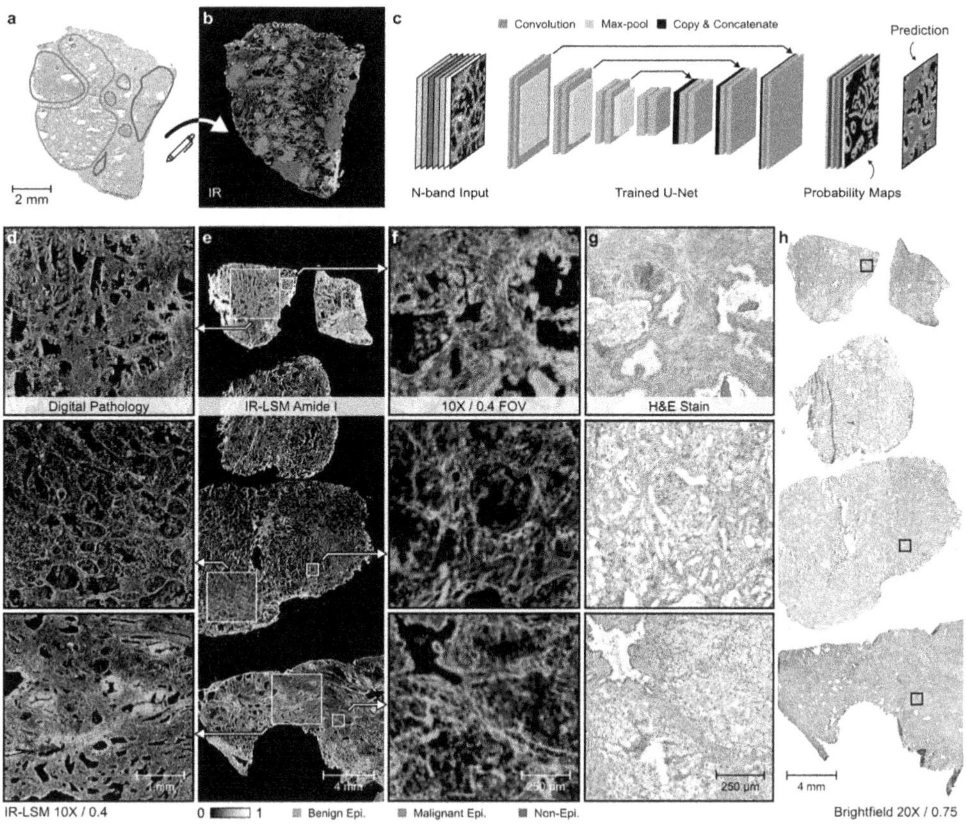

Figure 4.2. Visual comparison of prostate tumor segmentation. (a) Rough annotations guided by pathologists, (b) transferred from H&E to IR images on consecutive sections. (c) A DL model predicts epithelial malignancy using multispectral IR images. (d) The performance of the DL model is demonstrated on unstained samples with varying gland types, imaged using label-free IR technology. (e) Amide I images show target ROIs on full slides, (f) with 10× magnified views simulating screening. (g, h) Comparative H&E-stained parallel sections highlight corresponding ROIs. Reproduced with permission from a prior study [36] CC BY 4.0.

tissue samples for additional downstream analyses, such as immunohistochemistry or sequencing, without compromising their chemical or structural integrity. This opens new opportunities for integrating molecular-level analyses into routine workflows, further enriching the diagnostic capabilities of frozen labs. The ability to incorporate ML into the IR imaging pipeline also underscores its adaptability and scalability. As DL algorithms become more sophisticated, they can capture increasingly detailed spatial and textural features, enhancing the interpretative power of IR imaging. This synergy between advanced instrumentation and computational techniques positions QCL-IR imaging as a cornerstone for future innovations in pathology.

VS or stainless staining: In recent years, advancements in ML, and label-free imaging have come together, showing great potential to enhance the pathology [37, 52–58]. New DL methods are providing new means to use spatial-chemical data for AI to exceed current predictive and prognostic capabilities. A key advancement is the development of VS, which leverages DL to transform images from one modality or stain type into realistic representations of another [59–65]. This approach reduces the need for additional reagents and manual staining processes, potentially providing a faster, more cost-effective, and environmentally sustainable alternative to conventional methods. Among label-free technologies, chemical imaging stands out for VS due to its rich information content and quantitative measurement of tissue properties. These features not only provide an extensive (and redundant) information measure of tissue properties but also provide avenues to tackle such confounding effects as sample-thickness-dependent signals in label-free approaches. Further, the extensive data can be used to layer in multiple checks and balances to ensure that both the virtual inference and direct chemical measurement can be used to inform the status of the tissue, making it an excellent source for high-quality stain translations. Two techniques—stimulated Raman scattering (SRS) and infrared (IR) imaging—offer detailed chemical insights and can be used with minimal training, potentially enhancing both clinical diagnostics and research applications. Here we focus on IR imaging,

The process is relatively straightforward and has been relatively consistent since the first study [59]. In pathology, the use of haematoxylin and eosin (H&E) stains is commonly used to allow a visualization of tissue morphology using optical microscopy. In our approach, IR imaging data was recorded from unstained tissue and spectra contain the combined influences of molecular content of the sample, morphology and optical system. These features were used as input for statistical pattern recognition algorithms [66] (in this case, a neural network (NN) model) that related the IR input to molecular or dye parameters. The NN transforms the recorded spectroscopic data at every pixel into color values or staining intensity found in histological stains imaged using bright-field microscopy. The predicted stain or dye values can be used to generate a computed stain image that faithfully reproduces the staining pattern of H&E images that are important for recognition. However, H&E stains lack specificity in terms of the functional or molecular content of the tissue. Visualizing molecular content is significantly more expensive, time-consuming and difficult. We further evaluated molecularly-specific stains. IHC stains for cell types are often used in diagnostic imaging or for specific research purposes, for example, high molecular weight (HMW) cytokeratin (epithelial-type cell), vimentin (fibroblast-like cell), smooth muscle alpha actin (myo-like cell), P63 (myoepithelial cells), CD31 (endothelial cells) and Masson's Trichrome (MT) stain (collagen and keratin fibers), are commonly employed. A comparison of the physically stained and computationally stained images can be seen in figure 4.3. Using a combination of the staining results it is possible to subsequently deduce the cell types and/or molecular transformations present. The chemical content in spectroscopy, recorded once, can be used multiple times to relate to expression levels in tissue. Hence, the approach allows us to compute multiple stains from a single spectroscopic image for the same sample. Such a capability would be exceptionally useful when the tissue available is limited, e.g. in fine needle biopsies or spheroids in 3D cell culture. This capability also provides a quantitative method for histology, eliminating staining variance between sample replicates and providing

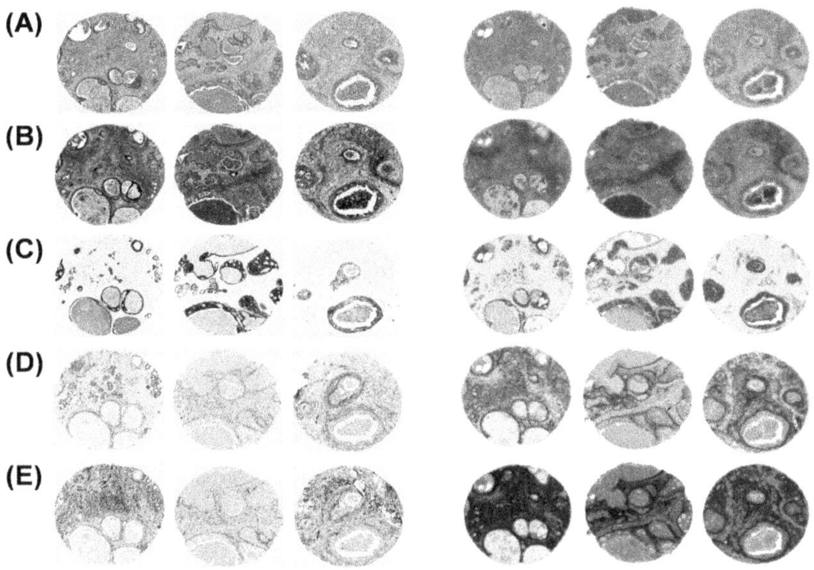

Figure 4.3. Molecular imaging (three sample panel on the left) can be reproduced by chemical imaging (right panel). In addition to H&E-stained imaged (a), we extend the concept of stainless staining to molecularly-specific stains, including (b) MT stain (collagen and keratin fibers) (b) High molecular Weight (HMW) cytokeratin (epithelial-type cell), (c) smooth muscle alpha actin (myo-like cell) and (d) vimentin (fibroblast-like cell). Each spot is 1.4 mm in diameter. Reproduced with permission from a prior study [59].

a means of quickly extracting a large range of histological information from a single tissue sample. The method can be equally applicable to fresh or FFPE-processed tissue and the use of only light preserves the tissue for further analyses.

Parallel to these efforts, stimulated Raman scattering (SRS) [54, 67–70] has emerged as a powerful complementary technique, bringing label-free, high-resolution chemical contrast to VS. SRS excels at distinguishing subtle biochemical variations within tissue, using nonlinear optical processes to achieve high-quality imaging with minimal sample preparation. Together, these advancements in IR and SRS techniques are setting new standards in spatial resolution, SNR, and speed, paving the way for VS that is both clinically practical and diagnostically robust. With these capabilities, chemical imaging stands as a transformative modality for VS, bridging raw spectral data and clinically actionable insights with precision and efficiency.

Hallucinations in VS: A major obstacle in VS lies in the issue of hallucinations—misrepresentations or inaccuracies in the generated images. These can stem from several challenges, including the inherently ambiguous nature of the translation task, limitations within DL frameworks that prevent convergence to the accurate mapping function, and the model's vulnerability to unfamiliar data outside its training distribution. These factors contribute to unpredictable results, raising concerns about reliability in clinical applications. For VS to be trusted, it is vital to provide a measure of diagnosis confidence by uncertainty estimation (UE). This aims to give pathologists an indication of which regions in the translated images are reliable. Among the various UE approaches proposed in literature, deep ensembles [71] is frequently cited the most competitive method [72], in which multiple models are trained under different DL random seeds and afterwards the predictive divergence is used to score uncertainty. This approach however imposes significant computational overhead from needing to train multiple models and performing multiple forward-passes during inference. While the former training cost is acceptable as it occurs offline, the latter is critical as it hinders the ability to perform VS in a timely manner. To address this specific issue, DL researchers proposed further constructing a single surrogate model emulating the statistics of the deep ensemble, termed ensemble distillation [73, 74]. Such an approach significantly reduces inference time as it only requires a single forward-pass using surrogate, while maintaining the high quality of the uncertainty achieved by deep ensembles. These benefits make such an approach an attractive solution in the realms of VS.

In this chapter, we inspect the feasibility of the ensemble distillation concept in VS over two distinct datasets. We start by training a deep ensemble of VS models to generate an example perceptual uncertainty map, using insights from prior research [75]. Next, we explore whether this perceptual uncertainty map can be distilled into a single model. Our findings indicate that this approach is indeed feasible.

4.2 Method

Datasets: We employ two distinct datasets as our test bed: (1) a paired dataset consisting of SRS source and H&E target images (termed VS dataset), and (2) unpaired dataset consisting of H&E source and MT targets (termed stain-to-stain, S2S dataset). Our VS dataset was procured in collaboration with Mayo Clinic, Rochester, MN, comprising fresh frozen prostate tissue samples from de-identified patients. These samples spanned clinically relevant Gleason grades from 3 + 3 to 5 + 5. We utilized the SRS data that has been published previously [70], which includes specific Raman shift frequencies of 2847, 2879, 2933, and 2979 cm^{-1}. Upon SRS imaging completion, the tissue sections were subjected to H&E staining, establishing the necessary ground truth for our VS framework. These H&E-stained whole slide images (WSIs) were subsequently captured with Nanozoomer scanners at 20x magnification, ensuring detailed high-resolution images. The creation of our training set involved extracting regions of interest (ROIs) from 25 frozen prostate samples, yielding a substantial collection of 4376 patches, each measuring 500 × 500 pixels. We earmarked 10% of these patches for validation. The test set was formulated from ROIs derived from two frozen prostate samples, resulting in a total of 385 patches, identical in dimensions to the training set. For the unpaired S2S, we utilized a publicly available resource [76]. In brief, WSIs were obtained from mouse liver tissue samples stained with H&E and MT using a Zeiss AxioScan scanner at 20x magnification. The training set contained approximately 26 000 tiles (each 256 × 256 pixels) extracted from WSIs for each staining type, with 10% set aside for validation. The test set comprised 1300 image tiles for each staining type, which were extracted from distinct histology sections.

Training details of deep ensembles: For both datasets, we train 50 virtual stainers to comprise our deep ensemble. This ensemble will be used to derive our perceptual uncertainty map, i.e., the label mask for the surrogate model, in later sections. Note, as our goal is to explore proof-of-concept of distillation, we purposely use a large ensemble to ensure convergent behavior. For both datasets, we adopt a least squares generative adversarial network (GAN) framework [77]. For the S2S task, we adopt a self-regularization loss to prevent the generator from adding clinically misleading information. For network architectures, we adopt the U-Net [51] for the generator and the multi-scale discriminator [78]. For VS, we first pre-train without the adversarial loss for 600 training iterations before commencing with it for an additional 30 000 iterations, which we found to yield more stable training. S2S was trained similarly but without the initial non-adversarial pre-training. For both VS and S2S, we employed a batch size of 10 using the Adam optimizer [79] set to an initial learning rate of 0.0001, scaled down by a factor of 0.97 after every 2000 iterations. Batch normalization (BN) [80] is also employed for stability. As for data augmentation, random affine transformations and Gaussian noise (just for SRS) were applied to enhance variability and robustness. We repeat this process 50 times but using different seeds to induce randomness in the network initialization, batch ordering, and augmentations.

Derivation of a perceptual uncertainty map: We proceed to utilize the predictive divergence amongst deep ensemble members to define a spatially resolved uncertainty map. The naïve approach of using the pixel-wise variance of the predicted target image is not helpful for decision-making as it is large for almost the entirety of the image frame, even in the absence of pathological differences (e.g., slight discrepancy in color or brightness), evident in figure 4.4. Clearly, there is a need for a more refined uncertainty representation. To this end, we leverage the deep features of pre-trained networks, which are known to correlate to the human visual perception [75]. Specifically, for each member, we extract the feature map at the last layer's internal activation of the ResNet50 model [81] upsampled to its original source/target image resolutions. Afterwards, we quantify the per-channel variance of the activations across ensemble members to derive a perceptual uncertainty (PU) map. The choice of ResNet50 is not a strict requirement but rather provides a defined distillation target. In this study, ResNet50 was selected based on comparative visual inspection; however, alternative feature extractors may be employed without compromising the approach. We show an example PU map in figure 4.4 where it is less sensitive to extraneous factors, and thus, serves as a more suitable uncertainty index to be learnt by distillation.

Uncertainty distillation: We finally train a surrogate model that upon receiving the source image predicts its associated PU map from 50 deep ensemble members. Prior to training, we first extract the training set's uncertainty map beforehand to avoid acquiring them on-the-fly, accelerating the training process. To leverage transfer learning, we set the architecture of the surrogate model to ResNet50, fine-tuning from its pre-trained weights. Additional layers randomly initialized are appended by the input and output to match the image source and uncertainty map dimensions, respectively. The training procedure is similar to that of section 2.2, but we perform

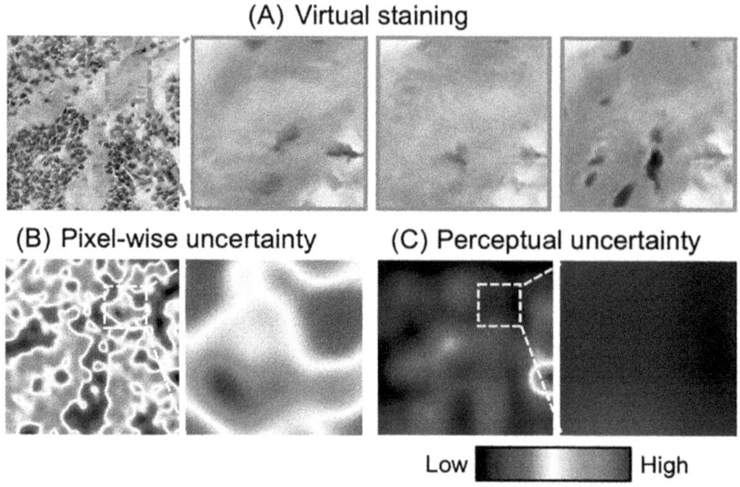

Figure 4.4. Conceptual visualization of the advantages of PU. (A) VS result with three magnified areas showcasing variations in the ensemble. (B) Pixel-wise uncertainty estimation. (C) PU estimation. Unlike the pixel-wise method, the perceptual index is less sensitive to uncertainties arising from factors like illumination, contrast, brightness, and minor local variances that are not crucial for pathology. The main patch measures 250 μm and magnified areas span 50 μm each.

early-stopping using a held-out validation set before ~8000 iterations to prevent overfitting. It is worth noting that the training of this surrogate is completely post-hoc and decoupled from the deep ensemble training. Likewise, we do not leak any test set information into the training of this surrogate. Once trained, this surrogate is used in place of the prohibitive deep ensemble whenever rapid uncertainty estimations are desired, shown schematically in figure 4.5.

4.3 Results and discussion

Distillation offers the best of both worlds: (1) the high-quality uncertainty of deep ensemble, and (2) rapid inference times, making it suitable for rapid trustworthy VS. One limitation is that a single surrogate may not be capable of expressing the uncertainty of the complex deep ensemble system. To investigate, we quantify the accuracy of the distilled surrogate over the test dataset using the l2-distance and dice score relative to the deep ensemble's 50-member uncertainty map. The l2-distance is simply the mean squared error between the two maps, whereas the dice score first thresholds them and quantifies the overlap between uncertain hot-spots. For comparison, we also evaluate these metrics when using the deep ensemble uncertainty comprised of 3, 5, 7, 10 members, randomly drawn from the initial pool of 50. Results are shown in table 4.1, and we observe that the surrogate achieves accuracies comparable to a deep ensemble consisting of five members. Thus, the inference cost benefit of the surrogate is five-fold. We also observe an improvement in stability compared to this ensemble, with nearly a ten-fold difference in some cases. It can thus be concluded that distillation is indeed feasible in the context of VS.

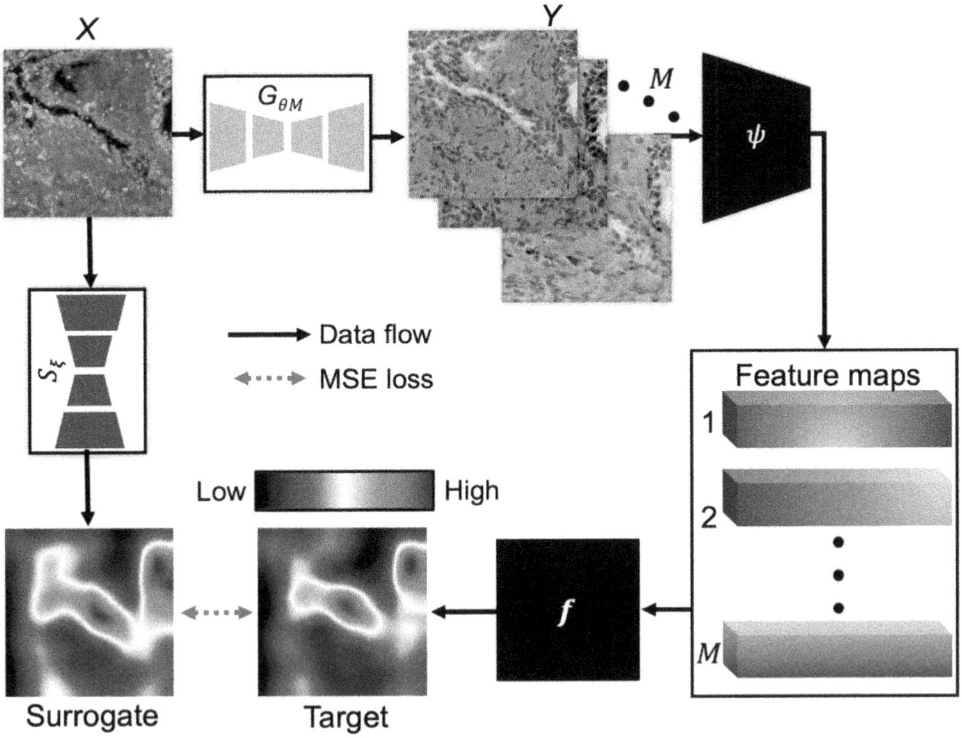

Figure 4.5. Schematic workflow. The process starts with the development of the deep ensemble virtual stainers to capture the dispersion in the feature space and quantify 'uncertainty'. Then, a surrogate network is utilized to estimate this prohibitive uncertainty directly from the source image during test time.

Table 4.1. Performance comparison. We show the mean (± std) of l2-squared distance and dice score (%) w.r.t. the ground-truth uncertainty map of the 50-member deep ensemble. The surrogate achieves comparable performance to a practical deep ensemble of ~5 members.

Dataset	Method	L2-squared (×1e−3)	Dice score %
VS	Deep ensemble (×3)	0.635 (± 0.067)	68.39 (±3.62)
	Deep ensemble (×5)	0.307 (± 0.018)	82.00 (±1.25)
	Deep ensemble (×7)	0.204 (± 0.014)	86.67 (±0.48)
	Deep ensemble (×10)	0.159 (± 0.014)	88.51 (±0.33)
	Surrogate	0.270 (± 0.011)	84.14 (±0.38)
S2S	Deep ensemble (×3)	0.201 (± 0.027)	59.97 (±5.24)
	Deep ensemble (×5)	0.089 (± 0.009)	76.89 (±3.59)
	Deep ensemble (×7)	0.060 (± 0.006)	81.16 (±1.54)
	Deep ensemble (×10)	0.051 (± 0.010)	83.66 (±0.78)
	Surrogate	0.125 (± 0.002)	76.02 (±0.33)

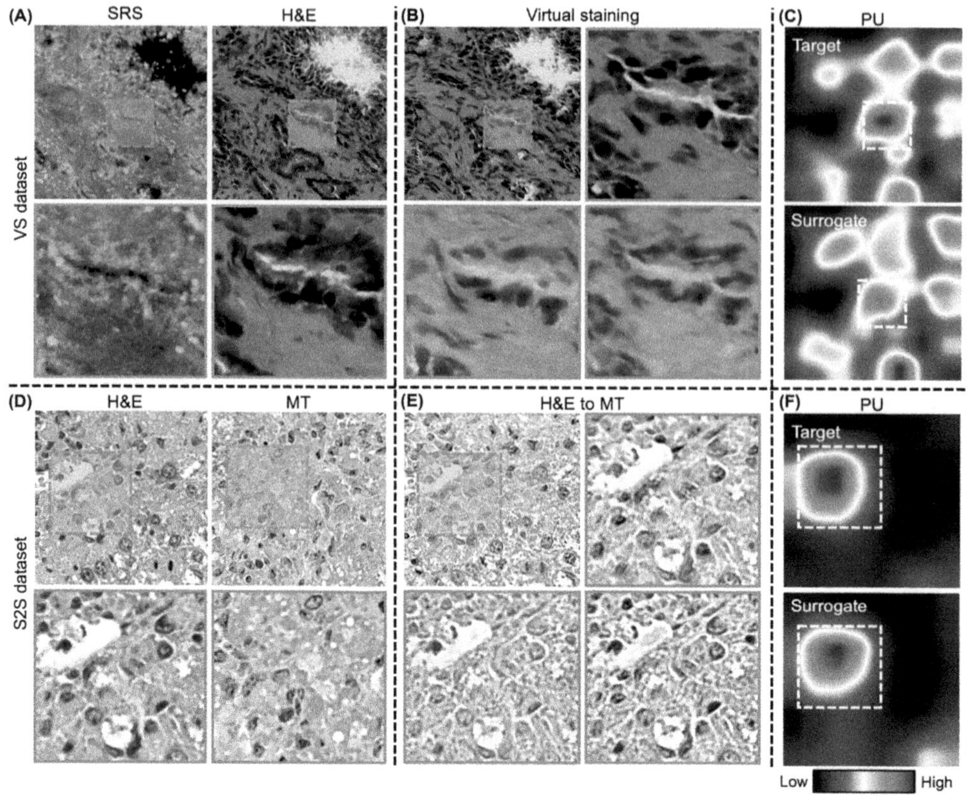

Figure 4.6. Visual results of proposed framework. (A) SRS and H&E images featuring zoomed-in sections. (B) Virtual stain visualization with three zoom-ins showcasing variations from multiple deep ensemble member. (C) Assessment of the PU. The top row represents the deep ensemble's ground-truth PU over 50 members (i.e., distillation target), while the bottom row illustrates the distillation via the surrogate model. (D) H&E and MT with detailed views. (E) Stain-to-stain translation depicted with three magnified views from different deep ensemble members. (F) PU analysis: Top row presents the target PU, and the bottom demonstrates distillation using the surrogate.

In figure 4.6, we further visualize our findings. In the top row of figure 4.6(A) and 4.6(D), the source image (SRS for VS, H&E for S2S) is juxtaposed with its target image (H&E for VS, MT for S2S). Note for the unpaired S2S, the target MT shows the data obtained at the nearest tissue section of the source H&E. We complement the images with a detailed zoom-in view in the bottom row. Figure 4.6(B) and 4.6(E) provides a large patch generated from one instance of the deep ensemble, accompanied by three magnified sections from distinct ensemble members from a high uncertainty region. Upon inspecting the zoomed-in areas, it is evident that the uncertainty arises from perceptual variations, e.g., the nuclear morphology and organization of glandular structures for VS's H&E and connective tissue morphology, nuclei shape and color for S2S's MT. These semantic nuances are effectively highlighted by the deep ensemble's 50-member PU map, shown in the top panel of figure 4.6(C) and 4.6(F). Lastly, it can be seen that the distilled 'surrogate's uncertainty map in the bottom panel shows strong agreement with this map, thus, proving the feasibility of distillation.

In figure 4.7, to further illustrate examples and meticulously inspect the performance of our models, we present visualizations comparing ground-truth uncertainty map, its surrogate prediction, and instances with varying levels of uncertainty. These are specifically demonstrated for both VS and S2S models, as shown in panels A and B, respectively. This comparative arrangement is particularly enlightening in regions of high uncertainty, where we observe significant perceptual variances in nuclear shape, organization, and count across individual deep ensemble members' outputs, indicating discernible perceptual discrepancies. Conversely, areas of low uncertainty exhibit remarkable consistency in outputs, reflecting a higher degree of certainty. Each segment in these visualizations is magnified to a scale of 50 × 50 μm, facilitating a detailed inspection of these subtle yet crucial differences in PU.

Finally, to ensure thoroughness, we highlight one primary limitation of our current approach. As depicted in figure 4.8, we present an SRS dataset that was compromised during recording. This anomaly is consistently exaggerated in all deep

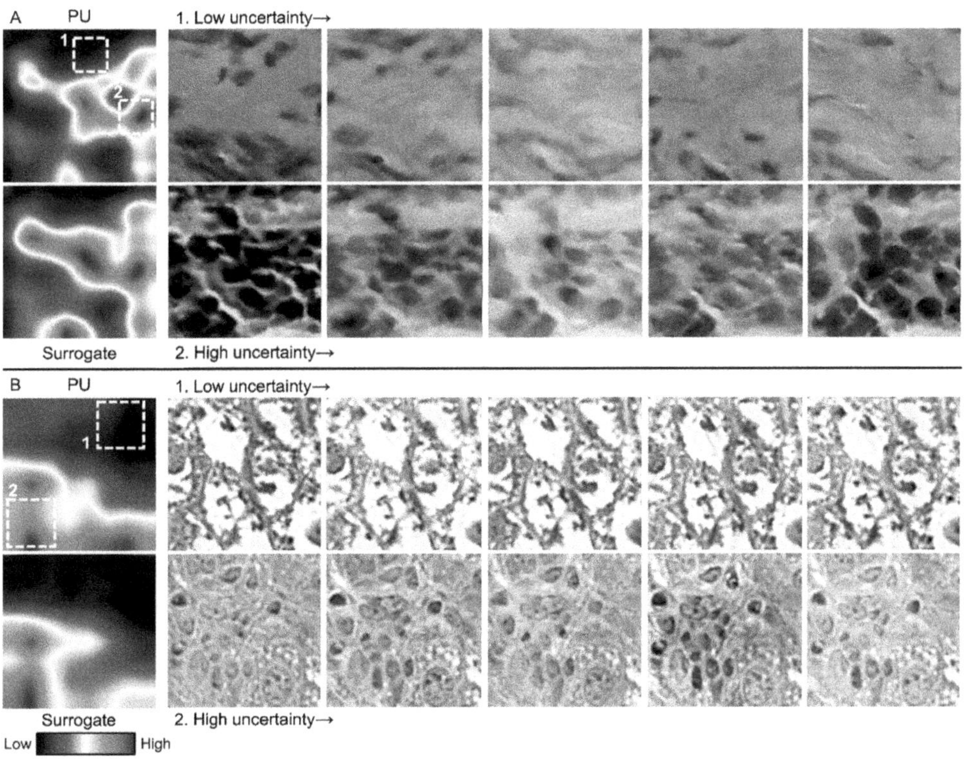

Figure 4.7. Visualization of the 50-member deep ensemble's uncertainty, its surrogate prediction, and examples with low and high uncertainty. (A) showcases these elements for VS models, while (B) represents them in the context of S2S models. The left column juxtaposes the target uncertainty with its surrogate. Subsequent columns display output from five deep ensemble members, emphasizing both low and high uncertainty regions. Each magnified segment measures 50 × 50 μm.

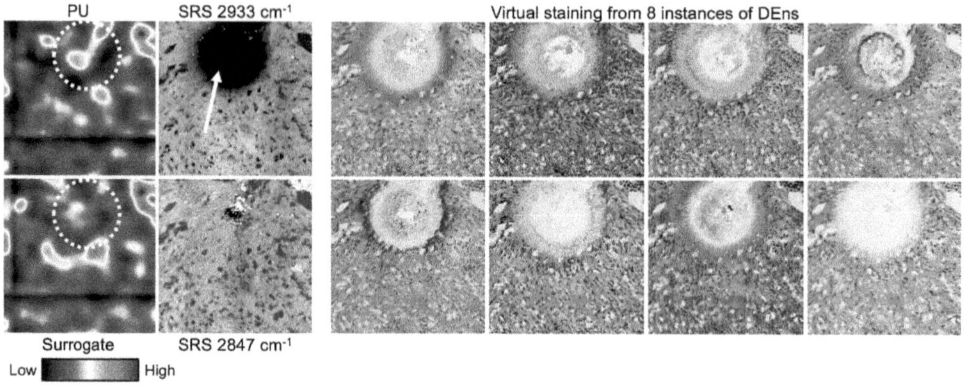

Figure 4.8. Failure Case. Presented here are the 50-member deep ensemble's uncertainty map, surrogate counterpart, SRS at 2933 and 2847 cm^{-1}, along with eight virtual stain images derived from eight distinct deep ensemble members. An arrow highlights an instrumental failure in the 2933 cm^{-1}. Remarkably, even with the evident perceptual differences in the generated VS images, both the uncertainty map and the surrogate failed to detect them, and thus, they did not signal increased uncertainty for this section. All the images are 500×500 μm.

ensemble members, leading to significant perceptual deviations in that specific area. However, the 50-member deep ensemble's uncertainty map fails to recognize these discrepancies, erroneously indicating low uncertainty. This issue may stem from the reliance on a pre-trained model like ResNet50, which uses ImageNet for training. While ImageNet is broadly applicable in many areas, it may not be entirely suitable for the specific nuances of histology contexts. We anticipate the utilization of foundational models pre-trained with histology patches to mitigate such artifacts.

4.4 Conclusions

This study was motivated by the need to assess confidence in VS, derived from chemical images, specifically for clinical applications, in a scalable manner. We demonstrated that by adopting distillation of state-of-the-art deep ensembles, we can achieve both high-fidelity uncertainty estimates while maintaining throughput, specifically accelerating inference time several-fold. Such enhancements are particularly valuable in the realm of histology, where both explainable and prompt VS is paramount to facilitate accurate diagnosis. By speeding up the process without compromising trustworthiness, we open doors for real-time applications, potentially changing the landscape of how histological examinations are conducted. We thus anticipate our study to be of value to the medical community to conclude, we discuss three future directions. One immediate task is to figure out a more histology-aware feature extractor to address the aforementioned limitation. Another avenue could be how to integrate these measures of uncertainty directly into the training regimen. By doing so, we could further enhance the quality and robustness of image-to-image translation models by less prioritizing of the reconstruction of semantically uncertain regions. Last, there is little-to-no work on how to propagate the uncertainty to downstream ML tasks. For example, given a virtually-stained

H&E translation and its corresponding uncertainty map, it would be desirable to predict, with foreknowledge of uncertainty, cancer grade or survival prediction. This work can serve to excite interest in both VS as well as its assurance, thereby providing a higher degree of confidence for practitioners to use both chemical imaging and AI-derived knowledge.

References

[1] Epstein J I 2010 An update of the Gleason grading system *J. Urol.* **183** 433–40

[2] Egevad L, Ahmad A S, Algaba F, Berney D M, Boccon-Gibod L, Compérat E *et al* 2013 Standardization of Gleason grading among 337 European pathologists *Histopathology* **62** 247–56

[3] Arvaniti E, Fricker K S, Moret M, Rupp N, Hermanns T, Fankhauser C *et al* 2018 Automated Gleason grading of prostate cancer tissue microarrays via deep learning *Sci. Rep.* **8** 12054

[4] Nagpal K, Foote D, Liu Y, Chen P-H C, Wulczyn E, Tan F *et al* 2019 Development and validation of a deep learning algorithm for improving Gleason scoring of prostate cancer *NPJ Digit. Med.* **2** 1–10

[5] Chung L W K, Baseman A, Assikis V and Zhau H E 2005 Molecular insights into prostate cancer progression: the missing link of tumor microenvironment *J. Urol.* **173** 10–20

[6] Chiarugi P, Paoli P and Cirri P 2014 Tumor microenvironment and metabolism in prostate cancer *Semin. Oncol.* **41** 267–80

[7] Barron D A and Rowley D R 2012 The reactive stroma microenvironment and prostate cancer progression *Endocr. Relat. Cancer* **19** R187–204

[8] Martin N E, Mucci L A, Loda M and Depinho R A 2011 Prognostic determinants in prostate cancer *Cancer J.* **17** 429–37

[9] Bello I O, Vered M, Dayan D, Dobriyan A, Yahalom R, Alanen K *et al* 2011 Cancer-associated fibroblasts, a parameter of the tumor microenvironment, overcomes carcinoma-associated parameters in the prognosis of patients with mobile tongue cancer *Oral Oncol.* **47** 33–8

[10] Dai J, Lu Y, Roca H, Keller J M, Zhang J, McCauley L K *et al* 2017 Immune mediators in the tumor microenvironment of prostate cancer *Chin. J. Cancer* **36** 29

[11] Sun W, Shi H, Yuan Z, Xia L, Xiang X, Quan X *et al* 2020 Prognostic value of genes and immune infiltration in prostate tumor microenvironment *Front. Oncol.* **10** 584055

[12] Ashida S, Orloff M S, Bebek G, Zhang L, Zheng P, Peehl D M *et al* 2012 Integrated analysis reveals critical genomic regions in prostate tumor microenvironment associated with clinicopathologic phenotypes *Clin. Cancer Res.* **18** 1578–87

[13] Bahmad H F, Jalloul M, Azar J, Moubarak M M, Samad T A, Mukherji D *et al* 2021 Tumor microenvironment in prostate cancer: toward identification of novel molecular biomarkers for diagnosis, prognosis, and therapy development *Front. Genet.* **12** 652747

[14] Adamaki M and Zoumpourlis V 2021 Prostate cancer biomarkers: from diagnosis to prognosis and precision-guided therapeutics *Pharmacol. Ther.* **228** 107932

[15] Rocco B, Sighinolfi M C, Bertoni L, Spandri V, Puliatti S, Eissa A *et al* 2020 Real-time assessment of surgical margins during radical prostatectomy: a novel approach that uses fluorescence confocal microscopy for the evaluation of peri-prostatic soft tissue *BJU Int.* **125** 487–9

[16] Milestones timeline: nature milestones in light microscopy https://nature.com/milestones/milelight/timeline.html
[17] Sammon C, Schultz Z D, Kazarian S, Barr H, Goodacre R, Graham D *et al* 2016 Spectral pathology: general discussion *Faraday Discuss.* **187** 155–86
[18] Diem M, Mazur A, Lenau K, Schubert J, Bird B, Miljković M *et al* 2013 Molecular pathology via IR and Raman spectral imaging *J. Biophotonics* **6** 855–86
[19] Nichols E F 1893 A study of the transmission spectra of certain substances in the Infra-red *Phys. Rev. (Series I)* **1** 1–18
[20] Blout E R and Mellors R C 1949 Infrared spectra of tissues *Science (1979)* **110** 137–8
[21] Steger W E, Messerschmidt R G, Harthcock M A (eds) 1989 Infrared microspectroscopy: Theory and applications *Practical Spectroscopy* vol 6 ed E G Brame Jr (New York; Basel: Marcel Dekker, Inc.) p 634
[22] Lewis E N, Gorbach A M, Marcott C and Levin I W 1996 High-fidelity fourier transform infrared spectroscopic imaging of primate brain tissue *Appl. Spectrosc.* **50** 263–9
[23] Fernandez D C, Bhargava R, Hewitt S M and Levin I W 2005 Infrared spectroscopic imaging for histopathologic recognition *Nat. Biotechnol.* **23** 469–74
[24] Reddy R K, Walsh M J, Schulmerich M V, Carney P S and Bhargava R 2013 High-definition infrared spectroscopic imaging *Appl. Spectrosc.* **67** 93–105
[25] Sreedhar H, Varma V K, Nguyen P L, Davidson B, Akkina S, Guzman G *et al* 2015 High-definition Fourier transform infrared (FT-IR) spectroscopic imaging of human tissue sections towards improving pathology *J. Vis. Exp.* **95** e52332
[26] Lotfollahi M, Berisha S, Daeinejad D and Mayerich D 2019 Digital staining of high-definition fourier transform infrared (FT-IR) images using deep learning *Appl. Spectrosc.* **73** 556–64
[27] Faist J, Capasso F, Sivco D L, Sirtori C, Hutchinson A L and Cho A Y 1994 Quantum cascade laser *Science (1979)* **264** 553–6
[28] Kole M R, Reddy R K, Schulmerich M V, Gelber M K and Bhargava R 2012 Discrete frequency infrared microspectroscopy and imaging with a tunable quantum cascade laser *Anal. Chem.* **84** 10366–72
[29] Tiwari S, Raman J, Reddy V, Ghetler A, Tella R P, Han Y *et al* 2016 Towards translation of discrete frequency infrared spectroscopic imaging for digital histopathology of clinical biopsy samples *Anal. Chem.* **88** 10183–90
[30] Yeh K, Kenkel S, Liu J N and Bhargava R 2015 Fast infrared chemical imaging with a quantum cascade laser *Anal. Chem.* **87** 485–93
[31] Kuepper C, Kallenbach-Thieltges A, Juette H, Tannapfel A, Großerueschkamp F and Gerwert K 2018 Quantum cascade laser-based infrared microscopy for label-free and automated cancer classification in tissue sections *Sci. Rep.* **8** 7717
[32] Bassan P, Weida M J, Rowlette J and Gardner P 2014 Large scale infrared imaging of tissue micro arrays (TMAs) using a tunable Quantum Cascade Laser (QCL) based microscope *Analyst* **139** 3856–9
[33] Kröger N, Egl A, Engel M, Gretz N, Haase K, Herpich I *et al* 2014 Quantum cascade laser–based hyperspectral imaging of biological tissue *J. Biomed. Opt.* **19** 111607
[34] Yeh K, Lee D and Bhargava R 2019 Multicolor discrete frequency infrared spectroscopic imaging *Anal. Chem.* **91** 2177–85

[35] Mittal S, Yeh K, Suzanne Leslie L, Kenkel S, Kajdacsy-Balla A and Bhargava R 2018 Simultaneous cancer and tumor microenvironment subtyping using confocal infrared microscopy for all-digital molecular histopathology *Proc. Natl. Acad. Sci. USA* **115** 651–60

[36] Yeh K, Sharma I, Falahkheirkhah K, Confer M P, Orr A C, Liu Y T *et al* 2023 Infrared spectroscopic laser scanning confocal microscopy for whole-slide chemical imaging *Nat. Commun. 2023* **14** 1–12

[37] Bhargava R 2023 Digital histopathology by infrared spectroscopic imaging *Annu. Rev. Anal. Chem.* **16** 205–30

[38] Tiwari S, Kajdacsy-Balla A, Whiteley J, Cheng G, Hewitt S M and Bhargava R 2021 INFORM: INFrared-based ORganizational measurements of tumor and its microenvironment to predict patient survival *Sci. Adv.* **7** eabb8292

[39] Krafft C, Steiner G, Beleites C and Salzer R 2009 Disease recognition by infrared and Raman spectroscopy *J. Biophotonics* **2** 13–28

[40] Pilling M and Gardner P 2016 Fundamental developments in infrared spectroscopic imaging for biomedical applications *Chem. Soc. Rev.* **45** 1935–57

[41] Lin H, Falahkheirkhah K, Kindratenko V and Bhargava R 2024 INSTRAS: INfrared Spectroscopic imaging-based TRAnsformers for medical image segmentation *Mach. Learn. Appl.* **16** 100549

[42] Tiwari S, Falahkheirkhah K, Cheng G and Bhargava R 2022 Colon cancer grading using infrared spectroscopic imaging-based deep learning *Appl. Spectrosc.* **76** 475–84

[43] Afara I O, Shaikh R, Nippolainen E, Querido W, Torniainen J, Sarin J K *et al* 2021 Characterization of connective tissues using near-infrared spectroscopy and imaging *Nat. Protoc.* **16** 1297–329

[44] Bird B, Miljkovi M, Remiszewski S, Akalin A, Kon M and Diem M 2012 Infrared spectral histopathology (SHP): a novel diagnostic tool for the accurate classification of lung cancer *Lab. Invest.* **92** 1358–73

[45] Lima C A, Correa L, Byrne H J and Zezell D M 2019 Label-free infrared spectroscopic imaging for characterization of necrotic tissue areas on cutaneous squamous cell carcinoma *Advanced Biomedical and Clinical Diagnostic and Surgical Guidance Systems XVII* **10868** (SPIE) 1086812

[46] Diem M 2015 *Modern Vibrational Spectroscopy and Micro-Spectroscopy. Modern Vibrational Spectroscopy and Micro-Spectroscopy: Theory, Instrumentation and Biomedical Applications* (John Wiley & Sons, Ltd)

[47] Holman H Y N, Martin M C, Blakely E A, Bjornstad K and Mckinney W R 2000 IR spectroscopic characteristics of cell cycle and cell death probed by synchrotron radiation based Fourier transform IR spectromicroscopy *Biopolymers, Biospectrosc. Sect.* **57** 329–35

[48] Gerwert K, Schörner S, Großerueschkamp F, Kraeft A, Schuhmacher D, Sternemann C *et al* 2023 Fast and label-free automated detection of microsatellite status in early colon cancer using artificial intelligence integrated infrared imaging *Eur. J. Cancer* **182** 122–31

[49] Evans C A and Suvarna S K 2006 Intraoperative diagnosis using the frozen section technique *J. Clin. Pathol.* **59** 334

[50] Jaafar H 2006 Intra-operative frozen section consultation: concepts, applications and limitations *Malays. J. Med. Sci.* **13** 4

[51] Ronneberger O, Fischer P and Brox T 2015 U-net: convolutional networks for biomedical image segmentation *Int. Conf. on Medical Image Computing and Computer-Assisted Intervention* pp 234–41

[52] Cao R, Nelson S D, Davis S, Liang Y, Luo Y, Zhang Y *et al* 2023 Label-free intraoperative histology of bone tissue via deep-learning-assisted ultraviolet photoacoustic microscopy *Nat. Biomed. Eng.* **7** 124–34

[53] Sun Y *et al* 2020 Real-time three-dimensional histology-like imaging by label-free nonlinear optical microscopy *Quant. Imaging Med. Surg.* **10** 2177

[54] Lu F K, Calligaris D, Olubiyi O I, Norton I, Yang W, Santagata S *et al* 2016 Label-free neurosurgical pathology with stimulated raman imaging *Cancer Res.* **76** 3451

[55] Lu F-K, Basu S, Igras V, Hoang M P, Ji M, Fu D *et al* 2015 Label-free DNA imaging *in vivo* with stimulated Raman scattering microscopy *Proc. Natl. Acad. Sci.* **112** 11624–9

[56] Pleitez M A, Khan A A, Soldà A, Chmyrov A, Reber J, Gasparin F *et al* 2020 Label-free metabolic imaging by mid-infrared optoacoustic microscopy in living cells *Nat. Biotechnol.* **38** 293–6

[57] Falahkheirkhah K, Yeh K, Mittal S, Pfister L and Bhargava R 2021 Deep learning-based protocols to enhance infrared imaging systems *Chemometr. Intell. Lab. Syst.* **217** 104390

[58] Schnell M, Mittal S, Falahkheirkhah K, Mittal A, Yeh K, Kenkel S *et al* 2020 All-digital histopathology by infrared-optical hybrid microscopy *Proc. Natl. Acad. Sci.* **117** 201912400

[59] Mayerich D, Walsh M J, Kadjacsy-Balla A, Ray P S, Hewitt S M and Bhargava R 2015 Stain-less staining for computed histopathology *Technology (Singap World Sci)* **3** 27–31

[60] Rivenson Y, Wang H, Wei Z, de Haan K, Zhang Y, Wu Y *et al* 2019 Virtual histological staining of unlabelled tissue-autofluorescence images via deep learning *Nat. Biomed. Eng.* **3** 466–77

[61] Xu Z, Moro C F, Bozóky B and Zhang Q 2019 GAN-based virtual Re-staining: a promising solution for whole slide image analysis arXiv:1901.04059 https://doi.org/10.48550/arXiv.1901.04059

[62] Rana A, Lowe A, Lithgow M, Horback K, Janovitz T, Da Silva A *et al* 2020 Use of deep learning to develop and analyze computational hematoxylin and eosin staining of prostate core biopsy images for tumor diagnosis *JAMA Netw. Open* **3** e205111

[63] Zimmermann E, Mukherjee S S, Falahkheirkhah K, Gryka M C, Kajdacsy-Balla A, Hasan W *et al* 2021 Detection and quantification of myocardial fibrosis using stain-free infrared spectroscopic imaging *Arch. Pathol. Lab Med.* **145** 1526–35

[64] Yoon C, Park E, Misra S, Kim J Y, Baik J W, Kim K G *et al* 2024 Deep learning-based virtual staining, segmentation, and classification in label-free photoacoustic histology of human specimens *Light Sci. Appl.* **13** 226

[65] Liu K, Li B, Wu W, May C, Chang O, Knezevich S *et al* 2023 VSGD-net: virtual staining guided melanocyte detection on histopathological images *2023 IEEE/CVF Winter Conf. on Applications of Computer Vision (WACV) (Piscataway, NJ)* (IEEE) pp 1918–27

[66] Bhargava R 2007 Towards a practical Fourier transform infrared chemical imaging protocol for cancer histopathology *Anal. Bioanal. Chem.* **389** 1155–69

[67] Hollon T C, Lewis S, Pandian B, Niknafs Y S, Garrard M R, Garton H *et al* 2018 Rapid intraoperative diagnosis of pediatric brain tumors using stimulated Raman histology *Cancer Res.* **78** 278

[68] Sarri B, Canonge R, Audier X, Simon E, Wojak J, Caillol F *et al* 2019 Fast stimulated Raman and second harmonic generation imaging for intraoperative gastro-intestinal cancer detection *Sci. Rep.* **9** 1–10

[69] Hollon T C, Pandian B, Adapa A R, Urias E, Save A V, Khalsa S S S *et al* 2020 Near real-time intraoperative brain tumor diagnosis using stimulated Raman histology and deep neural networks *Nat. Med.* **26** 52
[70] Falahkheirkhah K, Mukherjee S S, Gupta S, Herrera-Hernandez L, McCarthy M R, Jimenez R E *et al* 2023 Accelerating cancer histopathology workflows with chemical imaging and machine learning *Cancer Res. Commun.* **3** 1875–87
[71] Lakshminarayanan B, Pritzel A and Blundell C 2017 Simple and scalable predictive uncertainty estimation using deep ensembles *Adv. Neural Inform. Process. Syst.*
[72] Ovadia Y, Fertig E, Ren J, Nado Z, Sculley D, Nowozin S *et al* 2019 Can you trust your model's uncertainty? Evaluating predictive uncertainty under dataset shift arXiv:1906.02530 https://doi.org/10.48550/arXiv.1906.02530
[73] Lindqvist J, Olmin A, Lindsten F and Svensson L 2020 A general framework for ensemble distribution distillation *2020 IEEE 30th Int. Workshop on Machine Learning for Signal Processing (MLSP)* (Piscataway, NJ: IEEE) pp 1–6
[74] Malinin A, Mlodozeniec B and Gales M 2019 Ensemble distribution distillation *8th Int. Conf. on Learning Representations, ICLR 2020*
[75] Zhang R, Isola P, Efros A A, Shechtman E and Wang O 2018 The unreasonable effectiveness of deep features as a perceptual metric *Proc. of the IEEE Computer Society Conf. on Computer Vision and Pattern Recognition* 586–95
[76] Zingman I, Frayle S, Tankoyeu I, Sukhanov S and Heinemann F 2024 A comparative evaluation of image-to-image translation methods for stain transfer in histopathology *Proc. Mach. Learn. Res.* **227** 1509–25
[77] Mao X, Li Q, Xie H, Lau R Y K, Wang Z and Smolley S P 2016 Least squares generative adversarial networks *Proc. of the IEEE Int. Conf. on Computer Vision* 2813–21
[78] Wang T-C, Liu M-Y, Zhu J-Y, Tao A, Kautz J and Catanzaro B 2018 High-resolution image synthesis and semantic manipulation with conditional GANs *Proc. of the IEEE Conf. on Computer Vision and Pattern Recognition* pp 8798–807
[79] Kingma D P and Ba J 2015 Adam: a method for stochastic optimization *Int. Conf. for Learning Representations (ICLR)*
[80] Ioffe S and Szegedy C 2015 Batch normalization: accelerating deep network training by reducing internal covariate shift *Proc. of the 32nd Int. Conf. on Int. Conf. on Machine Learning*
[81] He K, Zhang X, Ren S and Sun J 2016 Deep residual learning for image recognition *Proc. of the IEEE Conference on Computer Vision and Pattern Recognition* pp 770–8

Chapter 5

Blood-based cancer diagnosis: role of spectroscopy

Panchali Saha and C Murali Krishna

Cancer remains a significant global health challenge due to the high mortality rates and complications arising from delayed diagnosis. Conventional detection methods, although sensitive, rely on morphological changes which appear much later than biochemical changes. These biochemical alterations can be identified through optical spectroscopy methods like infrared (IR), fluorescence and Raman spectroscopies, potentially facilitating earlier detection. This chapter reviews studies focused on optical spectroscopy methods for cancer detection with blood serum and plasma samples, published between 1997 and 2024. The opening section provides a summary of cancer statistics, current clinical cancer diagnostic methods, and the benefits of using blood-based tests for disease detection. A dedicated subsection explores common and advanced machine learning techniques which play a crucial role in spectroscopy-based diagnostic efforts. Further, the known limitations of conventional diagnostic methods are discussed, emphasizing the need for optical spectroscopy tools. The subsequent sections delve into the fundamentals of infrared, fluorescence, and Raman spectroscopy methods. The chapter provides an account of plasma-based studies of fluorescence spectroscopy as well as serum-based studies of IR and Raman spectroscopies. Additionally, the chapter offers insights into current challenges and outlook in cancer diagnosis through blood-based optical spectroscopy techniques

5.1 Introduction

Cancers pose a significant health, societal and economic challenge worldwide [1]. Globally, this group of diseases is responsible for high mortality rates, and leads to three in ten global premature deaths from non-communicable diseases [1]. In 2022, 9.7 million cancer-related deaths were estimated [1]. Early detection of cancers has proven to reduce mortality rates and economic burden [2]. This can be achieved by spreading awareness of the symptoms of various cancers, and highlighting the

doi:10.1088/978-0-7503-5949-8ch5

importance of consulting medical professionals regarding abnormal findings. Improved access to clinical services, especially in socio-economically challenged societies and the development of cost-efficient screening tools for mass screening of high-risk populations is of utmost importance. Indeed, screening and early detection efforts have led to significant decline in mortality rates for colorectal, cervical and breast cancers [3]. Visual screening of high-risk tobacco habitués for oral lesions also proved to be highly beneficial in a large-cohort clustered-randomized controlled trail conducted in India [4].

5.1.1 Brief overview of conventional cancer diagnosis

Cancer diagnosis typically involves a physical examination and a thorough review of the patient's medical history, wherein symptoms and risk factors are assessed, followed by various diagnostic tests [5]. Pathologists primarily rely on the morphology of cells to confirm diagnosis. Histological analysis, or tissue examination, is performed following a biopsy or excision of the suspected tumor. The biopsy site selection is highly crucial for accurate diagnosis [6, 7]. During surgery, frozen tissue sections are analyzed to ensure cancer-free margins, which are critical for determining if the entire tumor has been removed and guiding the surgical procedure [8].

For cancer detection, molecular pathology has several advantages over histology-based methods. While histology primarily focuses on the microscopic examination of tissue morphology and visible structural changes of cells, molecular pathology methods such as immunohistochemistry (IHC) and fluorescence *in situ* hybridization (FISH), gene sequencing examines cells for chromosomal aberrations, gene mutations, and biochemical changes indicative of specific cancer types [9]. These methods can enable the detection of cancer at earlier stages, often before morphological changes become evident. IHC is of immense importance in distinguishing between lymphoma, anaplastic carcinoma, sarcoma, and melanoma, which appear similar due to limited differentiation [10]. IHC is used identify features like cytokeratins in epithelial carcinoma, prostate-specific antigen (PSA) in metastatic prostate carcinoma, thyroglobulin in thyroid carcinoma, and desmin in myogenic carcinoma [10]. Cytology involves the study of cells for disease diagnosis and is widely used for cancer screening and biopsy. In addition to being less invasive than tissue biopsy, cytology methods are economical and yield quicker results. Brush cytopathology for colorectal [11] and upper gastrointestinal tract cancers [12] achieve results comparable to biopsy. Exfoliative cytology-based methods like pap smear for cervical cancer screening are used routinely in clinics [13]. Fine-needle aspiration cytology (FNAC) is employed for tumors that do not shed cells and is commonly used for diagnosing breast [14], thyroid [15], lymph node [16], and abdominal cancers [17]. Karyotyping is used for the identification of abnormality in the Philadelphia chromosome due to reverse translocations of chromosomes 9 and 22, in chronic myelogenous leukemia (CML) patients [18]. It has similar applications in Burkitt's lymphoma detection and colorectal adenocarcinoma [19, 20]. FISH uses fluorescent probes to detect specific DNA sequences on chromosomes, such as HER2 amplification in breast cancer or N-MYC amplification in neuroblastomas [21, 22].

Tumor markers include proteins, nucleic acids, antibodies, and peptides, which can be detected in body fluids like blood, urine, or saliva. PSA is a well-established marker for prostate cancer, while CEA (carcinoembryonic antigen) is used in diagnosing colorectal, bladder, breast, medullary thyroid and ovarian cancers [23, 24]. Mutations in the BRCA1 gene are linked to an increased risk of breast and ovarian cancers [25].

Imaging techniques play an essential role in detecting, staging, and monitoring cancer. Imaging modalities such as x-ray, computed tomography (CT), ultrasound (US), magnetic resonance imaging (MRI), single-photon emission computed tomography (SPECT), positron emission tomography (PET), are essential tools for cancer detection, biopsy guidance, staging, prognosis, monitoring therapy response, and detecting recurrence [26]. Electron microscopy allows for detailed visualization of cellular structures by passing a focused electron beam through tissue samples stained with heavy metals like uranium and lead. This technique provides highly magnified images, aiding in diagnosis by identifying specific cellular features such as tonofibrils in squamous cell tumors, and crystalline inclusions in certain sarcomas [27, 28].

5.1.2 Limitations of conventional diagnostic modalities

Conventional methods of cancer diagnosis by clinical examination followed by biochemical/microbiological/pathological tests rely on symptoms, and therefore diagnose an existing disease, which could contribute to late diagnosis, leading to poor prognosis. Tissue-based methods such as histology and IHC are not amenable to serial sampling and mass screening due to the invasive sample collection process, and are therefore unsuitable as screening tools. Cytology-based methods like FNAC and pap smear, although not as invasive as tissue biopsy, cause discomfort to patients. FISH and gene-sequencing methods are expensive. In addition to relying on morphological changes and symptoms, imaging techniques like MRI and CT scans can also be expensive [29]. Screening of individuals/populations at risk for cancers and early detection of the same have been proven to reduce mortality rates [2]. Since morphological changes could be rather late signs, diagnostics should be sensitive to biochemical changes. This is particularly applicable to diseases like cancers which are multi-step processes and usually pass through multiple stages, i.e., hyperplasia/metaplasia, dysplasia, carcinoma *in situ*, and eventually to invasive cancers [30]. During this process several biomolecules (tumor markers/biomarkers) are expressed which can be exploited to diagnose the pathological conditions. Therefore, there is a need for minimally-invasive methods which detect biochemical alterations that precede morphological changes and are suitable for serial sampling and mass screening. Optical spectroscopy methods such as fluorescence, IR and Raman spectroscopies using blood samples for investigations, are ideally suited for these applications. These methods can provide global biochemical information in the form of a 'molecular fingerprint' of a sample. Spectral data is amenable to model development by machine learning methods which achieve rapid, objective and accurate results.

5.1.3 Importance of serum-based diagnostics

Serum is the liquid component of blood, excluding blood cells and coagulation factors. Blood serum investigations for disease detection offer numerous advantages. One major benefit is its minimally-invasive collection process, which involves a simple blood draw. This makes it patient-friendly compared to tissue biopsies. Blood serum provides a comprehensive snapshot of a patient's systemic health, as it contains a wide array of biomarkers, including proteins, metabolites, lipids, electrolytes, cell-free nucleic acids, and other molecules that can indicate the presence of diseases. Due to ease of collection, transport and storage, serum is amenable to large-scale screening and serial sampling, contributing to more effective disease monitoring and management. Serology is vital for the detection of a variety of lifestyle-related conditions and infectious diseases. Serum biomarkers such as prostate-specific antigen (PSA) for prostate cancer and AFP for liver cancers are in clinical use [31]. Serum-based investigations provide a valuable, patient-friendly approach for disease detection and monitoring.

5.1.4 Role of machine learning methods in spectroscopy-based diagnostics

Objective disease diagnosis by spectral molecular signatures of body fluids is achieved using multivariate analysis which often incorporate machine learning algorithms. The aim of multivariate methods is to train models that distinguish seemingly similar patterns in pathological conditions and identify independent samples. Multivariate analysis can be unsupervised where no prior information is given and the method tries to establish relationships or trends in classification *de novo*. In the absence of preliminary information, unsupervised methods provide a first-hand estimate about the nature of data. Supervised learning methods are used to predict the association of new variables to one of the pre-existing groups.

Principal Component Analysis (PCA) is one of the most commonly used machine learning tools for spectroscopy data. PCA is a dimensionality reduction method that identifies the most significant variables, or 'principal components,' from a high-dimensional dataset [32]. PCA is often combined with supervised methods, such as linear discriminant analysis (LDA) [33]. LDA is the simplest classification method based on Bayes' formula. It is based on the assumptions of normal distribution and that the covariance matrices of the two (or more) groups are identical. LDA minimizes within-group variance and maximizes between-group variance. Support vector machines (SVMs) are another powerful machine learning tool commonly used for model development in spectroscopy-based cancer detection. It is a supervised learning algorithm that works by finding the hyperplane that best separates data into different classes while maximizing the margin between them [34]. Genetic algorithms (GAs) are also employed in spectroscopy for feature selection and optimization tasks, and are often combined with supervised methods such as SVM [35]. Partial least squares discriminant analysis (PLS-DA) is another widely used method in several spectroscopy studies for cancer detection. It is a supervised dimensionality reduction method that, unlike PCA, incorporates class labels in the analysis. It discovers latent variables that maximize the separation between different predefined groups in the data [36]. Deep learning, a discipline of artificial intelligence uses a machine learning method called artificial neural networks (ANNs) to extract patterns and make predictions from large datasets [37]. These advanced tools are being used with increasing popularity to analyze spectral data for the construction of highly accurate and objective models capable of rapid diagnosis.

5.2 Optical spectroscopy methods for cancer detection

Optical spectroscopy comprises a range of techniques that use light to study the interaction between electromagnetic radiation and matter thus providing insights into a sample's structure, composition, and electronic properties. These methods are based on the absorption, emission, or scattering of light. Optical spectroscopy methods include UV-Vis spectroscopy, which measures light absorption in the ultraviolet and visible regions; IR spectroscopy, used to study interaction of IR radiation with matter; Raman spectroscopy, which examines inelastic scattering of light, and fluorescence spectroscopy, which involves the emission of light by a substance that has absorbed photons, commonly used for detecting and analyzing fluorescent compounds. The present chapter focuses on fluorescence, IR and Raman spectroscopies for cancer diagnosis.

Numerous tissue-based and *in vivo* optical spectroscopy studies have achieved exemplary results in terms of accuracy [38–46]. As discussed before, tissue samples have the disadvantage of invasive collection procedure, making them unsuitable for mass-screening applications. *In vivo* examinations, though non-invasive, present significant infrastructural challenges in developing nations like India, as they require specialized equipment and stringent conditions that are difficult to maintain at tertiary clinics and health camps. In this regard, blood-based diagnosis utilizing spectroscopic techniques represents a promising frontier in the field of oncology, offering minimally-invasive, objective, rapid, and highly sensitive and specific methods for cancer detection and management. This involves the study of serum/plasma by methods such as fluorescence, IR, and Raman spectroscopies, which provide detailed molecular insights useful for diagnoses and therapeutic monitoring. Serum-based spectroscopic diagnostics hold the potential to revolutionize cancer detection and management by making early detection rapid and cost-efficient.

5.2.1 Fluorescence spectroscopy

Fluorescence is a form of luminescence that occurs when photons excite a molecule, elevating it to an electronic excited state. This process involves the absorption of photons, which promotes the molecule from its singlet ground state to a singlet excited state. As the molecule returns to its ground state, it emits a photon of lower energy, corresponding to a longer wavelength than the absorbed photon.

Fluorescence spectroscopy examines this emitted fluorescence by analyzing the fluorescent properties of the molecule.

Excitation and emission fluorescence spectra can be measured. An excitation spectrum is obtained by scanning the excitation wavelength while keeping the emission wavelength constant. An emission spectrum is recorded by scanning the emission wavelength at a constant excitation wavelength. Synchronous spectra can be acquired by simultaneously scanning the excitation and emission wavelengths. The spectra provide information on the absorption and emission properties of the sample, and are typically plotted as a function of counts (number of detected photons) against wavelength.

Most blood-based fluorescence spectroscopy investigations for cancer diagnosis have been performed on blood plasma. Plasma has identical composition to serum with the exception of clotting factors which are present in plasma and absent in serum.

Numerous studies have reported on the use of plasma-based fluorescence spectroscopy for cancer detection. In 1997, Madhuri *et al* published a pilot study for the characterization of blood plasma of both normal and oral carcinoma subjects [47]. Emission spectrum at 300 nm excitation exhibited differences among control and cancer subjects [47]. Analysis of fluorescence intensity ratios at 340 and 440 nm revealed that normal blood plasma exhibited a ratio value below 11, while tumor samples showed values exceeding 11. Furthermore, the ratio values for blood plasma obtained from cancer patients ranged from 11 to 28, with variations corresponding to the progression of malignancy [47]. Another study by the same group investigated native fluorescence characteristics of blood plasma in the visible spectral region, at 405 and 420 nm, to discriminate patients with different stages of oral malignancy from healthy subjects [48]. LDA models, validated by leave-one-out cross-validation were constructed using the fluorescence intensity ratios calculated at emission wavelengths [48]. LDA classified 94.7% of the original grouped cases and 93.7% of the cross-validated grouped cases. Further, in LDA across the normal, oral malignancy (including early and advanced stages) and liver diseases, 99% of the original grouped cases and 95.9% of the cross-validated grouped cases were correctly classified [48]. Similar analysis stratifying normal, early stage of oral cancer, advanced oral malignancy and liver diseases correctly classified 94.9% of the original grouped cases and 91.8% of the cross-validated grouped cases [48].

A study on the fluorescence characteristics of human blood plasma in the visible spectral range attempted to discriminate patients with colorectal cancer from subjects of a control population [49]. The study involved 169 controls, 143 colorectal adenocarcinomas patients (36 in the colon, 38 in the sigmoid colon and 69 in the rectum), 11 patients with local relapse, 10 familial adenomatous polyposis patients and 8 patients with single adenomas [49]. The intensity of a fluorescence emission peak around 615–635 nm, ascribed to endogenous porphyrins, was significantly different between colorectal cancer patients and control subjects. Reactive oxygen species (ROC) analysis resulted in an area under the curve of 0.72, comparable to the CEA test (figure 5.1) [49]. In another study, fluorescence spectroscopy excitation emission matrix (EEM) measurements were applied to human blood plasma samples

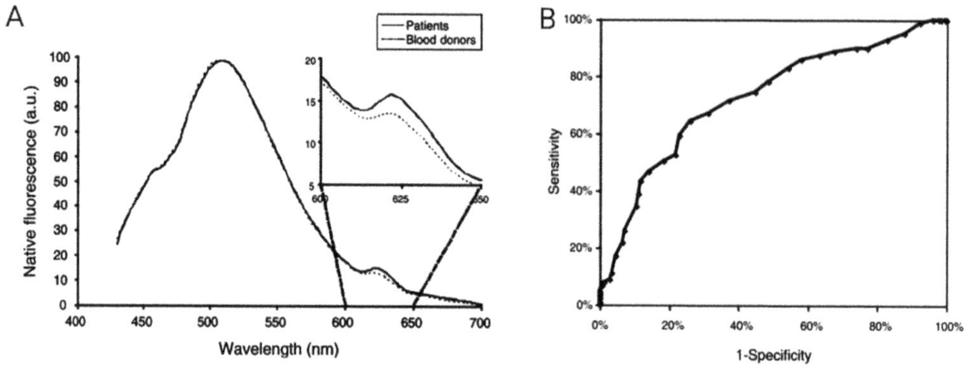

Figure 5.1. (A) Normalized fluorescence spectra of blood plasma of 169 blood donors (•••••) and 172 patients bearing colon diseases (——) at 405 nm excitation wavelength. (B) ROC analysis considering the whole set of colorectal patients versus blood donors. Reproduced from [49] Copyright 2007 SAGE Publications. Reprinted by permission of Sage Publications.

from a case-control study on colorectal cancer [50]. The study involved 308 participants, including colorectal cancer, adenomas, no-findings and non-malignant patients [50]. Parallel factor analysis (PARAFAC) was used to decompose the fluorescence EEMs, and both the pooled score matrix and raw spectra were utilized for discrimination models. The models achieved sensitivity and specificity values around 0.75 for distinguishing cancer from controls, though discrimination between different controls was poor [50]. PARAFAC revealed a blue shift in tryptophan emission in cancer patients. [50]. In 2017, Soares *et al* introduced a hierarchical classification method using plasma fluorescence to detect colorectal cancer (CRC), adenomas, and other non-malignant colorectal conditions [51]. They applied a feature selection algorithm to identify discriminant fluorescent wavelengths which were further used to train a binary SVM to identify CRC samples [51]. One-class SVM trained on healthy subjects was used to detect non-malignant findings [51]. Using a dataset with 12 341 wavelengths, the method achieved superior results, with sensitivity and specificity of 0.87 and 0.95 for CRC detection, and 0.60 and 0.79 for non-malignant findings [51].

The autofluorescence of blood components from healthy individuals and cancer patients with various types of cancer was analyzed using a steady-state spectro-fluorometer [52]. Patients with gastric cancer, breast cancer, and Hodgkin's lymphoma showed a distinct fluorescence band of high intensity at around 630 nm which was attributed to the porphyrin fluorophore [52]. Additionally, ratio fluorometry revealed a correlation with cancer stages, enabling the identification of early-stage cancer characteristics and the growth rates of certain cancers and benign tumors [52]. In their 2017 study, Pachaiappan *et al* explored the diagnosis of oral cancer using fluorescence polarization measurements at 405 nm excitation [53]. Fluorescence anisotropy values, derived from polarized fluorescence spectral data of both healthy and oral cancer subjects, were analyzed using a linear discriminant analysis-based ANN, yielding high diagnostic accuracy [53].

In a nutshell, blood plasma-based fluorescence spectroscopy has shown considerable promise in cancer diagnosis. Early work identifying oral carcinoma through fluorescence intensity ratios, achieved high classification accuracy of >90% with LDA models. Further studies successfully differentiated between normal, stages of oral malignancy, and liver disease, with up to 99% correct classifications. Fluorescence emission in the 615–635 nm range, attributed to endogenous porphyrins was used to great effect, to discriminate colorectal cancer patients from controls. Two separate studies revealed the efficacy of fluorescence spectroscopy of plasma for colorectal cancer diagnosis, with sensitivity and specificity values in the range of 75%–95%. In addition to the above, diagnostic potential of plasma-based fluorescence spectroscopy has shown diagnostic potential Hodgkin's lymphoma, breast and gastric cancers. Although fluorescence spectroscopy of blood is limited to native fluorophores such as reduced nicotinamide adenine dinucleotide (NADH), porphyrins and flavin adenine dinucleotide, and do not provide detailed information about the entire biomolecular milieu of the samples, the above investigations suggest that the method has potential for clinical translation.

5.2.2 Infrared spectroscopy

IR spectroscopy is a vibrational spectroscopy method based on the interaction of infrared light and matter. When a sample is exposed to IR radiation, a part of the radiation is absorbed while the remaining is transmitted. Two methods for acquiring IR spectra are FTIR (Fourier transform IR) spectroscopy and dispersive IR spectroscopy. In dispersive IR spectroscopy, a dispersive component such as a prism or grating is used to separate IR light into different wavelengths. The intensity of each wavelength is measured sequentially to construct the spectrum. FTIR spectroscopy employs an interferometer to measure the entire IR spectrum concurrently. The interferogram obtained undergoes Fourier-transformation to obtain the final spectrum. FTIR spectroscopy achieves faster results than dispersive IR spectroscopy as it measures the entire spectrum at once. It also has a higher signal-to-noise ratio, resulting in enhanced sensitivity, especially for weak signals. FTIR spectroscopy offers various sampling techniques, including transmission, reflection, and attenuated total reflectance (ATR). For blood-based measurements, FTIR is predominantly used due to its numerous benefits. ATR is a sampling methodology that involves direct examination of solid or liquid samples and eliminates the requirement for sample preparation. It uses total internal reflection to generate an evanescent wave that penetrates the sample, providing valuable molecular information.

Over the years, several studies have utilized FTIR spectroscopy combined with machine learning algorithms to distinguish cancer patients and healthy controls across various cancer types. Multiple breast cancer investigations have been reported. In 2010, Backhaus *et al* analyzed serum of 98 breast cancer patients and 98 healthy controls with FTIR spectroscopy [54]. Sensitivity and specificity of cluster analysis accounted for 98% and 95%, respectively, whilst a sensitivity of 92% and a specificity of 100% were determined with supervised ANNs [54]. The results were tested against 11 other diseases separately and 79% of breast cancer patients were successfully assigned to the correct class [54]. An FTIR spectroscopy study by Elmi *et al* on 43 each of breast cancer and healthy serum samples reported that the major spectral differences between the two groups were related to the differences in protein conformation in serum samples. The diagnostic accuracy, sensitivity, and specificity of PCA-LDA analysis for 3000–3600 cm^{-1} (NH stretching) were found to be 83%, 84%, 74% for the control and 80%, 76%, 72% for the breast cancer cases, respectively. Another study explored multivariate processing of spectra of serum (from 66 breast cancer patients and 80 healthy controls) obtained by ATR-FTIR spectroscopy [55]. In this study, an approach wherein a combination of PCA (figure 5.2) and principal component regression (PCR) were used for processing the IR spectra of blood serum [55]. They found that the range of 1306–1250 cm^{-1}, corresponding to functional groups of DNA and RNA in the spectrum of serum reported 92.3% sensitivity and 87.1% specificity using PCR [55]. Yang *et al* utilized FTIR spectroscopy to analyze serum samples from 114 non-cancer controls and 107 breast cancer patients at various stages [56]. To address sample imbalance, the synthetic minority oversampling technique (SMOTE) and random discarding methods were applied. Extreme learning machine (ELM), k-nearest neighbor (KNN), GA-SVM, particle swarm optimization-SVM (PSO-SVM), and grid search-SVM (GS-SVM) were explored for classification [56]. In oversampling, GS-SVM achieved the highest accuracy of 95.45%, while in under-sampling, GA-SVM reached 100% accuracy across all groups.

Ollesch *et al* investigated the efficacy FTIR transmission spectroscopy to study serum and plasma samples of urinary bladder cancer and suspected bladder cancer patients with inflammation [57]. Random forest (RF) models yielded high sensitivity but poor specificity [57]. In 2014, the team updated their results with multiple data analysis outputs on different datasets. RF classification outperformed the previous

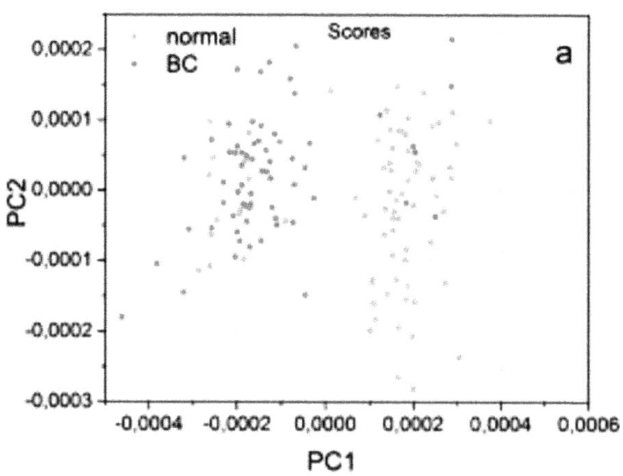

Figure 5.2. PCA scatter plot for 1305–1250 cm^{-1} region for normal and breast cancer sera. Reproduced with courtesy from [55], copyright (2020) Elsevier.

specificity values obtained, accounting for around 86%, and a high drop in sensitivity to 82% [57].

Maitra *et al* studied the urine, plasma, saliva and serum of oesophageal inflammation, Barrett's low-grade dysplasia, high grade dysplasia, oesophageal adenocarcinoma [58]. GA-QDA models of ATR-FTIR serum data achieved 100% performance for oesophageal adenocarcinoma using 13 wavenumbers in the range of 1435–1573 cm^{-1}, associated with methyl groups of proteins and Amide II absorption [58]. A different study investigated transmission FTIR spectroscopy for detecting oesophageal squamous cell carcinoma (ESCC) using serum and plasma samples [59]. Out of SVM, PC-LDA, decision tree (DT), KNN, ensemble algorithms (EA) and PLS-DA, the PC-LDA model achieved best results with 99.26% accuracy, 98.53% sensitivity, and 100% specificity for late-stage cancer detection; and 97.08% accuracy with 91.43% sensitivity for early-stage detection [59].

Several glioblastoma multiforme (GBM) investigations have been reported. Cameron *et al* studied, 41 lymphoma and 71 GBM serum samples with ATR-FTIR spectroscopy [60]. Out of RF, PLS-DA and SVM models, PLS-DA gave the best outcome in terms of specificity and sensitivity, at 90.1% and 86.3%, respectively [60]. A study employed mid-IR spectroscopy combined with algorithms such as PCA, SVM and DT to identify patients with glioma, to great effect, with the models achieving accuracies in the range of 87%–92% [61]. Qu *et al* have combined serum mid-IR spectroscopy with ensemble learning techniques to differentiate between healthy individuals and glioma patients [62]. particle swarm optimization-SVM (PSO-SVM), DT, logistic regression (LR), and RF along with adaptive boosting to enhance classification accuracy [62].

Giamougiannis *et al* employed ATR-FTIR spectroscopy on plasma, serum and urine, from 116 patients with ovarian cancer and 307 patients with benign gynecological conditions [63]. Further, they compared ovarian cancer patients without previous chemotherapy ($n = 71$) and those who had received neo-adjuvant chemotherapy-NACT ($n = 45$), separately with benign controls. Serum achieved 76% sensitivity and 98% specificity for ovarian cancer detection, whereas urine performed poorly [63]. Alcántara-Quintana *et al* studied HPV-associated anal cancers in men via one-drop- serum-based ATR-FTIR spectroscopy wherein they reported spectral alterations 1700–1100 and 1700–1400 cm^{-1} regions among the controls and the anal cancer group, attributable to the presence of proteins and nucleic acids [64]. High sensitivity ranging from 95.2% to 99.9% and a specificity ranging from 99.2% to 100% were obtained by chemometric models constructed for both regions [64]. Guo *et al* analyzed 252 samples from patients with liver, gastric, and colorectal cancers of various stages by serum-based ATR-FTIR spectroscopy, and created a two-dimensional second derivative spectrum dataset to capture IR molecular fingerprints [65]. The classification models, including PLS-DA and backpropagation (BP) neural networks, achieved high sensitivities and specificities, with overall accuracies exceeding 95% [65].

A study conducted by Duckworth *et al* in 2022 examined unfiltered human serum and its various molecular weight fractions using FTIR spectroscopy [66]. The team demonstrated the effective use of FTIR on the 10–30 kDa molecular weight fraction

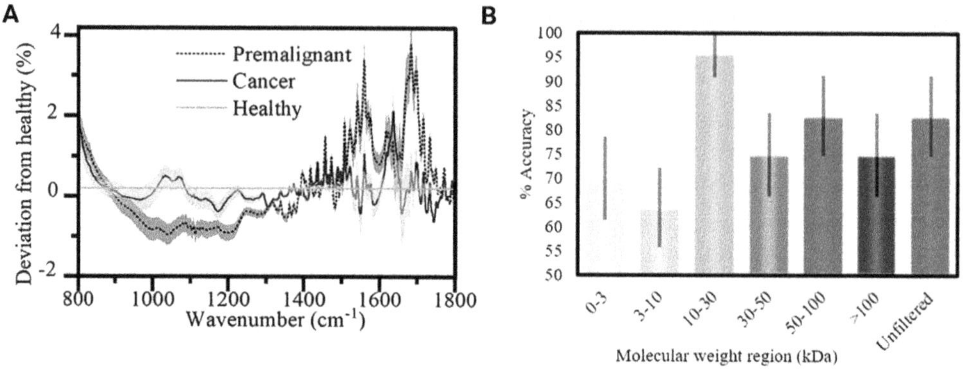

Figure 5.3. FTIR investigations of healthy, oral cancer and oral premalignant sera. (A) Average spectra of cancer, premalignant and healthy whole serum. Error in shaded region around each line shows level of distinction for each spectrum. (B) Classification accuracies between FTIR spectra of premalignant and cancer patients for different serum molecular weight subsets (molecular windows). The 95% confidence interval is shown by the gray lines over the bars. Reproduced with courtesy from [66] CC BY 4.0.

of human serum to differentiate between patients with premalignant conditions and those with oral cancer (figure 5.3). Linear PCA-SVM and LOOCV were used in this study for classification [66].

In summary, FTIR spectroscopy of blood serum has demonstrated significant potential of detection of various types of cancer. A review by Sala *et al* provides a comprehensive account of the different studies reported on biofluid-based FTIR spectroscopy investigations for cancer detection [67]. Particularly in breast cancer studies, alterations in nucleic acid-related spectral features were observed, and accuracy rates reached as high as 95%, with the use of sophisticated ANN models. Bladder cancer investigations have also yielded encouraging outcomes. In oesophageal cancer, changes in protein-related bands were detected, with PC-LDA models achieving high sensitivity. Similarly, studies on GBM have shown promising results, with PLS-DA models constructed from FTIR spectral data performing effectively. In ovarian cancer, though sensitivity was lower, high specificity was maintained. FTIR spectroscopy on the 10–30 kDa molecular weight fraction of human serum has proven effective in discriminating between premalignant and oral cancer patients. Moreover, FTIR spectroscopy investigations of rare anal cancers have produced remarkable results with sensitivity and specificity in the 95%–100% range, underscoring the efficacy of this technique.

5.2.3 Raman spectroscopy

Raman spectroscopy is a vibrational spectroscopy method that relies on the inelastic scattering of light. This phenomenon is known as the Raman effect and was named after its discoverer Sir C V Raman. Interaction of monochromatic light with a sample can lead to absorption, scattering, or reflection. While most scattered photons have the same frequency as the incident light (Rayleigh scattering), a minute fraction (one in ten million) scatter inelastically, exhibiting a different frequency from the incident photons—this is the Raman effect. A Stokes shift occurs when the scattered light's frequency is lower than the frequency of the incident photon, while an anti-Stokes shift happens when it's higher. The energy difference between incident and scattered photons (Raman shift) is expressed in wavenumbers (cm^{-1}). Raman scattered photon is generated when incident photon cause change in the vibrational state of a molecule. Since this frequency shift is unique to specific molecular vibration of the molecule, either by direct comparison of the spectra of known and unknown materials recorded consecutively or by comparison of the spectrum of the unknown compound with catalogs of reference spectra, identification of 'chemical moieties' provides a 'molecular fingerprint' of the sample.

IR and Raman spectroscopy are complementary methods: vibrations that are strong in IR spectra are typically weak in Raman spectra. Raman spectroscopy has several advantages such as non-destructiveness, minimal sample preparation, rapidity, objectivity, and negligible water interference, making it highly suitable for biological applications. Unlike IR spectroscopy, where water strongly absorbs light and interferes with the spectrum, Raman spectroscopy can be effectively utilized in aqueous solutions. Raman spectra provide crucial information about the chemical composition and molecular structure of a sample through the position and intensity of spectral features. While fluorescence spectroscopy of blood is limited to native fluorophores such as reduced nicotinamide adenine dinucleotide (NADH), porphyrins and flavin adenine dinucleotide, Raman spectroscopy is sensitive to all molecules with covalent bonds that experience changes in polarizability during vibrational transitions. As a result, Raman spectroscopy provides a more comprehensive snapshot of the various biomolecules in a blood serum or plasma sample. As each molecule produces a unique Raman spectrum and scattered light intensity is proportional to its relative abundance, Raman spectroscopy offers both qualitative and quantitative sample information. Due to its several advantages such as rapidity, no requirement for external labeling or sample processing, and objectivity, Raman spectroscopy is being pursued as potential alternative/adjunct screening/early diagnosis tool. Variants of conventional Raman spectroscopy such as resonance Raman spectroscopy, surface-enhanced Raman spectroscopy, stimulated Raman spectroscopy, spatially-offset Raman spectroscopy, confocal Raman microscopy have been studied extensively in recent years for various applications. A number of stimulated Raman and coherent anti-stokes Raman spectroscopy studies for cancer detection have investigated cells and tissue samples with significant outcomes. A subsequent chapter reviews the surface-enhanced Raman spectroscopy reports on cancer detection. The present chapter discusses conventional Raman spectroscopy and confocal Raman microscopy studies on serum samples for cancer diagnosis.

In 2007, Pichardo–Molina *et al* studied serum samples of 11 breast cancer patients and 12 healthy controls using Raman spectroscopy and analyzed the acquired Raman spectra by PCA and PC-LDA [68]. Bands attributable to proteins, phospholipids and polysaccharides were found to be significant [68]. A PC-LDA model constructed with smoothened and baseline corrected spectral data achieved 92.2 % sensitivity [68]. A subsequent RS study on sera of 23 triple-negative breast cancers patients, 22 HER2-positive breast cancers patients, and 30 healthy controls used pre-processed Raman spectra as the input of deep learning models [69]. A neural network language model (NNLM), bidirectional long-short-term memory network (BiLSTM), and convolutional neural network (CNN) achieved accuracy rates of 87.78%, 90.37%, and 91.11%, respectively [69]. In the same year, Li *et al* reported altered nucleic acids, carotenoids, amino acids, and lipid concentrations in serum Raman spectra of 171 invasive ductal carcinoma (IDC) and 100 healthy volunteers [70]. PCA was used to extract features followed by supervised model construction by LDA, SVM and NNLM [70]. The team concluded that the NNLM was the superior model [70]. Cao *et al* investigated serum Raman spectra of 87 cervical cancer patients, 60 breast cancer patients, and 78 healthy individuals and reported significant differences in bands attributable phenylalanine, tyrosine, β-carotene, amide III and olefinic stretch [71]. PC-LDA model's accuracy, precision, recall, and F1 score of the model were 92.90%, 92.62%, 92.10%, and 92.36%, respectively [71].

Multiple serum Raman spectroscopy studied on cancers of the gastrointestinal tract have been reported since 2012. Li *et al* reported a serum Raman study on 30 normal people, 46 colon cancer, and 44 rectum cancer patients. LDA models constructed using the PCs of the PCR and partial least square regression (PLSR) yielded accuracies of 88% and 83% [72]. In 2018, the development of a high-throughput serum Raman spectroscopy platform compared dry and liquid data acquisition of serum samples of 30 colorectal cancer patients and 30 matched controls, with 785 and 532 nm excitation wavelengths [73]. Fresh serum coupled with aluminium foil as substrate and 785 nm excitation achieved the best results in cross-validated PLS-DA model, with maximum sensitivity and specificity of 83% [73]. Liu *et al* studied Raman spectra of serum samples from patients with 93 gastric cancer patients, 92 colorectal cancer patients and 100 healthy individuals [74]. Cancer patients had significantly higher band areas at around 2923 cm^{-1}, corresponding to the presence of lipids and proteins [74]. This study revealed that PCA has a limited impact on the recognition results obtained using different recognition models [74]. Gated recurrent unit (GRU) algorithm and traditional machine learning methods were applied by the group to great effect [74]. Accuracy of identification of digestive tract tumors by SVM models was 84.72%, and 100% with GRU. GRU also identified the subtypes of gastric and colorectal cancers based on the degree of differentiation and stage, with high accuracy [74]. Raman measurements and ELİSA test to develop a prediction model based on machine learning methods were also examined [75]. In the post-surgery of gastric cancer patients ($n = 26$), an additional band at 1182 cm^{-1} was observed and the Raman intensity of amide III, II, I, and CH_2 proteins as well as lipids functional group was higher compared to the control group ($n = 44$). PCA using the 800 and 1800 cm^{-1} and the 2700 and 3000 cm^{-1} spectral ranges distinguished the two groups successfully. The vibrations at 1302 and 1306 cm^{-1} were characteristic for cancer patients. Deep neural networks and XGBoost algorithm achieved high classification accuracy of more than 95% [75].

A proof-of-concept serum RS study on hepatocellular carcinoma (HCC) samples by Taleb *et al* investigating 37 cirrhotic patients with HCC and 34 patients without HCC used two approaches-dried serum drops and freeze-dried serum [76]. Excitation wavelength of 785 nm was used in this study [76]. While PCA was not successful in differentiating the two groups, SVM with LOOCV was able to stratify the groups with overall accuracies of 84.5%–90.2% for dried serum drops and 86%–91.5% for freeze-dried serum [76].

Sahu *et al* published several reports on the efficacy of serum Raman spectroscopy for oral cancer detection. In their exploratory study of 2013, the group reported the findings of Raman studies on serum from 16 healthy control, 14 buccal mucosa cancer and 40 tongue cancer subjects [33]. Intense β-carotene bands were observed in all sera with the highest relative intensity in control samples [33]. Higher DNA and protein content were observed in the mean cancer spectra [33]. PC-LDA followed by LOOCV models were constructed for both spectra-and patient-wise analyses [33]. Both approaches were successful in classifying the groups and it was concluded that patient-wise was the preferred mode for prospective studies (figure 5.4) [33]. Another investigation involved 36 buccal mucosa, 33 tongue cancer patients and 17 healthy subjects wherein Raman spectra of sera were recorded using assembled Raman microprobe coupled with 40 × objective [77]. An average of three spectra recorded from each sample were subjected to PCA and PC-LDA followed by LOOCV. Cancer and normal groups could be stratified with ~78% classification efficiency [77]. Buccal

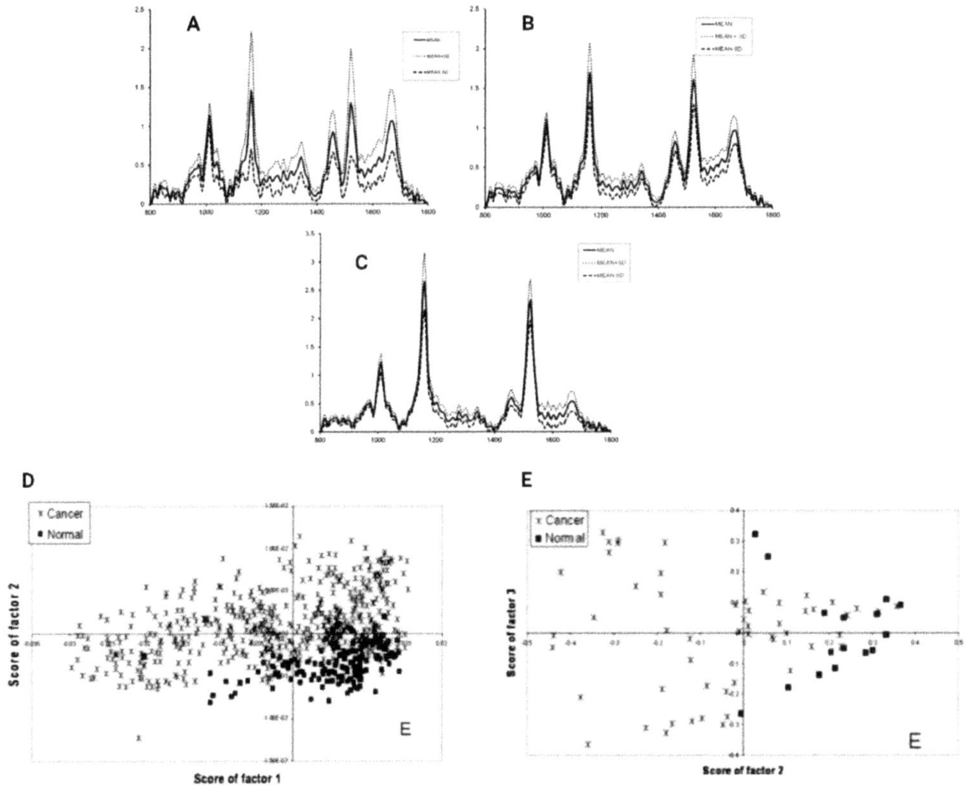

Figure 5.4. Mean and standard deviation spectra of (A) buccal mucosa cancer serum, (B) tongue cancer serum, (C) normal serum. PC-LDA for normal and cancer serum, (D) spectra-wise analysis, (E) sample-wise analysis. Reproduced from [33] wth permission from the Royal Society of Chemistry.

mucosa and tongue cancers were classified with ~68% accuracy [77]. Subsequently, the group evaluated the potential of serum RS in oral cancer screening, premalignant and cancer-specific detection using 328 subjects encompassing healthy controls, premalignant, disease controls, and oral cancer groups [77]. Alterations in amino acids, lipids, protein, DNA, and β-carotene were observed across the groups [77]. A patient-wise approach was adopted for analysis and PC-LDA models were constructed. Binary classification models among premalignant, disease control (non-oral cancer), oral cancer, and normal samples plus single four group model demonstrated the premalignant and specific cancer detection. The normal versus abnormal model achieved better sensitivity and specificity rates of 64% and 80%, comparable to standard screening approaches [77].

In 2014, González–Solís *et al* studied serum samples of 19 cervical cancer patients, three pre-cancer subjects, and 20 healthy volunteer controls [78]. Higher amounts of carotenoids and protein components were reported in the control spectra [78]. Glutathione and tryptophan were higher in the cancer spectra [78]. They also noted that weak tryptophan bands at 545, 760, and 1174 cm^{-1} and amide III bands between 1234 and 1290 cm^{-1} seemed to disappear and decrease in the cervical cancer samples, respectively [78]. A study by Ullah *et al* investigated serum Raman spectroscopy ovarian cancer screening [79]. SVM models achieved 90% sensitivity, 100% specificity, 100% positive predictive value and 87.5% negative predictive value [79]. In another study, the performances of Raman spectroscopy of blood plasma, serum and ascitic fluid for ovarian cancer detection, in 18 cancer patients and 20 controls were compared [80]. Ascitic fluid outperformed plasma and serum in unsupervised and supervised discrimination models [80].

Wang *et al* studied the Raman spectra of the sera of peripheral venous blood with a LabRAM HR 800 confocal Micro Raman spectrometer of 14 healthy volunteers (control group), 23 patients with stage I non-small cell lung cancer (NSCLC) (stage I group), 24 patients with stage II NSCLC (stage II group), 19 patients with stage III NSCLC (stage III group), 11 patients with stage IV NSCLC (stage IV group), using the patient-wise mean spectra approach [81]. The Raman spectra of the five groups were analyzed by analysis of variance (ANOVA), PCA, LDA, and cross-validation. The control group exhibited the highest peak intensity, while the stage III/IV group showed the lowest intensities at 848, 999, 1152, 1446, and 1658 cm^{-1} [81]. LDA revealed varying levels of diagnostic accuracy: for healthy individuals, the sensitivity was 86% and specificity 95%; for stage I NSCLC, 65% sensitivity and 94% specificity; for stage II, 75% sensitivity and 88% specificity; and for stage III/IV, 87% sensitivity and 93% specificity [81]. The overall accuracy rate achieved was 92%, correctly identifying 71 out of 77 cases [81]. In a subsequent study, FTIR and Raman serum spectra were acquired from samples of 45 healthy controls, 44 NSCLC, 38 glioma and 37 esophageal cancer patients. Low-level fusion and feature fusion on the spectral, followed by SVM, convolutional neural network-long-short term memory (CNN-LSTM) and the multi-scale convolutional fusion neural network (MFCNN) were used [82]. Fused models achieved improved results by about 10% compared to spectral models based on individual methods. [82].

Corriea *et al* aimed to identify the differences in the Raman spectra of serum samples with normal and altered PSA values and correlate these differences by PCA and PLSR [83]. Discriminating and quantitative models employing PCA and PLS were developed after obtaining 270 spectra from 91 non-altered PSA samples and 51 spectra from 17 samples with altered PSA, and standardizing the spectra to area under the curve [83]. PCA achieved >85% sensitivity and >75% specificity. PLS achieved ~98% sensitivity and lower specificity [83]. The quantitative PLS regression model yielded a good correlation between PSA values and the spectral features [83].

Song *et al* studied papillary thyroid carcinoma (PTC) and papillary microcarcinoma (PMC) detection using serum Raman spectroscopy in 16 PTC and 31 PMC patients [84]. Synthetic minority oversampling technique (SMOTE) and PCA were used for pre-processing and dimensionality reduction, respectively [84]. Single DT classifier and RF built on the idea of boosting ensemble and the adaptive boosting (Adaboost) model built on the idea of bagging ensemble explored for classification resulted in accuracies of 75.38%, 81.54%, and 84.61%, respectively [84]. Su *et al* explored serum Raman spectroscopy for rapid screening of cholangitis and cholangiocarcinoma (CCA) in 49 patients with cholangitis, 38 patients with CCA, and 55 healthy volunteers. SVM classification models with LOOCV achieved ~90% accuracies [85].

Overall, Raman spectroscopy has demonstrated significant efficacy for cancer diagnosis through numerous studies across various cancer types. The earliest investigations on breast cancer serum samples achieved 92.2% sensitivity using PCA and PC-LDA models, while more advanced deep learning techniques showed over 90% accuracy in distinguishing subtypes such as triple-negative and HER2-positive breast cancers. Studies on cervical and colorectal cancers further highlighted the efficacy of serum-based Raman spectroscopy, with PC-LDA and PLS-DA models reporting accuracy rates nearing 92%. For hepatocellular carcinoma, freeze-dried serum yielded considerable accuracy in SVM models. Investigations into oral cancer across multiple studies emphasized the effectiveness of serum Raman spectroscopy, with PC-LDA models achieving good classification efficiencies. The diagnostic capabilities of serum Raman spectroscopy have been explored in ovarian, NSCLC and colorectal cancers with significant success. These studies highlight the evolving role of serum Raman spectroscopy in cancer diagnostics, with progressively refined techniques and computational models enhancing accuracy and early detection.

5.3 Spectroscopy in blood-based cancer diagnosis: perspectives and challenges

In the field of oncology, optical spectroscopy methods have shown potential for early diagnosis, improving diagnostic sensitivity and specificity. However, there is a lack of uniformity in protocols for sample collection, storage of samples, instrument settings, and spectral pre-processing, which can lead to erroneous results. Construction of machine learning models ideally require large sample sizes to avoid overfitting. Many of the studies report investigations on small sample sizes with no test sets, inadvertently leading to overfitted classification models with exaggerated results. Serum composition and quality can be influenced by sample collection methodology, processing and storage conditions. The more crucial challenge is that of data transportability. Development of software to make data amenable to analysis across different instrument platforms for seamless application in clinics, is necessary for commercialization and routine clinical applications. Despite challenges, the remarkable results reported in the numerous studies discussed in the previous sections indicate the promise these methods hold for clinical translation as stand-alone/adjunct tools for screening and early diagnosis of cancer.

References

[1] Bray F, Laversanne M, Sung H, Ferlay J, Siegel R L, Soerjomataram I and Jemal A 2024 Global cancer statistics 2022: GLOBOCAN estimates of incidence and mortality worldwide for 36 cancers in 185 countries *CA Cancer J. Clin.* **74** 229–63

[2] Bannister N and Broggio J 2016 Cancer survival by stage at diagnosis for England (experimental statistics): adults diagnosed 2012 2013 and 2014 and followed up to 2015. 2016 Produced in collaboration with Public Health England https://backup.ons.gov.uk/wp-content/uploads/sites/3/2016/06/Cancer-survival-by-stage-at-diagnosis-for-England-experimental-statistics-Adults-diagnosed-2012-2013-and-2014-.pdf

[3] Loud J T and Murphy J 2017 Cancer screening and early detection in the 21st century *Semin. Oncol. Nurs.* **33** 121–8

[4] Sankaranarayanan R, Ramadas K, Thomas G, Muwonge R, Thara S, Mathew B and Rajan B 2005 Effect of screening on oral cancer mortality in Kerala, India: a cluster-randomised controlled trial *Lancet* **365** 1927–33

[5] Rosenzweig P F-B M Q, Gardner F M D and Griffith B 2014 The history and physical in cancer care: a primer for the oncology advanced practitioner *J. Adv. Pract. Oncol.* **5** 262–8

[6] Stevenson P and Rodins K 2018 Improving diagnostic accuracy of skin biopsies *Aust. J. Gen. Pract.* **47** 216–20

[7] Okada K 2016 Points to notice during the diagnosis of soft tissue tumors according to the 'Clinical Practice Guideline on the Diagnosis and Treatment of Soft Tissue Tumors' *J. Orthop. Sci.* **21** 705–12

[8] Wasif M, Mughal A, Hussain M, Zaidi M, Awan M S, Sidddique S, Awan O, Ghaloo S K and Suahil A 2022 The utility of frozen sections in the evaluation of clear margins in oral squamous cell carcinomas: a cross-sectional study from a tertiary care center *Cureus* **14** e22308

[9] Wenzel C, Herold S, Wermke M, Aust D E and Baretton G B 2021 Routine molecular pathology diagnostics in precision oncology *Dtsch. Arztebl. Int.* **118** 255–61

[10] Hawes D, Shi S R, Dabbs D J, Taylor C R and Cote R J 2009 Immunohistochemistry *Modern Surgical Pathology* (Elsevier) pp 48–70

[11] Brouwer R, MacDonald A, Matthews R, Gunn J, Monson J R and Hartley J E 2009 Brush cytology for the diagnosis of colorectal cancer *Dis. Colon Rectum* **52** 598–601

[12] Kaur S, Sharma R, Kaushal V, Gulati A and Sharma B 2016 Diagnostic accuracy of endoscopic brush cytology in malignancies of upper gastrointestinal tract: a prospective study of 251 patients in North India *J. Cancer Res. Ther.* **12** 681

[13] Sachan P L, Singh M, Patel M L and Sachan R 2018 A study on cervical cancer screening using pap smear test and clinical correlation *Asia-Pac. J. Oncol. Nurs.* **5** 337–41

[14] Kazi M, Suhani , Parshad R, Seenu V, Mathur S and Haresh K P 2017 Fine-Needle Aspiration Cytology (FNAC) in breast cancer: a reappraisal based on retrospective review of 698 cases *World J. Surg.* **41** 1528–33

[15] Hajmanoochehri F and Rabiee E 2015 FNAC accuracy in diagnosis of thyroid neoplasms considering all diagnostic categories of the Bethesda reporting system: a single-institute experience *J. Cytol.* **32** 238

[16] Wilkinson A R, Mahore S D and Maimoon S A 2012 FNAC in the diagnosis of lymph node malignancies: a simple and sensitive tool *Indian J. Med. Paediatr. Oncol.* **33** 21–4

[17] Ahmad S S, Akhtar K, Akhtar S, Abrari A, Khalid M and Mansoor T 2006 Ultrasound guided fine needle aspiration biopsy of abdominal masses *JK Science* **8** 200–4

[18] Quintás-Cardama A and Cortes J E 2006 Chronic myeloid leukemia: diagnosis and treatment *Mayo Clin. Proc.* **81** 973–88

[19] Bardi G, Sukhikh T, Pandis N, Fenger C, Kronborg O and Heim S 1995 Karyotypic characterization of colorectal adenocarcinomas *Genes Chromosomes Cancer* **12** 97–109

[20] Aukema S M *et al* 2015 Sequential karyotyping in Burkitt lymphoma reveals a linear clonal evolution with increase in karyotype complexity and a high frequency of recurrent secondary aberrations *Br. J. Haematol.* **170** 814–25

[21] Ishikawa T, Kobayashi M, Mai M, Suzuki T and Ooi A 1997 Amplification of the c-erbB-2 (HER-2/neu) gene in gastric cancer cells. Detection by fluorescence *in situ* hybridization *Am. J. Pathol.* **151** 761–8

[22] Shapiro D N, Valentine M B, Rowe S T, Sinclair A E, Sublett J E, Roberts W M and Look A T 1993 Detection of N-myc gene amplification by fluorescence *in situ* hybridization. Diagnostic utility for neuroblastoma *Am. J. Pathol.* **142** 1339–46

[23] Dilek O N, Arslan Kahraman D İ and Kahraman G 2024 Carcinoembryonic antigen in the diagnosis, treatment, and follow-up of focal liver lesions *World J. Gastrointest. Surg.* **16** 999–1007

[24] Gao X, Porter A T, Grignon D J, Pontes J E and Honn K V 1997 Diagnostic and prognostic markers for human prostate cancer *Prostate* **31** 264–81

[25] King M-C, Marks J H and Mandell J BNew York Breast Cancer Study Group 2003 Breast and ovarian cancer risks due to inherited mutations in BRCA1 and BRCA2 *Science* **302** 643–6

[26] Hussain S, Mubeen I, Ullah N, Shah S S U D, Khan B A, Zahoor M, Ullah R, Khan F A and Sultan M A 2022 Modern diagnostic imaging technique applications and risk factors in the medical field: a review *Biomed. Res. Int.* **2022** 5164970

[27] Battifora H and Applebaum E L 1979 Electron microscopy in the diagnosis of head and neck tumors *Head Neck Surg.* **1** 202–12

[28] Tanaka N, Sugihara K, Odajima T, Mimura M, Kimijima Y, Ichinose S, Tanaka N, Sugihara K, Mimura M and Kimijima Y 2002 Oral squamous cell carcinoma: electron microscopic and immunohistochemical characteristics *Med. Electron. Microscop.* **35** 127–38

[29] Reyes-Santias F, García-García C, Aibar-Guzmán B, García-Campos A, Cordova-Arevalo O, Mendoza-Pintos M, Cinza-Sanjurjo S, Portela-Romero M, Mazón-Ramos P and Gonzalez-Juanatey J R 2023 Cost analysis of magnetic resonance imaging and computed tomography in cardiology: a case study of a university hospital complex in the euro region *Healthcare* **11** 2084

[30] Klein J D and Grandis J R 2010 The molecular pathogenesis of head and neck cancer *Cancer Biol. Ther.* **9** 1–7

[31] Hanif H, Ali M J, Susheela A T, Khan I W, Luna-Cuadros M A, Khan M M and Lau D T-Y 2022 Update on the applications and limitations of alpha-fetoprotein for hepatocellular carcinoma *World J. Gastroenterol.* **28** 216–29

[32] Jolliffe I T and Cadima J 2016 Principal component analysis: a review and recent developments *Philos. Transact. A Math. Phys. Eng. Sci.* **374** 20150202

[33] Sahu A, Sawant S, Mamgain H and Krishna C M 2013 Raman spectroscopy of serum: an exploratory study for detection of oral cancers *Analyst* **138** 4161–74

[34] Mohamed A E 2017 Comparative study of four supervised machine learning techniques for classification *Int. J. Appl. Sci. Technol.* **7** 5–14

[35] Devos O, Downey G and Duponchel L 2014 Simultaneous data pre-processing and SVM classification model selection based on a parallel genetic algorithm applied to spectroscopic data of olive oils *Food Chem.* **148** 124–30

[36] Lasalvia M, Capozzi V and Perna G 2022 A comparison of PCA-LDA and PLS-DA techniques for classification of vibrational spectra *Appl. Sci.* **12** 5345

[37] Houston J, Glavin F G and Madden M G 2020 Robust classification of high-dimensional spectroscopy data using deep learning and data synthesis *J. Chem. Inf. Model.* **60** 1936–54

[38] Malini R, Venkatakrishna K, Kurien J, Pai K M, Rao L, Kartha V B and Krishna C M 2006 Discrimination of normal, inflammatory, premalignant, and malignant oral tissue: a Raman spectroscopy study *Biopolymers* **81** 179–93

[39] Sahu A, Deshmukh A, Hole A R, Chaturvedi P and Krishna C M 2016 In vivo subsite classification and diagnosis of oral cancers using Raman spectroscopy *J. Innov. Opt. Health Sci.* **9** 1650017

[40] Singh S P, Deshmukh A, Chaturvedi P and Murali Krishna C 2012 In vivo Raman spectroscopic identification of premalignant lesions in oral buccal mucosa *J. Biomed. Opt.* **17** 1050021

[41] Malik A, Sahu A, Singh S P, Deshmukh A, Chaturvedi P, Nair D, Nair S and Murali Krishna C 2017 In vivo Raman spectroscopy–assisted early identification of potential second primary/recurrences in oral cancers: an exploratory study *Head Neck* **39** 2216–23

[42] Singh S P, Sahu A, Deshmukh A, Chaturvedi P and Krishna C M 2013 In vivo raman spectroscopy of oral buccal mucosa: a study on malignancy associated changes (MAC)/ cancer field effects (CFE) *Analyst* **138** 4175–82

[43] Chowdary M V P, Kumar K K, Kurien J, Mathew S and Krishna C M 2006 Discrimination of normal, benign, and malignant breast tissues by Raman spectroscopy *Biopolymers* **83** 556–69

[44] Chwirot B W, Chwirot S, Jedrzejczyk W, Jackowski M, Raczyńska A M, Winczakiewicz J and Dobber J 1997 Ultraviolet laser-induced fluorescence of human stomach tissues: detection of cancer tissues by imaging techniques *Lasers Surg. Med.* **21** 149–58

[45] Krishna C M, Sockalingum G D, Bhat R A, Venteo L, Kushtagi P, Pluot M and Manfait M 2007 FTIR and Raman microspectroscopy of normal, benign, and malignant formalin-fixed ovarian tissues *Anal. Bioanal. Chem.* **387** 1649–56

[46] Kaznowska E, Depciuch J, Szmuc K and Cebulski J 2017 Use of FTIR spectroscopy and PCA-LDC analysis to identify cancerous lesions within the human colon *J. Pharm. Biomed. Anal.* **134** 259–68

[47] Madhuri S, Aruna P, Summiya Bibi M I, Gowri V S, Koteeswaran D and Ganesan S 1997 Ultraviolet fluorescence spectroscopy of blood plasma in the discrimination of cancer from normal *Proc. SPIE 2982, Optical Diagnostics of Biological Fluids and Advanced Techniques in Analytical Cytology* (SPIE) https://doi.org/10.1117/12.273649

[48] Madhuri S, Vengadesan N, Aruna P, Koteeswaran D, Venkatesan P and Ganesan S 2007 Native fluorescence spectroscopy of blood plasma in the characterization of oral malignancy *Photochem. Photobiol.* **78** 197–204

[49] Lualdi M, Colombo A, Leo E, Morelli D, Vannelli A, Battaglia L, Poiasina E and Marchesini R 2007 Natural fluorescence spectroscopy of human blood plasma in the diagnosis of colorectal cancer: feasibility study and preliminary results *Tumori. J.* **93** 567–71

[50] Lawaetz A J, Bro R, Kamstrup-Nielsen M, Christensen I J, Jørgensen L N and Nielsen H J 2012 Fluorescence spectroscopy as a potential metabonomic tool for early detection of colorectal cancer *Metabolomics* **8** 111–21

[51] Soares F, Becker K and Anzanello M J 2017 A hierarchical classifier based on human blood plasma fluorescence for non-invasive colorectal cancer screening *Artif. Intell. Med.* **82** 1–10

[52] Masilamani V, Al-Zhrani K, Al-Salhi M, Al-Diab A and Al-Ageily M 2004 Cancer diagnosis by autofluorescence of blood components *J. Lumin.* **109** 143–54

[53] Pachaiappan R, Prakasarao A, Manoharan Y, Dornadula K and Singaravelu G 2017 Oral cancer detection based on fluorescence polarization of blood plasma at excitation wavelength 405 nm *Proc. SPIE 10060, Optical Biopsy XV: Toward Real-Time Spectroscopic Imaging and Diagnosis* R R Alfano and S G Demos (SPIE) p 100601D

[54] Backhaus J, Mueller R, Formanski N, Szlama N, Meerpohl H G, Eidt M and Bugert P 2010 Diagnosis of breast cancer with infrared spectroscopy from serum samples *Vib. Spectrosc.* **52** 173–7

[55] Sitnikova V E, Kotkova M A, Nosenko T N, Kotkova T N, Martynova D M and Uspenskaya M V 2020 Breast cancer detection by ATR-FTIR spectroscopy of blood serum and multivariate data-analysis *Talanta* **214** 120857

[56] Yang B, Chen C, Chen C, Cheng H, Yan Z, Chen F, Zhu Z, Zhang H, Yue F and Lv X 2021 Detection of breast cancer of various clinical stages based on serum FT-IR spectroscopy combined with multiple algorithms *Photodiagnosis Photodyn. Ther.* **33** 102199

[57] Ollesch J, Drees S L, Heise H M, Behrens T, Brüning T and Gerwert K 2013 FTIR spectroscopy of biofluids revisited: an automated approach to spectral biomarker identification *Analyst* **138** 4092–102

[58] Maitra I, Morais C L M, Lima K M G, Ashton K M, Date R S and Martin F L 2019 Attenuated total reflection Fourier-transform infrared spectral discrimination in human bodily fluids of oesophageal transformation to adenocarcinoma *Analyst* **144** 7447–56

[59] Chen H, Li X, Zhang S, Yang H, Gao Q and Zhou F 2022 Rapid and sensitive detection of esophageal cancer by FTIR spectroscopy of serum and plasma *Photodiagnosis Photodyn. Ther.* **40** 103177

[60] Cameron J M *et al* 2019 Developing infrared spectroscopic detection for stratifying brain tumour patients: glioblastoma multiforme *vs.* lymphoma *Analyst* **144** 6736–50

[61] Chen F, Meng C, Qu H, Cheng C, Chen C, Yang B, Gao R and Lv X 2021 Human serum mid-infrared spectroscopy combined with machine learning algorithms for rapid detection of gliomas *Photodiagnosis Photodyn. Ther.* **35** 102308

[62] Qu H, Wu W, Chen C, Yan Z, Guo W, Meng C, Lv X, Chen F and Chen C 2021 Application of serum mid-infrared spectroscopy combined with an ensemble learning method in rapid diagnosis of gliomas *Anal. Methods* **13** 4642–51

[63] Giamougiannis P, Morais C L M, Rodriguez B, Wood N J, Martin-Hirsch P L and Martin F L 2021 Detection of ovarian cancer (± neo-adjuvant chemotherapy effects) via ATR-FTIR

spectroscopy: comparative analysis of blood and urine biofluids in a large patient cohort *Anal. Bioanal. Chem.* **413** 5095–107

[64] Alcántara-Quintana L E, López-Mendoza C M, Rodríguez-Aguilar M, Medellín-Castillo N, Mizaikoff B, Flores-Ramírez R, Galván-Romero V S and Díaz de León-Martínez L 2022 One-drop serum screening test for anal cancer in men via infrared attenuated total reflection spectroscopy *Anal. Chem.* **94** 15250–60

[65] Guo S, Wei G, Chen W, Lei C, Xu C, Guan Y, Ji T, Wang F and Liu H 2022 Fast and deep diagnosis using blood-based ATR-FTIR spectroscopy for digestive tract cancers *Biomolecules* **12** 1815

[66] Duckworth E, Hole A, Deshmukh A, Chaturvedi P, Chilakapati M K, Mora B and Roy D 2022 Improving vibrational spectroscopy prospects in frontline clinical diagnosis: Fourier transform infrared on buccal mucosa cancer *Anal. Chem.* **94** 13642–6

[67] Sala A, Anderson D J, Brennan P M, Butler H J, Cameron J M, Jenkinson M D, Rinaldi C, Theakstone A G and Baker M J 2020 Biofluid diagnostics by FTIR spectroscopy: a platform technology for cancer detection *Cancer Lett.* **477** 122–30

[68] Pichardo-Molina J L, Frausto-Reyes C, Barbosa-García O, Huerta-Franco R, González-Trujillo J L, Ramírez-Alvarado C A, Gutiérrez-Juárez G and Medina-Gutiérrez C 2007 Raman spectroscopy and multivariate analysis of serum samples from breast cancer patients *Lasers Med. Sci.* **22** 229–36

[69] Zeng Q, Chen C, Chen C, Song H, Li M, Yan J and Lv X 2023 Serum Raman spectroscopy combined with convolutional neural network for rapid diagnosis of HER2-positive and triple-negative breast cancer *Spectrochim. Acta A Mol. Biomol. Spectrosc.* **286** 122000

[70] Li H, Wang S, Zeng Q, Chen C, Lv X, Ma M, Su H, Ma B, Chen C and Fang J 2022 Serum Raman spectroscopy combined with multiple classification models for rapid diagnosis of breast cancer *Photodiagnosis Photodyn. Ther.* **40** 103115

[71] Cao Y, Xiong J, Du Y, Tang Y and Yin L 2024 Raman spectroscopy combined with multivariate statistical algorithms for the simultaneous screening of cervical and breast cancers *Lasers Med. Sci.* **39** 68

[72] Li X, Yang T and Li S 2012 Discrimination of serum Raman spectroscopy between normal and colorectal cancer using selected parameters and regression-discriminant analysis *Appl Opt* **51** 5038–43

[73] Jenkins C A, Jenkins R A, Pryse M M, Welsby K A, Jitsumura M, Thornton C A, Dunstan P R and Harris D A 2018 A high-throughput serum Raman spectroscopy platform and methodology for colorectal cancer diagnostics *Analyst* **143** 6014–24

[74] Liu K, Liu B, Wang Y, Zhao Q, Wu Q and Li B 2023 Evaluation of Raman spectroscopy combined with the gated recurrent unit serum detection method in early screening of gastrointestinal cancer *Analyst* **148** 6061–9

[75] Guleken Z *et al* 2023 An application of raman spectroscopy in combination with machine learning to determine gastric cancer spectroscopy marker *Comput. Methods Programs Biomed.* **234** 107523

[76] Taleb I *et al* 2013 Diagnosis of hepatocellular carcinoma in cirrhotic patients: a proof-of-concept study using serum micro-Raman spectroscopy *Analyst* **138** 4006

[77] Sahu A, Sawant S, Talathi-Desai S and Murali Krishna C 2015 Raman spectroscopy of serum: a study on oral cancers *Biomed. Spectrosc. Imaging* **4** 171–87

[78] González-Solís J L, Martínez-Espinosa J C, Torres-González L A, Aguilar-Lemarroy A, Jave-Suárez L F and Palomares-Anda P 2014 Cervical cancer detection based on serum sample Raman spectroscopy *Lasers Med. Sci.* **29** 979–85

[79] Ullah I, Ahmad I, Nisar H, Khan S, Ullah R, Rashid R and Mahmood H 2016 Computer assisted optical screening of human ovarian cancer using Raman spectroscopy *Photodiagnosis Photodyn. Ther.* **15** 94–9

[80] Giamougiannis P, Morais C L M, Grabowska R, Ashton K M, Wood N J, Martin-Hirsch P L and Martin F L 2021 A comparative analysis of different biofluids towards ovarian cancer diagnosis using Raman microspectroscopy *Anal. Bioanal. Chem.* **413** 911–22

[81] Wang H, Zhang S, Wan L, Sun H, Tan J and Su Q 2018 Screening and staging for non-small cell lung cancer by serum laser Raman spectroscopy *Spectrochim. Acta A Mol. Biomol. Spectrosc.* **201** 34–8

[82] Leng H *et al* 2023 Raman spectroscopy and FTIR spectroscopy fusion technology combined with deep learning: a novel cancer prediction method *Spectrochim. Acta A Mol. Biomol. Spectrosc.* **285** 121839

[83] Correia N A, Batista L T A, Nascimento R J M, Cangussú M C T, Crugeira P J L, Soares L G P, Silveira Jr L and Pinheiro A L B 2020 Detection of prostate cancer by Raman spectroscopy: a multivariate study on patients with normal and altered PSA values *J. Photochem. Photobiol.* B **204** 111801

[84] Song H, Dong C, Zhang X, Wu W, Chen C, Ma B, Chen F, Chen C and Lv X 2022 Rapid identification of papillary thyroid carcinoma and papillary microcarcinoma based on serum Raman spectroscopy combined with machine learning models *Photodiagnosis Photodyn. Ther.* **37** 102647

[85] Su N, Dawuti W, Hu Y and Zhao H 2022 Noninvasive cholangitis and cholangiocarcinoma screening based on serum Raman spectroscopy and support vector machine *Photodiagnosis Photodyn. Ther.* **40** 103156

Chapter 6

Raman spectroscopy: a potential tool for cancer analysis

Phularida Amulraj, Jayasree Kumar, Murali Krishna Chilakapati, Hemanth Noothalapati and Rajapandiyan Panneerselvam

Cancer is a major global health concern owing to the impact of delayed diagnosis and escalating mortality rates. Consequently, traditional cancer screening methods are being re-examined, propelling researchers to explore new technologies for early diagnosis with improved precision and effectiveness. Raman spectroscopy, a powerful analytical technique, is utilized for its ability to provide valuable insights into the molecular composition and structural alterations of cancerous tissues through photon scattering. Surface-enhanced Raman spectroscopy (SERS), which enhances the sensitivity of Raman spectroscopy using plasmonic nanoparticles, has emerged as a powerful technique for cancer analysis, particularly for biomarker identification. This chapter begins with the basics of Raman spectroscopy and SERS along with related techniques like tip-enhanced Raman spectroscopy (TERS) and shell-isolated nanoparticle-enhanced Raman spectroscopy (SHINERS). We then describe the different types of substrates used in SERS for bioanalysis as well as the fabrication method of novel SERS substrates ideal for cancer diagnosis. This chapter also highlights how Raman spectroscopy and SERS have been applied to detect common cancers, including breast, lung, colorectal, prostate, and oral cancer. Finally, we discuss the current challenges and exciting possibilities in the field, such as advancements in instruments, nanoparticle design, integration with other analytical methods, and combining these techniques with artificial intelligence and machine learning.

6.1 Introduction

Cancer is one of the most fatal diseases, causing more than 10 million deaths annually worldwide [1]. According to current estimates, the global population is

doi:10.1088/978-0-7503-5949-8ch6

projected to reach approximately 8.3 billion by the year 2025. Additionally, the World Health Organization (WHO) has predicted that by 2040, the annual number of new cancer cases could exceed 28.9 million [2]. In 2022, India reported over 14.1 lakh additional cases of cancer and roughly 9.1 lakh cancer-related deaths, according to the WHO's latest global cancer burden estimates. The International Agency for Research on Cancer (IARC), reports that oral and lung cancers are the most common types in men, accounting for 15.6% and 8.5% of new cases, respectively, while breast and cervical cancers are the most common in women, accounting for nearly 27% and 18% of new cases, correspondingly [3].

Cancer is a genetic disease that stems from alterations in the cellular DNA sequences. These changes can arise from a variety of sources, including DNA damage [4], errors during cell division [5], or inherited genetic mutations [6, 7]. Cancers are not limited to specific locations, but can develop in various areas of the body, including the lungs, breasts, lymph nodes, blood, connective tissues, and skin, leading to diverse clinical presentations and treatment approaches. Figure 6.1 illustrates the most prevalent types of cancer and the corresponding samples analyzed for their detection. Several factors, including heredity [8], age [9], smoking [10], prolonged sun exposure [11], radiation exposure [12], viral infections [13], the use of hormonal drugs [14], lifestyle choices [15], consumption of contaminated carcinogenic foods [16], exposure to harmful substances [17], polymers [18], and certain chemicals [19], contribute to the onset of cancer and are recognized as risk factors [20]. However, many cancer-related deaths occur due to ignorance of symptoms, which are often non-specific, making timely diagnosis challenging but

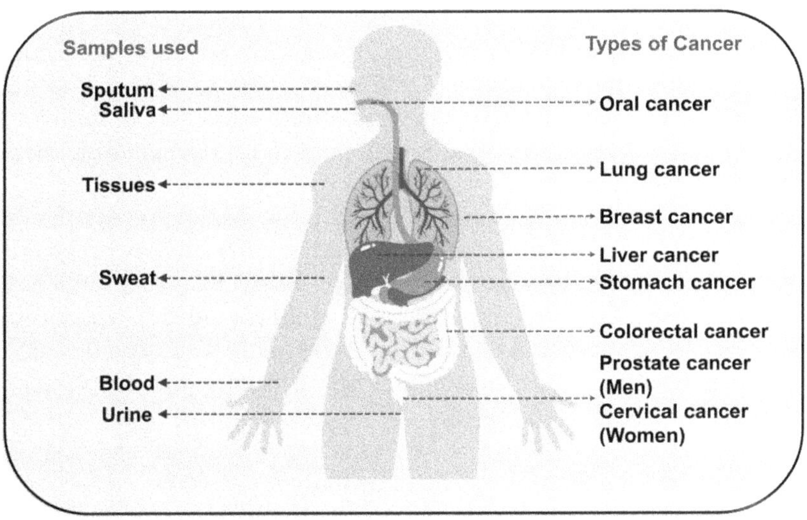

Figure 6.1. Schematic representation of prevalent cancer types and the samples used for detection (drawn using Canva).

crucial for effective treatment. It is widely acknowledged that identification of cancer at an early stage can lead to much better treatment results and survival rates, which emphasizes the importance of rapid detection [21–24].

Early stage cancer diagnosis is a crucial concern in medical research and clinical practice, highlighting the importance of rapid cancer screening pathways that guide appropriate therapies based on marker detection. This underscores the role of primary care in biomedical research to provide effective solutions. Cancer screening enables early detection, enhances treatment effectiveness, and improves survival rates by identifying cancer before it spreads, potentially reducing treatment intensity and recovery time. The challenge lies in diagnosing cancer early because of subtle or absent symptoms, making regular population screening a viable approach to address the imperative need for affordable and sensitive diagnostic analytical methods for early detection [25–27].

Physical examinations [28], laboratory tests [29], blood tests [30], endoscopies [31], medical histories [32], and symptom analyses [33] are some of the traditional methods used in cancer diagnosis. Imaging methods include x-rays [34], ultrasound [35], magnetic resonance imaging (MRI) [36], computerized tomography [37], and positron emission tomography [38] scans; other analytical methods include biopsy [39], mass spectrometry,[40], Raman spectroscopy [41], Fourier transform infrared spectroscopy [42], fluorescence spectroscopy [43], nuclear magnetic resonance (NMR) spectroscopy [44], radiology [45] etc. However, there are drawbacks to the diagnostic methods currently in use, such as tissue biopsy, in which a sample of tissue or cells from a suspected tumor or abnormal growth is removed for microscopic examination. Although this is the most accurate way to diagnose cancer and identify its type and grade, the process is intrusive and entails a risk of infection, bleeding, and other consequences [46]. With the use of next-generation sequencing [47], large DNA or RNA segments may be quickly sequenced, making it possible to identify genetic changes and mutations linked to cancer [47]. Yet it is a very expensive procedure, and it is less sensitive and can miss low-frequency mutations, especially in samples with low tumor content. Imaging-based techniques may not always distinguish between benign and malignant growths [48, 49].

Additionally, some imaging techniques such as radiology involve radiation exposure and may not be suitable for certain individuals such as pregnant women. It is believed that non-radiation methods, such as MRI [50] and ultrasonic scanning [51], are ineffective in identifying minimal residual illness [50–52], whereas stool- and blood-based laboratory tests have insufficient sensitivity and accuracy [25, 26, 53]. Spectroscopic methods, such as fluorescence spectroscopy, face drawbacks such as restricted tissue penetration and lack of specificity with fluorescent markers, potentially leading to false positives and challenges in quantification. Similarly, the limitations of NMR spectroscopy lie in its inability to detect early stage cancers, its low sensitivity in discerning subtle tissue variations, the necessity for meticulous sample preparation, and the high cost and specialized expertise required for clinical implementation.

Among these different diagnostic methods, Raman spectroscopy has become a vital analytical tool for early cancer diagnosis, offering noninvasive analysis and detailed biochemical insights [54]. It exhibits high sensitivity and specificity in distinguishing between benign and malignant tissues, as evidenced in skin and breast tissue studies [55, 56]. Moreover, its efficacy extends to head and neck cancers, demonstrating accurate tumor grading and treatment assessment [57]. Interestingly, the application of Raman spectroscopy extends to liquid biopsy samples for cancer diagnosis in its initial phases, and advances such as SERS, greatly increase the accuracy and precision of the analysis of cancer biomarkers [56–58]. Raman spectroscopy is becoming a more promising diagnostic technique for early cancer detection as a result of ongoing improvements, especially in SERS and its interaction with nanotechnology [58–61].

In this chapter, we cover the evolution of Raman spectroscopy, its development alongside SERS, TERS, and SHINERS, and the different substrates used in SERS applications. Subsequently, we discuss the diagnostic potential of Raman spectroscopy and SERS in diverse cancer types. The most common types of cancer based on the SCOPUS data are illustrated in figure 6.2, showing the top ten cancer cases in 2020 as percentages. We also review the potential impact of advancements in nanomaterials, development of Raman spectroscopy instruments, integration with complementary analytical techniques, and combination with artificial intelligence and machine learning (AI-ML) to improve the timely detection of cancer and increase patient survival rates.

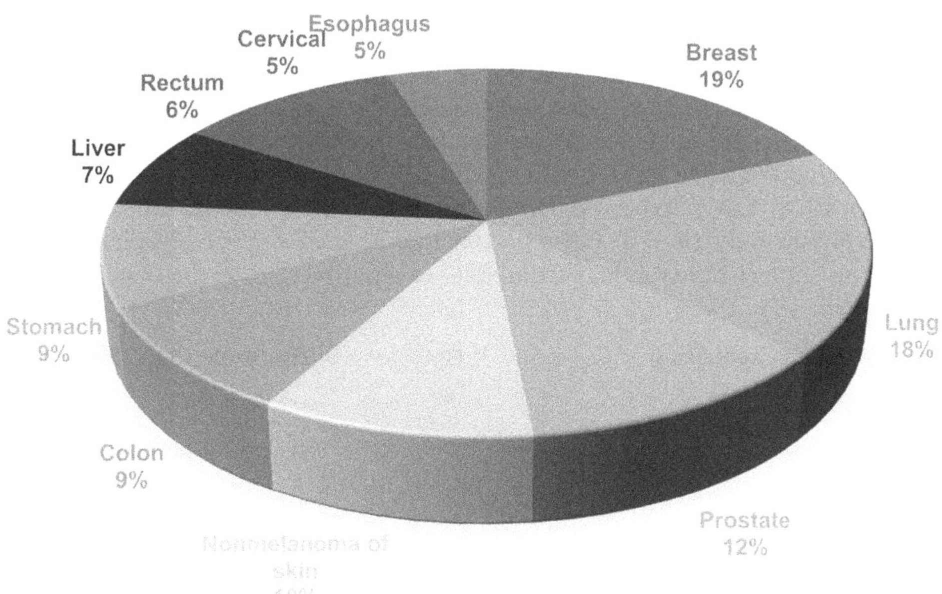

Figure 6.2. The ten most common types of cancer worldwide in 2020 (represented by percentage) [1].

6.2 Raman spectroscopy and its developments

6.2.1 Raman spectroscopy and surface-enhanced Raman spectroscopy

The Raman effect, the inelastic scattering of light, is a scientific phenomenon that was discovered by two Indian physicists, Chandrasekhara Venkata Raman, and Kariamanickam Srinivasa Krishnan in 1928. The notable contributions of Raman resulted in the effect bearing his name, which earned him the Nobel Prize in 1930 for this significant discovery [62]. The Raman effect occurs when a monochromatic laser interacts with a molecule, causing it to scatter photons inelastically. The vibrational energy levels that provide fingerprint information of the molecule are matched by the energy transfer between the laser and molecule. Initially hindered by its low sensitivity, Raman spectroscopy has faced limited adoption in the scientific community. However, with the discovery of lasers in the 1960s, the sensitivity of Raman spectroscopy has significantly improved. As a result, researchers have started using it extensively for analyzing bulk samples [63]. The advantage of this methodology is its capacity to analyze the unique Raman spectra of molecules without requiring sample modification or labeling. Raman spectroscopy has a significant benefit over other analytical techniques such as infrared spectroscopy due to its lack of interference with water and carbon dioxide under atmospheric conditions, and over mass spectroscopy, as it is non-destructive. It is also minimally invasive, accurate, reproducible, high-resolution, label-free, and cost-effective [64, 65].

Despite its numerous advantages, Raman spectroscopy is regarded as a weak scattering technique with only one in a million inelastically scattered incident photons. Consequently, detecting low concentrations of analyte molecules using Raman spectroscopy is challenging. The significant breakthrough occurred in 1974 when Fleischmann, Hendra, and McQuillan first observed the SERS effect while examining the pyridine Raman spectra on an electrochemically roughened silver electrode [66]. Figure 6.3 provides a schematic illustration of Raman and SERS scattering of the pyridine molecule. Researchers initially credited this improvement to the increased electrode surface area resulting from the electrochemical roughening process. In 1977, Van Duyne and Jeanmarie discovered a substantial enhancement factor, approximately 10^5–10^6 times greater than that of a single pyridine molecule in solution. Further research and theoretical calculations led to the conclusion that

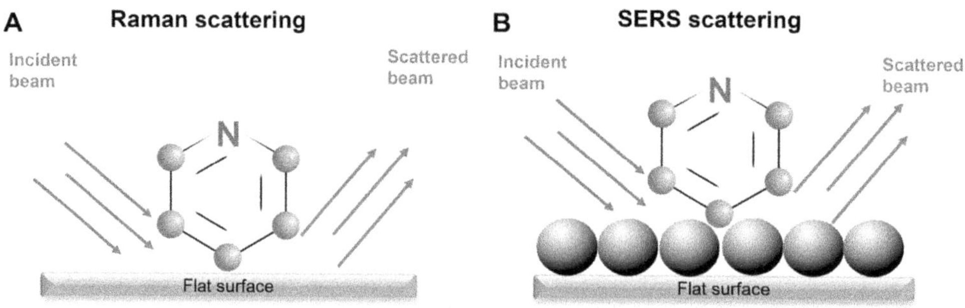

Figure 6.3. Schematic representation of (A) Raman scattering and (B) SERS scattering of pyridine molecule.

the roughened electrode surface generated a heightened electric field within the electrochemical double-layer region. This enhancement subsequently increased the Raman scattering cross-section of adsorbed pyridine molecules [67]. Albrecht and Creighton also contributed to the understanding of the enhancement effect in 1977, elucidating that it was due to the electronic coupling of molecules adsorbed on roughened metal surfaces [68]. The attribution of the Raman signal enhancement to surface plasmon resonance effect on silver (Ag) and copper (Cu) colloids was first reported by Moskovits in 1978 [69]. It was further solidified in 1979 by Creighton *et al* through experiments with silver (Ag) and gold (Au) colloids [70]. This groundbreaking series of observations and discoveries laid the foundation for the field of SERS and significantly contributed to the understanding of the underlying mechanisms.

Two enhancement mechanisms, chemical enhancement and electromagnetic enhancement, have been proposed to account for the SERS enhancement effect [71]. Due to the amplification of electromagnetic radiation by plasmonic nanostructures, specifically localized surface plasmon resonance (LSPR), electromagnetic enhancement is considered more significant than chemical enhancement [72–75]. Conversely, the charge transfer effect between the analyte molecules and the SERS substrate causes a significant change in the polarizability of the molecule, which causes chemical enhancement [74, 76–80]. During the 1980s, the use of roughened metal electrodes for SERS measurements became common, but it resulted in a lack of reproducibility and reliability in this technique [72]. Ag and Au are preferred for SERS because of their favorable electronic structures, surface morphologies, and interactions with the analytes. By contrast, Cu is more reactive and typically exhibits weaker SERS signals. Transition metals such as Pd, Pt, Rh, Ru, Co, Fe, and Ni are widely used, but they generally exhibit weaker SERS enhancements ($10^{-1}-10^{-3}$) [72]. Single-molecule SERS measurements were made possible in 1997 by Rieder *et al* [81], Kneipp *et al* [82] making SERS the first vibrational spectroscopy method to reach ultrahigh sensitivity at this scale.

SERS holds significant promise in biological applications because of its unique advantages, offering exceptional specificity for identifying and characterizing biomolecules based on their Raman fingerprints coupled with remarkable specificity that permits the detection of molecules at low concentrations, even within complex biological samples. Furthermore, SERS allows multiplexed detection, enabling simultaneous analysis of multiple analytes within a single sample [83–87]. With the ability to provide subcellular resolution, SERS is well suited for studying cellular processes and interactions at the nanoscale, including live-cell imaging [82, 88]. It also enables high-resolution bioimaging, offering insights into cellular structures and dynamics with enhanced spatial resolution. SERS has applications in protein analysis [89], DNA/RNA detection [90], biosensing [91], drug delivery [92], pathogen detection [93], cancer diagnostics [94], and point-of-care testing [95]. The versatility makes SERS, a valuable tool for biomedical research and contributing to advancements in understanding and treating complex diseases across various disciplines [58, 89, 96–99]. Figure 6.4(A) illustrates the growth curve of Raman spectroscopy and SERS in cancer detection. The increasing number of publications on both Raman spectroscopy and SERS indicates the widespread adoption of these

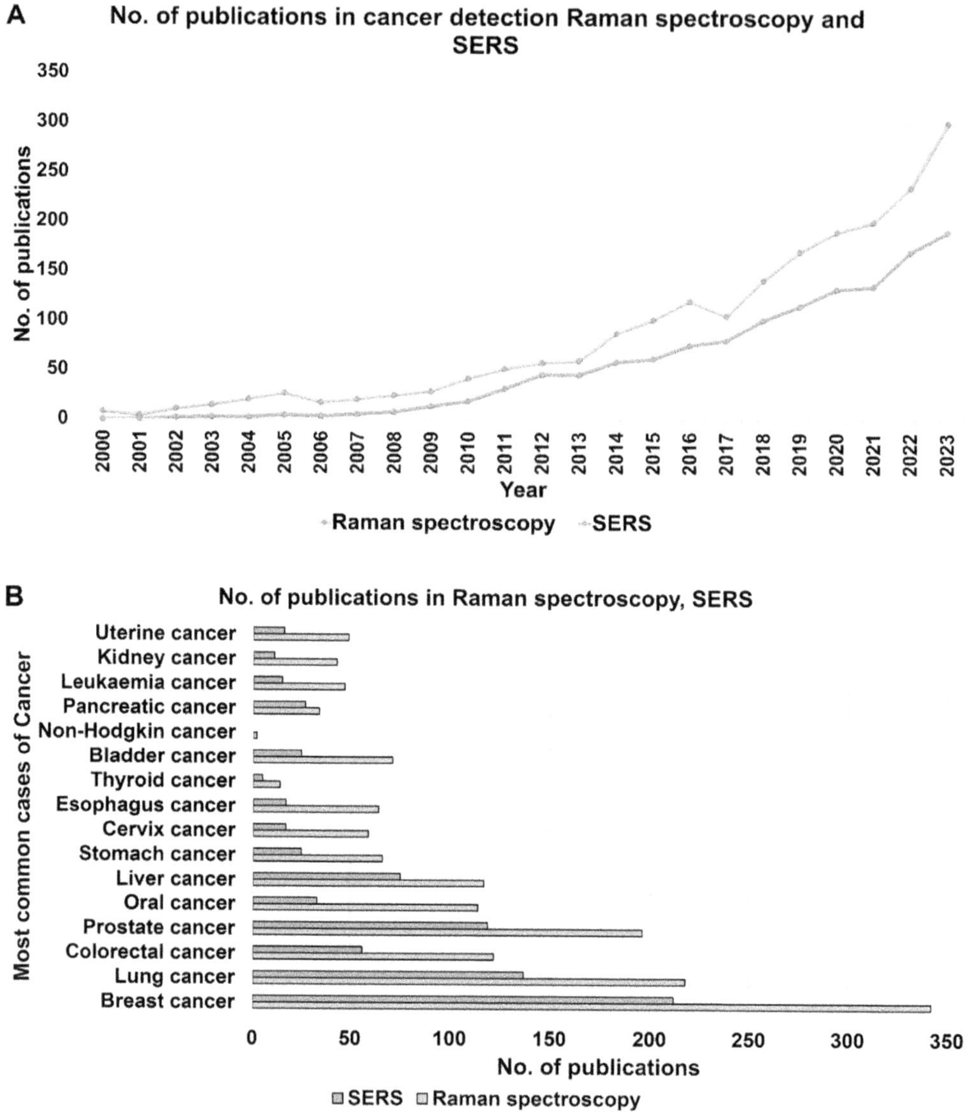

Figure 6.4. (A) The number of publications retrieved from SCOPUS using the keywords 'Cancer detection, Raman spectroscopy' and 'Cancer detection, SERS' from the years 2000–2023 and (B) Cancer types with the highest number of publications retrieved from SCOPUS using the keywords 'name of the cancer detection, Raman spectroscopy' and 'name of the cancer detection, SERS.'

techniques in cancer detection. These data were obtained using SCOPUS with search keywords such as 'Cancer detection, Raman spectroscopy' and 'Cancer detection, SERS.' Figure 6.4(B) highlights the most common types of cancer with the highest publication frequency from 2000 to 2023, revealing that breast cancer is the most extensively studied. This chapter discusses the five most frequently reported types of cancer, based on the number of publications.

6.2.2 Tip-enhanced Raman spectroscopy and shell-isolated nanoparticle-enhanced Raman spectroscopy

TERS was reported in 2000 by four different groups [100–103], although Wessel proposed the idea of TERS in 1985 [104]. TERS was developed by combining Raman spectroscopy and scanning probe microscopy to analyze surfaces beyond the diffraction limit of light. It progresses through various stages, including the integration of plasmonic and near-field optics, to attain a higher sensitivity and selectivity in chemical imaging. Using a silver/gold-coated sharp nanotip, TERS improves Raman signals with spatial resolution at the nanometer scale, allowing for a thorough examination of biological molecules and structures at the nanoscale [105–107].

Typically, SERS utilization is constrained by three primary issues: material, morphology, and molecular specificity. In 2010, Tian *et al* introduced the SHINERS technique, which addresses a few limitations of SERS and TERS by utilizing shell-isolated nanoparticles to non-intrusively enhance the Raman signal, enabling broader material analysis with enhanced reliability [108–112]. In SHINERS technique, each plasmonic nanoparticle is coated with a thin layer of silica or alumina. In this setup, each nanoparticle functions as a gold tip in the TERS system, effectively bringing thousands of TERS tips to the substrate surface for simultaneous probing. The primary advantage of this shell-isolated mode is its significantly enhanced detection sensitivity and wide range of practical applications for various materials with different morphologies. Both techniques offer label-free detection, enabling direct observation of biological processes without the need for chemical labels or dyes [110, 113].

In 2016, Xiao *et al* utilized TERS to discern the human integrin receptors $\alpha5\beta1$ and $\alpha v\beta3$ within a cancer cell membrane. Their approach involved employing cyclic arginine-glycine-aspartic acid peptide-conjugated Au nanoparticles as probes [114]. Researchers have developed a reversible cycle of phosphorylation and dephosphorylation for TERS measurements in a research study. The downstream binding domain Src homology region 2, which is linked to cancer cell invasion signaling, is subsequently connected to this reversible TERS sensing. As confirmed in a cell model, this approach has the benefit of easily detecting nanotags and shows good sensitivity [115].

Zheng *et al* developed the Au@SiO_2 SHINERS technology to improve the accuracy of Raman spectra. This technology was first used to identify and describe various breast tissue types, including invasive ductal carcinoma, fibroadenoma, ductal carcinoma *in situ*, and normal breast tissues [116]. They discovered that discrete DNA and β-carotene bands could distinguish malignant tissues from other types [116]. In addition, a unique approach using SHINs and a microfluidic device with an integrated photovoltaic-based SERS-active platform enabled noninvasive cancer screening and predictive treatment [117]. This method allowed for label-free, simultaneous separation and analysis of circulating tumor cells (CTCs) in blood specimens with high specificity and sensitivity. Principal component analysis (PCA) was used to identify significant variations in SHINERS data among renal cell carcinoma, cervical carcinoma, and blood cells [117].

6.3 Different types of substrates in SERS

The sensitivity of SERS detection is crucial for cancer diagnosis, because the concentration of cancer biomarkers in biological samples is typically low. Therefore, it is essential to develop analytical methods that are capable of examining ultralow analyte concentrations in real samples. SERS enhancement is influenced by several factors, including Raman instrument parameters; the structure and concentration of the analytes; and the size, shape, morphology, and nature of the plasmonic nanostructures. One strategy to increase the sensitivity is to develop SERS substrates with improved uniformity and reproducibility to detect ultralow concentrations of analytes [118, 119]. SERS substrates for cancer detection can be broadly categorized into colloidal substrates (nanoparticles in suspension) and planar substrates (nanoparticles attached to a solid substrate). These substrates are typically fabricated using bottom-up or top-down methods. Various SERS substrates that are suitable for cancer detection are discussed in the following section.

6.3.1 Planar substrates for cancer detection

Planar substrates are solid surfaces used for creating nanostructures through nanoparticle deposition or self-assembly, providing hotspot locations for analyte adsorption [120, 121]. Large-scale production methods, such as thin-layer deposition [122], lithography [123], and nanoimprinting [124] render planar substrates suitable for commercial applications. Functionalization with specific molecules or coatings enables the selective capture of target analytes, facilitating detection even in complex sample matrices [125]. Shin *et al* created an array chip with aggregated Au nanoparticles on glass functionalized using 3-Aminopropyltriethoxysilane (APTES) and ethanoic acid. This chip was designed to detect six types of early stage cancers: liver, pancreas, stomach, lung, breast, and colon. Figure 6.5(A) illustrates each chip, which features ten detecting locations [126]. In an alternative approach, a 3D-stacked Ag nanowires-glass fiber filter (AgNWs-GFF) sensor was developed for diagnosing prostate and pancreatic cancer. Figure 6.5(B) (i) and (ii) show the scanning electron microscopy (SEM) images of Ag nanowires, which were vacuum-filtered onto a glass fiber filter and densely stacked, creating a structure with nanogaps and nanojunctions that significantly enhanced the SERS effect. Using rhodamine B, the results showed that the enhancement factor (EF) and limit of detection (LOD) were 1.77×10^7 and 1.77 nM, respectively [127].

A flexible 3D plasmonic cluster SERS platform was developed using hybrid bio-ink-based blood plasma from patients with cancer and healthy individuals using a bottom-up methodology. The primary aim of this study is to develop a diagnostic tool for accurately detecting breast cancer using label-free SERS analysis of blood, coupled with an AI-based classification approach, as shown in figure 6.5(C) (i) and (ii) with the vertical 3D structure, with nanoholes from metallic nanoparticles, that enhances SERS sensitivity by providing effective binding sites for analyte capture in hot spots, enabling simultaneous measurement of multiple analytes [128]. Wu *et al* synthesized peptide-functionalized SERS nanotags targeting PD-L1 using AuNPs and 4-mercaptophenylboronic acid for signal enhancement by utilizing $Ti_3C_2T_x$

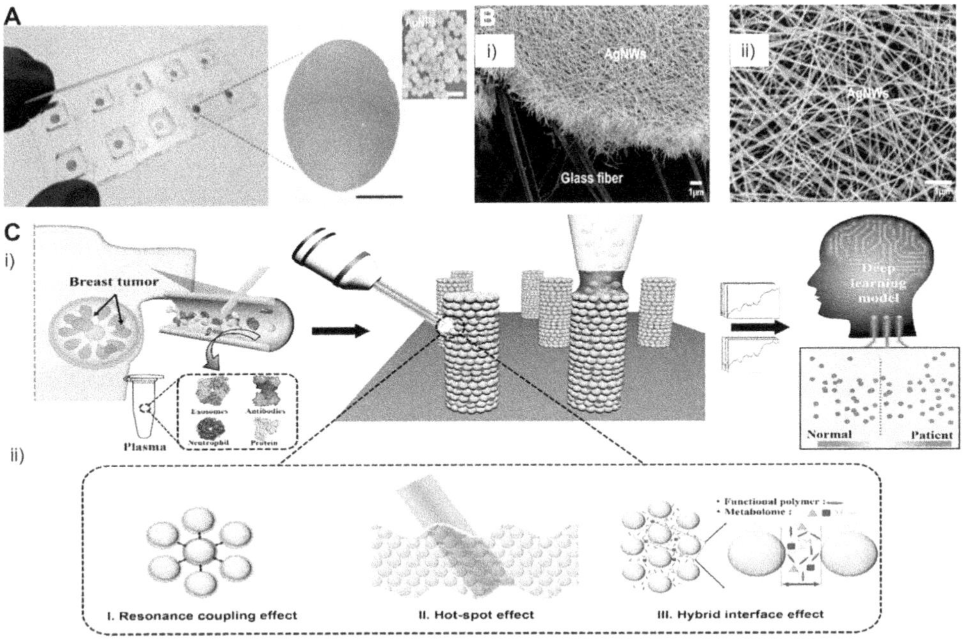

Figure 6.5. (A) AuNPs coated with APTES-functionalized cover glass, enhancing SERS. Reproduced from [126], CC BY 4.0. (B) (i) and (ii) SEM image of AgNWs layered on the GFF sensor. Reproduced with permission from [127], copyright (2021) American Chemical Society. (C) (i) CNN deep learning analyzes 3D plasmonic clusters, which are made of metabolome and self-assembling nanoparticles, for the diagnosis of breast cancer and (ii) Images showing the three benefits of 3D clusters. Reproduced with permission from [128], copyright (2024) American Chemical Society.

M*X*ene nanosheets for substrate modification, enabling specific PD-L1 recognition and SERS detection of labeled exosomes [129].

6.3.2 Colloidal substrates for cancer detection

Colloidal substrates involve nanoparticles mixed with liquid analytes, offering a high surface area for molecule–substrate interactions and reproducibly enhancing SERS signals. Although tailored for specific applications, they are simpler and more accessible than lithographically patterned substrates. In a study distinguishing benign from malignant breast cancers, SERS spectra using Ag nanoparticles synthesized according to Leopold and Lendl's method effectively differentiated between the two types based on saliva protein samples [130]. Additionally, blood plasma samples from 60 cervical cancer patients and 50 healthy volunteers were collected, processed to remove blood cells, incubated, and analyzed via SERS on an aluminum plate within three hours. The study demonstrates the Raman scattering and signal enhancement of human plasma facilitated by silver nanoparticles [131].

As shown in figure 6.6, a magnetic SERS immunoassay using Fe_3O_4 nanorings (R-Fe_3O_4) was developed for sensitive and selective detection of interleukin-6 (IL-6), a tumor marker for primary liver cancer. The strong magnetism of R-Fe_3O_4

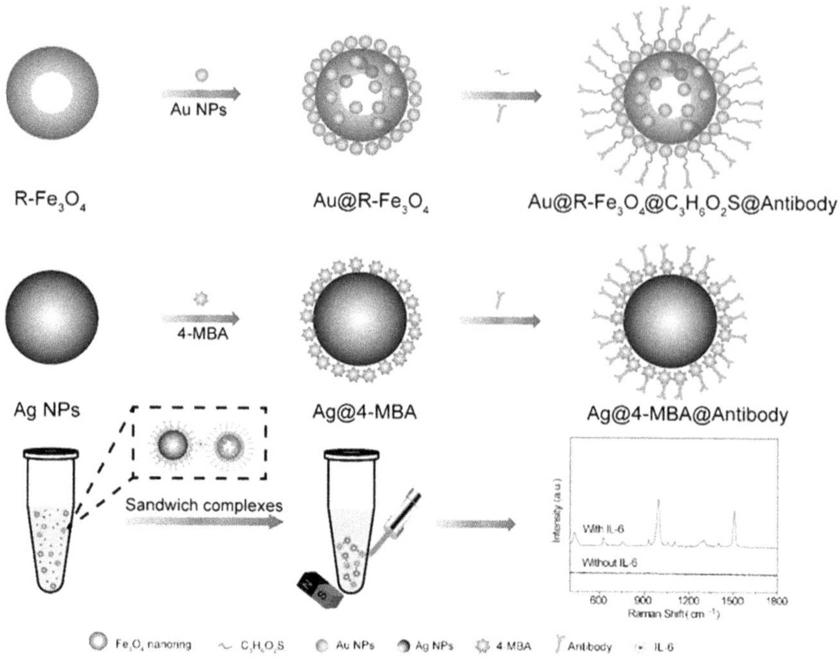

Figure 6.6. Scheme of IL-6 detection procedure by the magnetic SERS immunoassay based on R-Fe_3O_4. Reproduced with permission from [132], copyright 2022, with permission from Elsevier B.V. All rights reserved.

enriched target molecules at low concentrations, while its ring structure facilitated the deposition of metal particles, enhancing the Raman signal. The assay enabled quantitative IL-6 detection in the range of 0.1–1000 pg ml^{-1}, with a detection limit of 0.028 pg ml^{-1}. This method demonstrated high selectivity for IL-6 in serum samples and holds significant potential for early cancer diagnosis and medical applications [132]. Silver colloids, synthesized at a diameter of 35 nm using silver nitrate and hydroxylamine hydrochloride, facilitated high-quality SERS spectra of saliva proteins via membrane protein purification, revealing cancer-related alterations. Using PCA combined with linear discriminant analysis (PCA-LDA), the study achieved 70.7% sensitivity and 70.3% specificity for diagnosing nasopharyngeal carcinoma, showing promise for noninvasive clinical screening [133].

6.4 Different types of cancer detected using Raman spectroscopy and SERS

Although numerous types of cancer exist, this chapter specifically focuses on the application of Raman spectroscopy to five types of cancer which have been extensively discussed based on their publication frequency from 2000 to 2023. These five cancers are among the most prevalent cancers worldwide and affect a substantial number of individuals.

6.4.1 Breast cancer

Breast cancer is the most common cancer worldwide, causing 585 000 deaths and 2.3 million new cases in 2022 [134]. Current diagnostic and treatment methods, such as mammography, lumpectomy, and radiation therapy, are often painful and invasive [135]; hence, developing noninvasive, cost-effective, and pain-free diagnostic techniques is crucial. In a study on breast cancer, patients were monitored during various chemotherapy stages and their blood serum was analyzed using Raman spectroscopy combined with PCA. This approach identified glutathione as a potential biomarker for breast cancer, suggesting a minimally invasive diagnostic method [136]. SERS technology guided real-time tumor removal in mouse mammary tumor virus promoter (MMTV)-polyoma virus middle T (PyMT) mice expressing the PyMT antigen (figure 6.7(A)). Liposomal hyaluronan (HA)-SERS-nanoparticles were applied to tumors, incubated for 15 min, and washed. A 1:1 mixture of liposome-S440 SERS-PEG and liposome-S421 SERS-HA improved specificity despite initial non-specific nanoparticle retention with S440. The S421/S440 intensity ratio accurately identified tumor locations, with higher ratios indicating HA binding to CD44 in tumors. Post-surgery, Raman and ratiometric Raman (S421/S440) imaging (figure 6.7(B)) confirmed complete tumor eradication, supported by

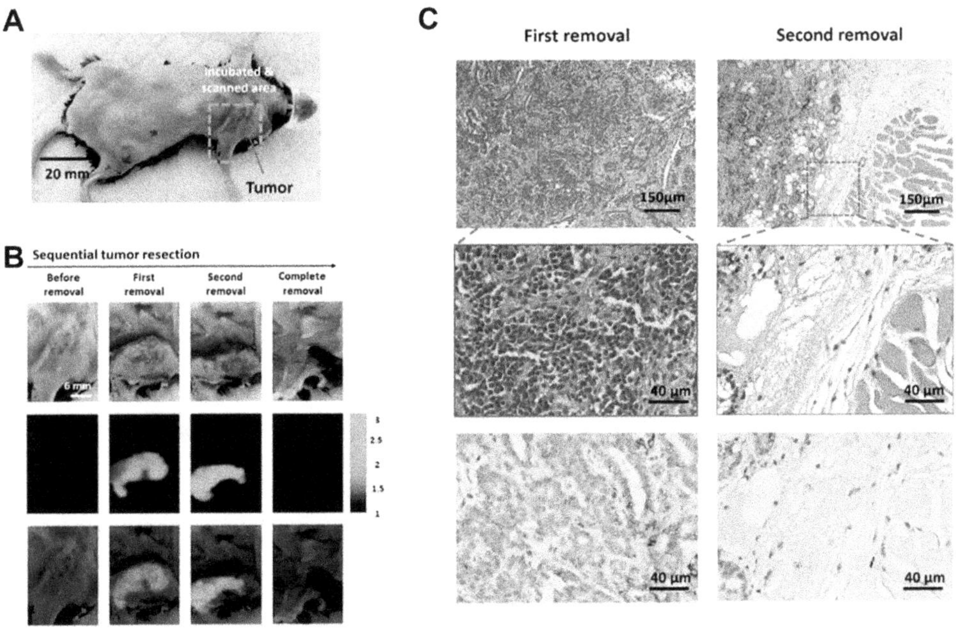

Figure 6.7. Raman-guided surgery using liposome-S421 SERS-HA and liposome-S440 SERS-PEG: (A) Pre-surgery photograph of the tumor-bearing mouse, (B) Sequential tumor resection: Photographs of the tumor area, ratiometric Raman (S421/S440) images, and overlaid ratiometric images with pre- and post-surgery tumor photographs, and (C) H&E and IHC images of resected tumors: H&E images (10*X* and 40*X* magnification) and CD44 IHC images (40*X* magnification). Reproduced with permission from [137] CC BY 4.0.

histopathological and immunohistochemical analyses including hematoxylin & eosin (H&E) staining (figure 6.7(C)) [137].

Murali *et al* developed Raman label-SERS-nanotags with monoclonal antibodies for simultaneous detection of breast tissue biomarkers human epidermal growth factor receptor2 (HER2), progesterone receptor (PR), and estrogen receptor (ER). The SERS analysis identified distinct peaks at 580, 1084, and 440 cm^{-1}, validating their presence. The method accurately distinguished receptor-positive and-negative areas in images, demonstrating its potential for comprehensive biomarker detection in single samples [138]. Researchers achieved successful detection of breast cancer using noninvasive samples such as urine in which urine samples were mixed with Au colloids and SERS spectra were measured, revealing specific and subtle changes in biomolecules present in cancerous urine samples [139].

6.4.2 Lung cancer

Lung cancer is among the most prevalent and deadly malignant tumors globally, and poses a severe threat to human health. Standard diagnostic techniques, such as physical examinations, biopsies, and imaging, are invasive and time-consuming, highlighting the need for early diagnosis methods to increase the survival rate of cancer patients [140, 141]. Addressing this need, Yuan *et al* devised a microfluidic technique with Au core-Ag shell nanoparticles to directly detect extracellular vesicles (EVs) in plasma. In this method, plasma samples are applied to a nanomixing device, allowing for the specific capture and labeling of EVs associated with lung cancer. Through SERS, this assay enables the multiplex detection of the canonical EV marker CD63, as well as the lung cancer-associated markers long pentraxin-3 and thrombospondin-1 [142]. Researchers have used SERS to distinguish lung cancer cell-derived exosomes from healthy ones in blood serum at the individual vesicle level. Figure 6.8(A) outlines the synthesis and surface modification of a porous gold SERS chip formed by the self-assembly of gold nanoparticles into a three-dimensional pore structure. The chip was functionalized with 11-

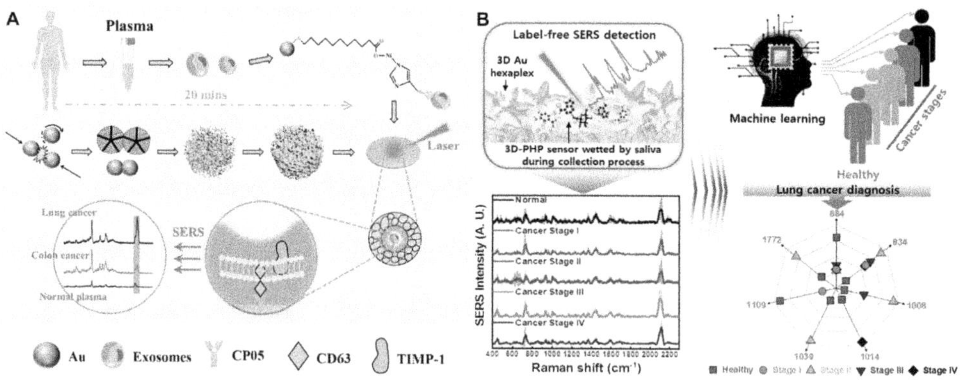

Figure 6.8. (A) Diagrammatic representation of the discovery of EV characteristics related to lung cancer for lung cancer screening. Reproduced from [143] CC BY 4.0. (B) Schematic illustration of the 3D-PHP sensor for the detection of human saliva and diagnosis of lung cancer. Reproduced from [145] CC BY 4.0.

mercaptoundecanoic acid-Ni^{2+}-His-CP05 polypeptide for specific exosome capture, targeting cancer-derived exosomes via high CD63 affinity [143]. In pleural fluid samples for lung cancer detection, SERS measurements on isolated cells dropped onto an Ag-coated silicon nanopillar SERS substrate achieved 85% accuracy in classification using partial least squares-discriminant analysis (PLS-DA), with an area under the curve value of 0.93, 87% sensitivity, and 83% specificity [144].

Noninvasive saliva samples were employed for quick on-site diagnosis of lung cancer using three-dimensional plasmonic hexaplex nanostructures coated on a paper substrate (3D-PHP). Metabolite compounds such as tyrosine, cadaverine, phenylalanine, hippuric acid, and tryptophan are found in higher concentrations in patients with advanced stages of the disease compared to those with benign conditions when the disease reaches its later stages (III and IV), as shown in figure 6.8(B) [145]. The SERS method was applied to identify lung cancer in urine samples, using adenosine as a biomarker, where magnetically assisted Fe_3O_4/Au/Ag nanocomposites and the azo coupling reaction enabled rapid and selective detection of trace levels of adenosine while simultaneously eliminating urea interference [146]. Zhang *et al* made use of dendritic Ag nanocrystals pre-grafted with the Raman-active probe molecule p-amino thiophenol (4-ATP) to sensitively capture and detect gaseous aldehyde molecules which serve as biomarkers for lung cancer at parts per billion levels through nucleophilic addition reaction [147].

6.4.3 Colorectal cancer

Colorectal cancer (CRC), a cancer of the colon or rectum, is one of the most widespread forms of cancer worldwide. In the early stages, many individuals may not exhibit any symptoms as the condition progresses [148]. SERS experiments were conducted on normal and cancerous human colon tissues to analyze epithelial layers using Ag colloids to enhance SERS signals in solid tumors or within cells. The resulting SERS spectra from colon cancer tissues displayed tissue heterogeneity, with predominant bands at 1138, 1269, 1452, 1495, 1572, and 2934 cm^{-1} [149]. Serum samples from CRC patients were used to identify protein biomarkers (hnRNP A1 and S100P) using a novel lab-on-chip (LoC-SERS) technology that makes use of an aptamer-functionalized Au nanocrown array, as shown in figure 6.9. Between CRC patients and healthy individuals, there were notable variations in the spectral peaks at 1176 cm^{-1} (S100P) and 1367 cm^{-1} (hnRNP A1). The LOD for S100P and hnRNP A1 was found to be 0.057 pg ml^{-1} and 0.031 pg ml^{-1}, respectively, falling between 10^{-6} and 10^{-12} g ml^{-1} [150]. A very sensitive label-free method of detecting the CRC protein marker NDKA was developed by employing Cr^{3+} ions to aggregate Au@Ag nanoparticles (ICNPs) and for the first time, concentration-dependent SERS spectra were observed. By taking advantage of the aggregating interaction between Au@Ag ICNPs and the SERS substrates of the protein analyte, this approach shows great promise for accurate and sensitive detection of CRC protein markers [151].

A recent research initiative focused on overcoming the challenge of identifying gaseous compounds using SERS by implementing a plasmonic metal-organic

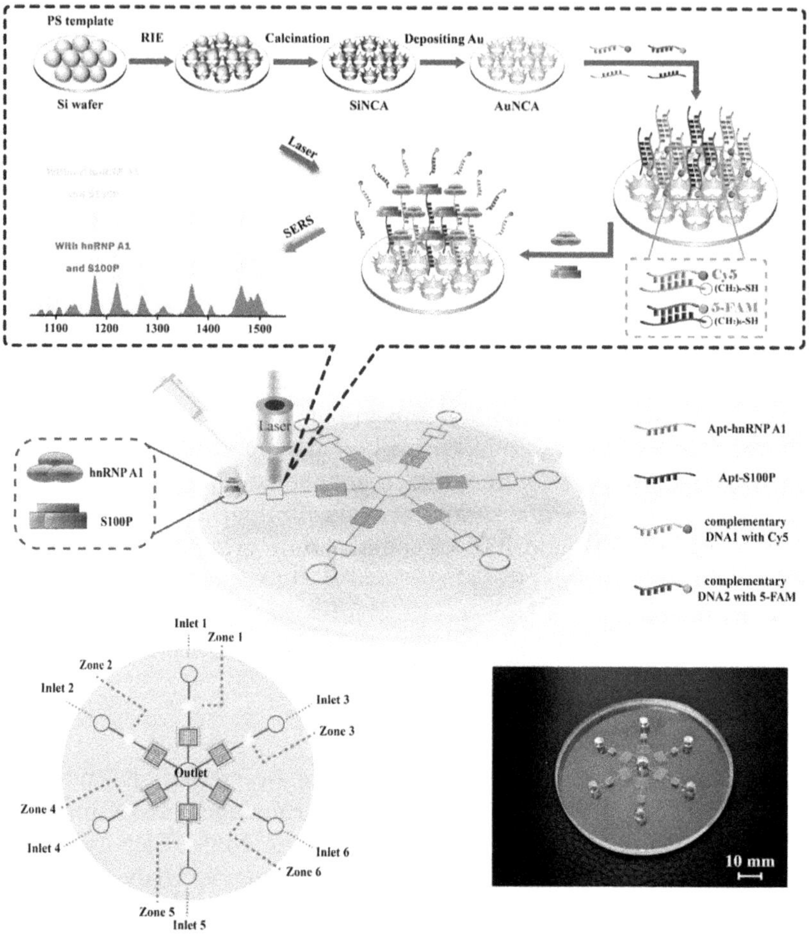

Figure 6.9. Diagram showing the picture, functional information, and LoC-SERS platform for multiplex biomarker detection. Reproduced from [150], copyright 2023, with permission from Elsevier B.V.

framework (MOF) film on flexible paper. This innovative MOF film, equipped with micro-nanopores, effectively captured simulated gaseous molecules to facilitate precise SERS spectral analysis [152]. Circulating miRNAs are promising CRC biomarkers for early diagnosis. An inverse molecular sentinel probe using a plasmonic bimetallic nanostar biosensing platform was developed to enhance the SERS detection capabilities. The probe achieved ultrasensitive detection with LOD values of 6.8 and 16.7 zmol for two targeted miRNA sequences [153]. A study suggests piR-31 143 as a potential biomarker for CRC detection due to higher blood concentrations in patients compared to healthy controls. A novel photoelectrochemical biosensor using hybrid MoS_2@ReS_2/Ti_3C_2 and duplex-specific nuclease signal amplification significantly enhanced CRC biomarker detection sensitivity in human blood [154]. Fousková *et al* introduced a unique *in vivo* tissue diagnosis technique for colorectal cancer using Raman spectroscopy. Spectral analysis revealed significant increases in the diseased tissues. Multivariate analysis improved accuracy in distinguishing normal tissue, benign lesions, and cancerous tissue, promising faster endoscopic diagnostic procedures [155].

6.4.4 Prostate cancer

Globally, prostate cancer is the most common cancer in men, and because of the lack of effective treatments for advanced metastatic prostate cancer, early detection and intervention are essential [156]. In the first clinical trial using Raman spectroscopy, researchers conducted analyses of freshly extracted *ex vivo* biopsy cores from prostate cancer tissue. They employed PLS-DA and support vector machining models to classify Gleason patterns 3, 4, and 5 as cancerous prostate tissues and to distinguish between benign and malignant prostate tissues. This study indicated a potential decrease in β-carotene levels under malignant conditions [157]. As shown in figure 6.10(A), a particular type of immunostructure was introduced for ultralow-level prostate-specific antigen (PSA) detection. It was made of Ag nanoparticle/porous carbon (Ag NP/PorC) films as the immunosubstrate and Ag NCs as the immunoprobes. The measured PSA levels in patients were approximately 11.3 ng ml^{-1}, compared to 1.23 and 0.015 ng ml^{-1} for normal cases, respectively [158]. PSA is crucial for early prostate cancer detection and monitoring, and SERS-based aptasensors, utilizing polystyrene colloidal sphere shell@Ag shell arrays, are designed to detect PSA biomarkers in serum samples. This novel sensor achieves high selectivity, spectrum consistency, and sensitivity through PSA aptamers, patterned Ag substrates, and SERS of methylene blue [159].

Peng *et al* developed a SERS-lateral flow immunoassay (LFA) platform with internal standard calibration for prostate cancer biomarkers, showing improved repeatability (1.65-fold) and sensitivity (3.5-fold). Figure 6.10(B) illustrates the

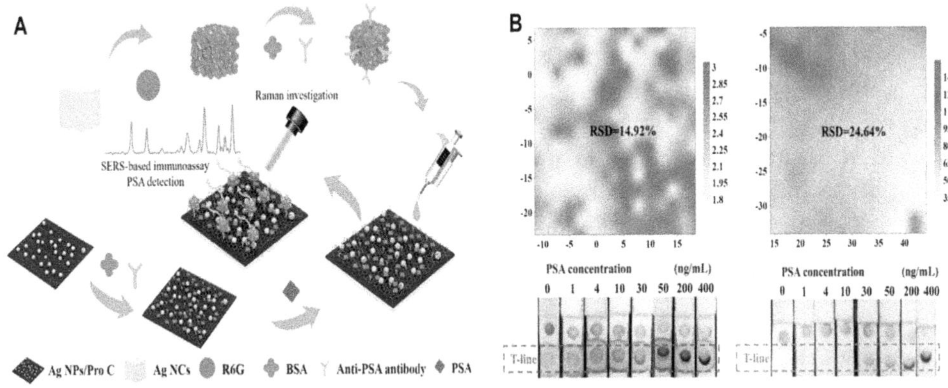

Figure 6.10. (A) Diagram of the Ag NC and Ag NP/PorC film-based SERS-type Immunoassay for ultrasensitive detection of antigen-specific to the prostate. Reproduced with permission from [158], copyright (2023) American Chemical Society. (B) Comparison of performance between the conventional SERS-LFA and self-calibrating SERS-LFA platforms includes Raman mapping based on the I_{1073}/I_{1312} ratio from the self-calibrating platform and I_{1073} from the conventional platform, along with combined optical images. Reproduced from [160], copyright 2023, with permission from Elsevier B.V. All rights reserved.

SERS spectrum mapping based on signal intensity ratios at 1073 and 1312 cm^{-1} for the self-calibrated platform compared to the conventional SERS-LFA at 1073 cm^{-1}. At a PSA concentration of 50 ng ml^{-1}, the relative standard deviations were 14.92% and 24.64%, respectively [160]. A SERS-based biosensor detects both total prostate-specific antigen (t-PSA) and free prostate-specific antigen (f-PSA). The immunocapture substrate used 4-MBA and t-PSA antibodies, which altered the Raman frequencies upon interaction. Specific capture of f-PSA employs MBA-modified SERS substrates with immunocolloidal Au-(f-PSA) antibodies. This method distinguishes prostate cancer patients by elevated t-PSA levels with less than 25% f-PSA in serum [161]. Ge *et al* employed silver nanoparticle substrates and deep learning algorithms to detect pancreatic cancer in blood plasma. Their PCA-multilayer perceptron algorithm achieved a classification accuracy exceeding 90%, outperforming PCA-LDA. This method holds potential for streamlining preprocessing stages in clinical applications [162].

6.4.5 Oral cancer

Oral cancer, which encompasses malignancies of the lip, various oral tissues, and the oropharynx, is the 13th most prevalent cancer globally. Treatment options such as surgery, radiation, chemotherapy, immunotherapy, and targeted therapy are available for managing oral cancers [163]. Despite advancements, the 30-year survival rate for oral squamous cell carcinoma remains below 50% [164]. However, early stage malignancies have a higher chance of successful treatment, highlighting the critical role of early detection and intervention in improving patient survival and reducing mortality [165, 166]. A promising biomarker for oral cancer diagnosis, S100 calcium-binding protein P (S100P) mRNA, was identified in a saliva-focused study. Gold nanoparticles were linked to oligonucleotides and malachite green isothiocyanate served as a Raman reporter molecule, SERS measurements of saliva samples from healthy groups (T1, T3, T21) and oral squamous cell carcinoma (OSCC) patients (M1, M5, M7) showed significantly higher levels of S100P mRNA in oral cancer patients (× Mann–Whitney test: $p < 0.05$), which were approximately three times higher than those in healthy controls [167]. Through SERS analysis of blood serum samples with Ag nanoparticles, researchers employed SERS to distinguish oral cancer patients from normal subjects. The intensities of some SERS peaks, such as phenylalanine and phospholipids, were higher in the oral cancer spectra than in the healthy spectra. Patients with oral cancer showed larger amounts of DNA and protein in their SERS mean spectra [168].

Opiorphin, identified in saliva as a potential biomarker for oral cancer, was analyzed using SERS after 3 kDa filtration and combined with plasmonic Ag nanoparticles. Filtering at 30 kDa preserved key peak ratios (720, 1000, 1250, and 1650 cm^{-1}), as illustrated in figure 6.11(A), enhancing the adsorption of small proteins onto Ag SERS nanopillars [169]. Esophageal cancer progression from Barrett's esophagus to adenocarcinoma cells was studied using single-cell Raman spectroscopy and microfluidic techniques. As shown in figure 6.11(B), Raman spectra from live single cells of cancerous (OE19), healthy (HET-1A), and Barrett's (CP-A to CP-D) lines were averaged over 100 cells and normalized to

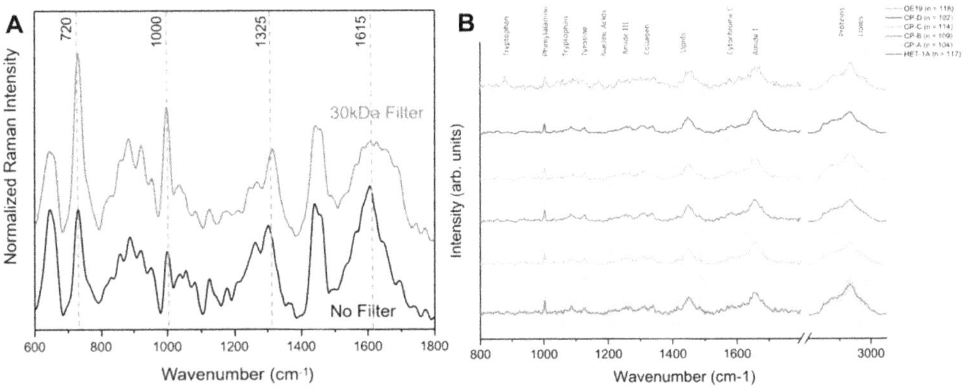

Figure 6.11. (A) Mean saliva SERS spectra pre-filtration (black) and post-filtration (red) utilizing a 30 kDa cut-off. Reproduced from [169] CC BY 4.0. (B) Single-cell Raman spectra showing the progression from healthy esophageal epithelia to esophageal adenocarcinoma, with key bands highlighted and spectra normalized to the Amide I band at 1656 cm^{-1}. Reproduced from [170] CC BY 4.0.

the Amide I peak at 1656 cm^{-1}. Increased aromatic amino acids were observed, with OE19 showing a tryptophan shoulder at 1009 cm^{-1}. The spectra mapped the transition from healthy squamous epithelia to cancer, revealing key spectral changes linked to abnormal membrane composition in cancer cells [170]. A novel study introduced SERS for diagnosing oral and oropharyngeal squamous cell carcinoma by analyzing salivary exosomes, achieving up to 79.3% sensitivity with PC-LDA analysis. SERS measurements showed preserved exosome integrity during dehydration, revealing distinct vibrational bands for thiocyanate, proteins, and nucleic acids in cancerous versus control groups [171]. Table 6.1 provides an overview of recent SERS-based strategies for cancer detection, outlining the relationship between cancer type, biomarker used, and the corresponding plasmonic substrate.

6.5 Future directions

Raman spectroscopy and SERS have become prominent tools in cancer analysis for detecting biomarkers. As highlighted in the previous sections, these techniques enable accurate differentiation between cancer patients and healthy individuals through noninvasive methods. However, challenges related to the sensitivity, repeatability, and reliability, particularly for low-concentration samples, limit their broad application. The following section explains these potential limitations and discusses future directions for improvement.

6.5.1 Development in nanostructures

The development of novel nanostructures and nanoparticles has significantly increased sensitivity and specificity, driving advances in SERS technology and greatly enhancing cancer diagnosis [118, 187, 188]. Progress in nanotechnology allows for the precise fabrication of nanostructures with controlled characteristics, which is essential for the effective application of SERS in biomedical analysis,

Table 6.1. Summary of SERS-based detection approaches for various cancer types, highlighting the sample type, cancer marker, marker type, SERS substrate, nanoparticle composition, laser source, and detection method.

S. No.	Cancer type	Sample type	Cancer marker	Markertype	SERS substrate	Nanoparticle	Laser source	Detection type	References
1	Liver cancer, colonic cancer, esophageal cancer, nasopharyngeal cancer, gastric cancer	Blood serum	—	Noninvasive	Planar	Ag colloid	785 nm	Direct	[172]
2	Nasopharyngeal cancer	Saliva	Protein	Noninvasive	Colloidal	Ag colloid	785 nm	Direct	[173]
3	Rectal cancer	Blood serum	—	Noninvasive	Colloidal	Ag colloid	632.8 nm	Direct	[174]
4	Oral squamous cell cancer	Saliva and desquamated oral cells	—	Noninvasive	Colloidal	Ag-coated silicon nanopillar	785 nm	Direct	[175]
5	Hepatocellular carcinoma	Blood serum	Alpha-fetoprotein	Noninvasive	Planar	Au@Ag nanorods	785 nm	Direct	[176]
6	Lung cancer	Exhaled breath	4-Ethylbenz aldehyde	Noninvasive	Planar	GSPs@ZIF-8	—	Direct	[177]
7	Gastric cancer	Saliva	Amino acids	Noninvasive	Planar	Graphene oxide nanoscrolls wrapped with gold nanoparticles	785 nm	Direct	[178]
8	Pancreatic cancer, ovarian cancer	Serum	Protein	Noninvasive	Planar	Au nanoshells	785 nm	Indirect	[179]
9	Renal cell carcinoma	Blood serum	Purinic metabolites	Noninvasive	Planar	Ag colloids	785 nm	Direct	[180]
10	Pancreatic cancer	Blood serum	CA19–9	Noninvasive	Planar	Ag nanogap shells	532 nm	Indirect	[181]
11	Bladder cancer in rat	Urine	EpCAM	Noninvasive	Planar	Au-coated ZnO	785 nm	Direct	[182]
12	Breast cancer	Blood serum	Protein	Noninvasive	Colloidal	Polyethylene glycol (PEG)-coated silver nanocubes	—	Direct	[183]
13	Oral cancer	Saliva	Protein, amino Acids and thiocyanate	Noninvasive	Planar	Au colloids	785 nm	Direct	[184]
14	Bladder cancer	Blood serum	—	Noninvasive	Planar	Ag colloids	785 nm	Direct	[185]
15	Cervical cancer	Blood serum	B7-H6	Noninvasive	Planar	Au colloids	785 nm	Direct	[186]

particularly in cancer diagnostics [187]. Various substrates, including nanorods [189], nanopyramids [190], nanoflowers [191, 192], nanotriangles [193], nanocages [194], nanocubes [195], etc, have been designed for cancer diagnostic applications. Beyond traditional nanostructures, Janus Au and Ag substrates [196], reduced graphene oxide [197], metal oxides [198], nanohybrid substrates [199], and DNA-assisted assembly of core-satellite nanostructures [200, 201] play crucial roles in achieving high and reproducible SERS effects for molecular detection and bio-marker attachment [199]. Additionally, advancements in heterogeneous mesoporous coatings and solvent-free techniques for producing SERS-active platforms further enhance the detection capabilities for trace molecules [201, 202].

Fe_3O_4-Au hybrid nanoparticles labeled with 4-ATP and anti-CEA antibodies (anti-CEA/4-ATP/Fe_3O_4-Au) serve as SERS tags, while anti-CEA-coated AuNPs (anti-CEA/Au) act as SERS substrates for detecting low-abundance CEA-positive cancer cells, such as A549 lung cancer cells. These structures generate SERS hot spots on cell surfaces, amplifying the 4-ATP signal for sensitive CEA detection, even at very low cell levels (<10 cells ml^{-1}) [204]. Figure 6.12(A) illustrates magnetic

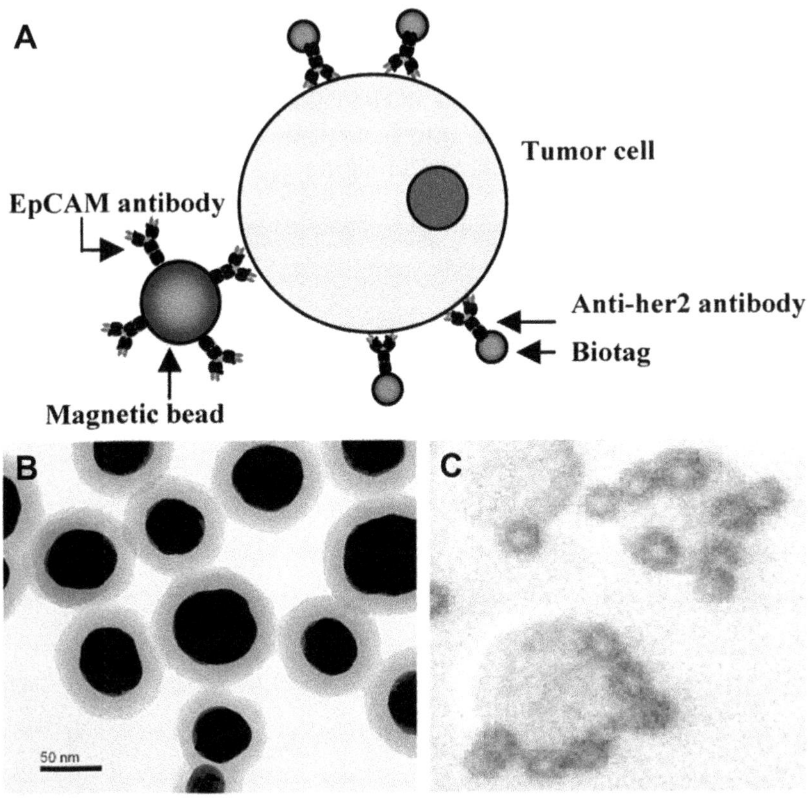

Figure 6.12. (A) Schematic illustration of the ternary immuno-complex formed by nanoplex biotags and magnetic bead conjugates binding to a model tumor cell, (B) TEM image of Nanoplex biotags, and (C) Small magnetic beads attached to SKBR3 cells. Reproduced with permission from [203], copyright (2008) American Chemical Society.

beads conjugated with anti-EpCAM antibodies and SERS tags linked to anti-HER2 antibodies to target tumor cells. These Nanoplex biotags, composed of magnetic beads with epithelial cell-specific antibodies and SERS tags with anti-HER2 antibodies, facilitated the direct detection and isolation of circulating tumor cells (CTCs) from whole human blood. Figure 6.12(B) displays a TEM image of the nanoplex biotags, while figure 6.12(C) shows small magnetic beads attached to SKBR3 cells [203]. Qian *et al* developed biocompatible PEGylated Au nanoparticles that showed significant optical enhancements for *in vivo* tumor detection, highlighting the potential for molecular imaging and targeted therapy. This research advances the creation of safe, effective gold nanoparticles for precise *in vivo* applications in therapy and imaging [94].

6.5.2 Development in Raman instruments

Recent advancements in Raman spectroscopy instrumentation have significantly improved cancer detection by integrating multiple spectroscopic techniques to enhance diagnostic accuracy, such as a multimodal optical cancer detection system combining diffuse reflectance, Raman, and intrinsic fluorescence spectroscopy [119, 205]. Innovations like stand-off [206] and transmission Raman spectroscopy [207] have further boosted sensitivity and expanded clinical applications, making Raman spectroscopy increasingly indispensable in clinical diagnostics and cancer treatment [205–211]. Optical fibers integrated into a medtronic brain biopsy device enable precise tissue measurement, as shown in figure 6.13 with angled tips for side

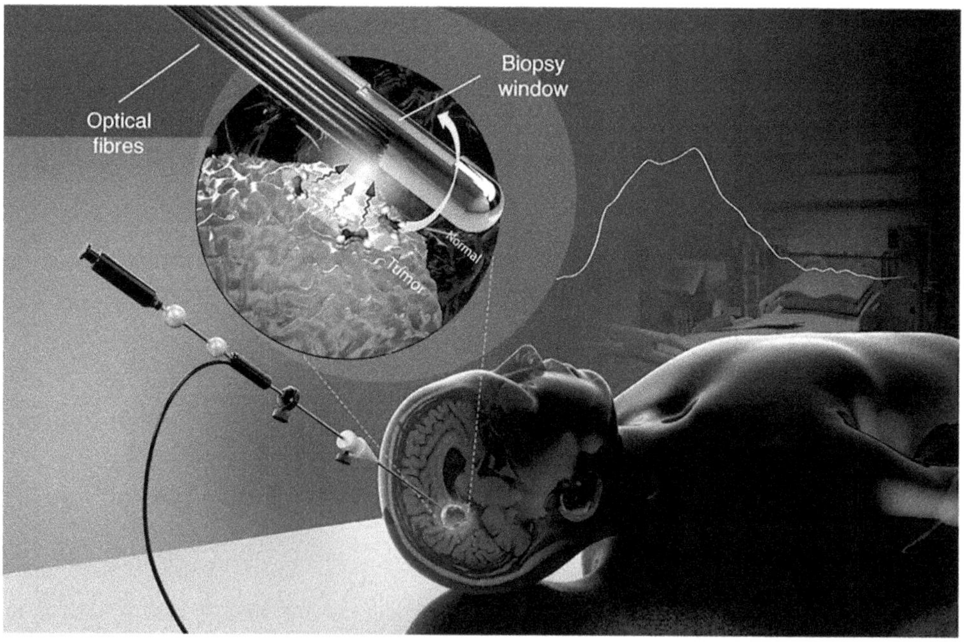

Figure 6.13. Diagram of an optical core needle biopsy displaying beveled fibers for detection and lighting and a magnified tip with a biopsy window. Reproduced from [212] CC BY 4.0.

illumination. This system demonstrated effective cancer detection in human and swine brain biopsy models using a 671 nm diode laser and spectrometer detection through the same fiber. Future research aims to refine statistical models for improved cancer detection reliability and compatibility with standard clinical procedures [212].

In vivo Raman spectroscopy with fiber-optic probes is challenging because of the strong background signals. A single unfiltered optical fiber configuration, using commercially available silica core-silica-clad fibers with a black nylon jacket, was used for high-wavenumber tissue characterization. *In vitro* tests on pig brain tissue confirmed the system's ability to reduce background signals and produce high-quality data efficiently [213]. The SpectroPen, a portable device, enhances real-time tumor detection during surgery using near-infrared light, improving fluorescence and Raman signal examination by eliminating silica Raman peaks and reducing excitation light [214]. *In vitro* and *ex vivo* experiments validated its detection limits and effectiveness in animal tissues, while *in vivo* tests on mice precisely identified tumors, improving surgical outcomes [214].

6.5.3 Integration of Raman spectroscopy with other analytical techniques

The potential to improve cancer biomarker detection and diagnostic precision through the integration of Raman equipment with other analytical techniques is promising [215, 216]. Combining SERS with mass spectroscopy or nuclear magnetic resonance, for instance, offers complementary data, enabling more accurate characterization of cancerous tissues and overcoming some limitations of SERS [217]. LoC-SERS, a pump-free microfluidic device, measures D-proline (D-Pro) and D-alanine (D-Ala) levels linked to gastric cancer using a D-amino acid (D-AA) oxidase-mediated cascade reaction. As illustrated in figure 6.14(A–C), it employs magnetic nanoparticles (MNPs) with boronic acid probes for quick and precise SERS nanolabeling of D-Pro and D-Ala in saliva. Polyethyleneimine and 3-mercaptophenylboronic acid were used to synthesize Fe_3O_4@Au MNPs (SAuMNPs) and SERS nanolabels for H_2O_2 detection, producing a new SERS peak at 882 cm^{-1}. The capillary pump design of the device, along with micro-channels treated to be hydrophilic, enabled automatic fluid flow and the mixing of saliva samples with SERS nanolabels in the reaction area [218].

A label-free SERS approach for lung cancer differentiation in blood utilizes machine learning with self-positioning on a hydrophobic-hydrophilic (DHH) platform. The DHH platform's molecular detection capabilities enhanced serum analysis, validated by liquid chromatography with tandem mass spectrometry (LC-MS) and nanosep [219]. Innovative hyphenated techniques combine targeted mass spectrometry and parallel reaction monitoring assays for ovarian cancer biomarker detection in serum with SERS spectra validated by LC-MS/MS analysis [220]. Integrating SERS with photothermal therapy, photodynamic therapy, or drug delivery systems extends its clinical utility for both diagnostics and treatment. These advancements promise improved cancer detection, early diagnosis, tailored treatments, and better patient outcomes [215, 216, 221].

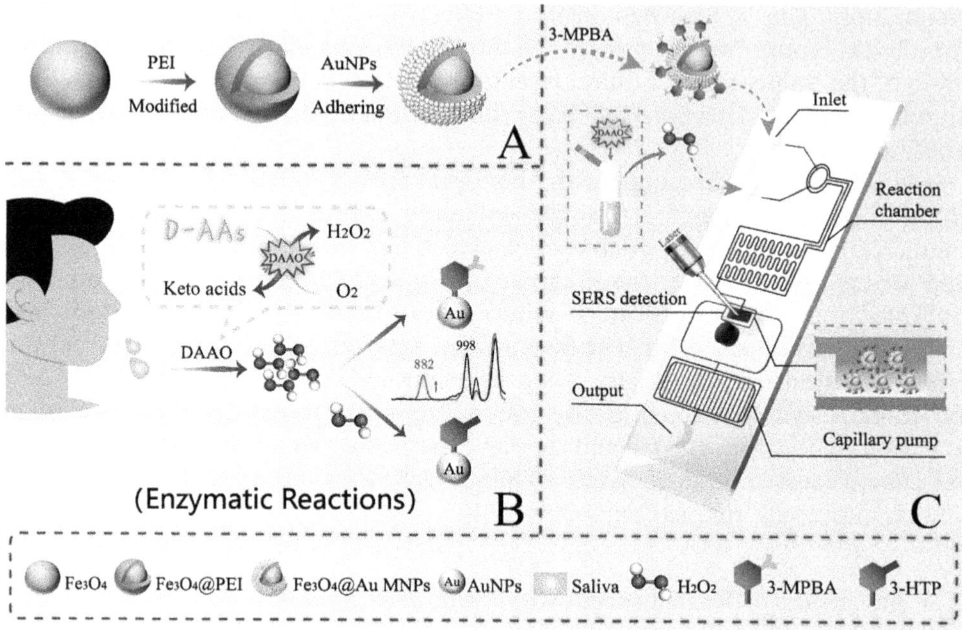

Figure 6.14. (A) Fe_3O_4@Au MNPs synthesis procedure, (B) schematic of the enzymatic reaction, and (C) LoC-SERS device detecting D-AAs in the saliva of gastric cancer patients. Reproduced from [218], copyright 2024, with permission from Elsevier B.V. All rights reserved.

6.5.4 SERS with artificial intelligence and machine learning

Combining Raman spectroscopy with AI and ML has revolutionized cancer detection by enhancing its precision and efficacy. AI and ML algorithms decode complex datasets, predict disease progression, and provide real-time decision-making support. Integrating Raman spectroscopy and SERS with AI and ML enables data fusion with other imaging modalities, thereby enhancing the diagnostic specificity. In recent studies on cervical tissues, CNN accurately classified seven tissue types with high accuracy using derivative models and pre-processed Raman data [222]. A label-free serum analysis platform (figure 6.15(A–D)) classified cervical cancer stages using binary weight robust PCA (BWRPCA), two-layer nearest neighbor (TLNN) model, and SERS. Ag-AuNRs on indium tin oxide glass with polydimethylsiloxane create a microarray chip for precise serum detection and SERS spectra. It achieved 91.2% classification accuracy with high diagnostic sensitivity and specificity [223].

AI and ML algorithms significantly enhance Raman spectroscopy-based cancer detection by improving sensitivity and specificity, ensuring reproducibility and reliability across laboratories [211]. Their ability to learn continuously from new data advances research and clinical applications in cancer detection and personalized medicine, potentially transforming diagnostics and patient care [224].

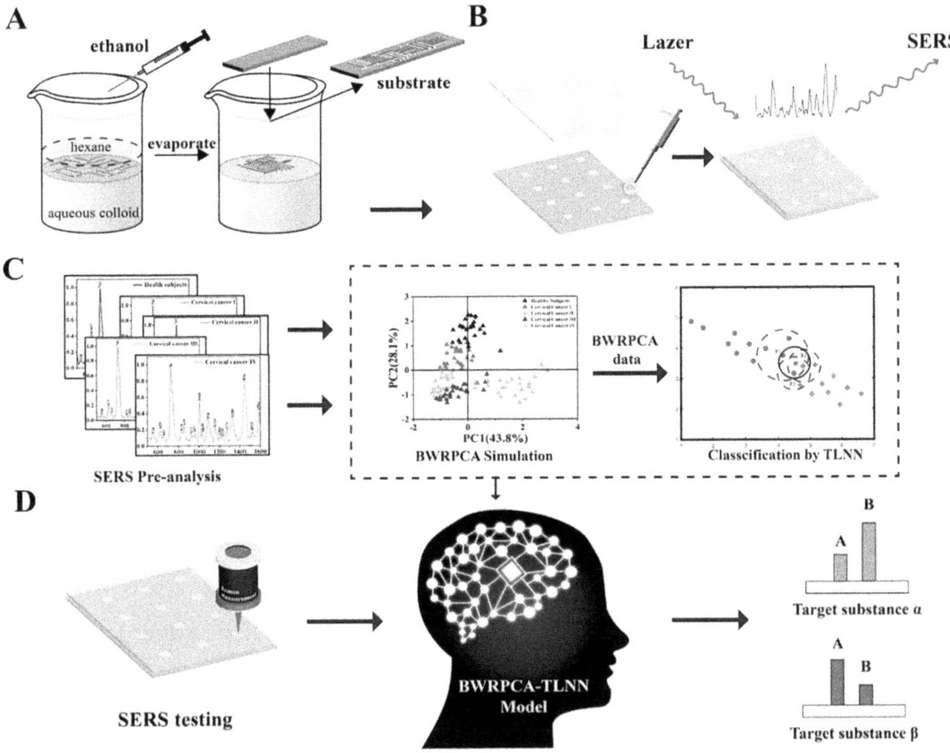

Figure 6.15. Diagram of the label-free SERS serum analysis platform for cervical cancer stages: (A) Ag-AuNR substrate synthesis, (B) microarray chip fabrication and SERS spectra measurement, (C) and (D) Serum SERS spectra analysis with the BWRPCA-TLNN model. Reproduced from [223], copyright 2023, with permission from Elsevier B.V. All rights reserved.

6.6 Conclusion

This chapter covers the fundamental principles of Raman spectroscopy and SERS as well as the development of Raman spectroscopy instruments and the introduction of related techniques such as TERS and SHINERS. We also elaborate on the various SERS substrates used for cancer analysis. Additionally, we discuss the common types of cancer and the diverse substrates and nanomaterials used in their detection methods, including M*X*enes and functionalized plasmonic nanomaterials. Furthermore, we addressed the current challenges in cancer diagnosis and proposed future directions to overcome these limitations. These include advancements in nanostructure design, instrument technology, and the integration of AI-ML techniques, which have the potential to enhance the sensitivity and specificity of Raman spectroscopy for analyzing cancer biomarkers and tissues.

Acknowledgments

The authors thank SRM University-AP, Andhra Pradesh for providing the SEED funding.

References

[1] Sung H *et al* 2021 Global cancer statistics 2020: GLOBOCAN estimates of incidence and mortality worldwide for 36 cancers in 185 countries *CA. Cancer J. Clin.* **71** 209–49

[2] Vázquez-Iglesias L *et al* 2024 SERS sensing for cancer biomarker: approaches and directions *Bioact. Mater.* **34** 248–68

[3] The Economic Times 2024 14.1 lakh new cancer cases, 9.1 lakh deaths in India: WHO *The Economic Times* 12–4

[4] Basu A K 2018 DNA damage, mutagenesis and cancer *Int. J. Mol. Sci.* **19** 1050

[5] Teschendorff A E 2024 On epigenetic stochasticity, entropy and cancer risk *Philos. Trans. R. Soc. B Biol. Sci.* **379** 20230054

[6] Stratton M R, Campbell P J and Futreal P A 2009 The cancer genome Michael *Nature* **458** 719–24

[7] Novikov N M, Zolotaryova S Y, Gautreau A M and Denisov E V 2021 Mutational drivers of cancer cell migration and invasion *Br. J. Cancer* **124** 102–14

[8] Öfverholm A, Karlsson P and Rosén A 2024 The experience of receiving a letter from a cancer genetics clinic about risk for hereditary cancer *Eur. J. Hum. Genet.* **32** 539–44

[9] White M C *et al* 2014 Age and cancer risk: a potentially modifiable relationship *Am. J. Prev. Med.* **46** S7–15

[10] Doll R, Peto R, Boreham J and Sutherland I 2005 Mortality from cancer in relation to smoking: 50 Years observations on British doctors *Br. J. Cancer* **92** 426–9

[11] Savoye I *et al* 2018 Patterns of ultraviolet radiation exposure and skin cancer risk: the E3N-SunExp Study *J. Epidemiol.* **28** 27–33

[12] Shimizu Y *et al* 2010 Radiation exposure and circulatory disease risk: Hiroshima and Nagasaki atomic bomb survivor data, 1950–2003 *Brit. Med. J.* **340** 193

[13] Moore P S and Chang Y 2010 Why do viruses cause cancer? Highlights of the first century of human tumour virology *Nat. Rev. Cancer* **10** 878–89

[14] Lipsett B 1979 Interaction of drugs, hormones, and nutrition in the causes of cancer *Cancer* **43** 1967–81

[15] Huxley R R *et al* 2009 The impact of dietary and lifestyle risk factors on risk of colorectal cancer: a quantitative overview of the epidemiological evidence *Int. J. Cancer* **125** 171–80

[16] Abnet C C 2007 Carcinogenic food contaminants *Cancer Invest* **25** 189–96

[17] Chequer F M D, Venâncio V P, Bianchi M L P and Antunes L M G 2012 Genotoxic and mutagenic effects of erythrosine B, a xanthene food dye, on HepG2 cells *Food Chem. Toxicol.* **50** 3447–51

[18] Leber A P 2001 Human exposures to monomers resulting from consumer contact with polymers *Chem. Biol. Interact.* **135–136** 215–20

[19] Cohen L and Jefferies A 2019 Environmental exposures and cancer: using the precautionary principle *Ecancermedicalscience* **600** 1–9

[20] Kaur B, Kumar S and Kaushik B K 2022 Recent advancements in optical biosensors for cancer detection *Biosens. Bioelectron.* **197** 113805

[21] Huang L *et al* 2020 Machine learning of serum metabolic patterns encodes early-stage lung adenocarcinoma *Nat. Commun.* **11** 3556

[22] Ott J J, Ullrich A and Miller A B 2009 The importance of early symptom recognition in the context of early detection and cancer survival *Eur. J. Cancer* **45** 2743–8

[23] Hassan A and Al Moaraj A M H A 2022 The role of Artificial Intelligence in entrepreneurship *Lect. Notes Netw. Syst.* **423 LNNS** 530–42

[24] Kiviat N B and Critchlow C W 2002 Novel approaches to identification of biomarkers for detection of early stage cancer *Dis. M.* **18** 73–81

[25] Marrugo-Ramírez J, Mir M and Samitier J 2018 Blood-based cancer biomarkers in liquid biopsy: a promising non-invasive alternative to tissue biopsy *Int. J. Mol. Sci.* **19** 1–21

[26] Levenson V V 2007 Biomarkers for early detection of breast cancer: what, when, and where? *Biochim. Biophys. Acta—Gen. Subj.* **1770** 847–56

[27] McGuire S 2016 World Cancer Report 2014. Geneva, Switzerland: World Health Organization, International Agency for Research on Cancer, WHO Press, 2015 *Adv. Nutr.* **7** 418–9

[28] Kösters J P and Gøtzsche P C 2003 Regular self-examination or clinical examination for early detection of breast cancer *Cochrane Database Syst. Rev.* **2010** CD003373

[29] Burd E M 2016 Human papillomavirus laboratory testing: the changing paradigm *Clin. Microbiol. Rev.* **29** 291–319

[30] Chen X *et al* 2020 Non-invasive early detection of cancer four years before conventional diagnosis using a blood test *Nat. Commun.* **11** 1–10

[31] Tajiri H *et al* 2002 Routine endoscopy using a magnifying endoscope for gastric cancer diagnosis *Endoscopy* **34** 772–7

[32] Grover S, Stoffel E M, Bussone L, Tschoegl E and Syngal S 2004 Physician assessment of family cancer history and referral for genetic evaluation in colorectal cancer patients *Clin. Gastroenterol. Hepatol.* **2** 813–9

[33] Walter F M *et al* 2015 Symptoms and other factors associated with time to diagnosis and stage of lung cancer: a prospective cohort study *Br. J. Cancer* **112** S6–S13

[34] Alsharif A M, Abdul Sani S F and Moradi F 2020 x-ray diffraction method to identify epithelial to mesenchymal transition in breast cancer tissue *IOP Conf. Ser.: Mater. Sci. Eng.* **785** 012044

[35] Siddiqui M M *et al* 2015 Comparison of MR/ultrasound fusion-guided biopsy with ultrasound-guided biopsy for the diagnosis of prostate cancer - *J. Am. Med. Assoc.* **313** 390–7

[36] Saslow D *et al* 2007 American cancer society guidelines for breast screening with MRI as an adjunct to mammography *Obstet. Gynecol. Surv.* **62** 458–60

[37] Mourtzakis M *et al* 2008 A practical and precise approach to quantification of body composition in cancer patients using computed tomography images acquired during routine care *Appl. Physiol. Nutr. Metab.* **33** 997–1006

[38] Staging P, Non O F, Cancer S L and Tomography W P 2000 Preoperative staging of non-small-cell lung cancer with positron-emission tomography *N. Engl. J. Med.* **343** 254–7

[39] Plowman E K *et al* 2014 Prostate cancer detection with magnetic resonance-ultrasound fusion biopsy: the role of systematic targeted biopsies *Laryngoscope* **122** 884–92

[40] Rodland K D 2004 Proteomics and cancer diagnosis: the potential of mass spectrometry *Clin. Biochem.* **37** 579–83

[41] Stone N, Kendall C, Smith J, Crow P and Barr H 2004 Raman spectroscopy for identification of epithelial cancers *Faraday Discuss.* **126** 141–57

[42] Gajjar K *et al* 2013 Fourier-transform infrared spectroscopy coupled with a classification machine for the analysis of blood plasma or serum: a novel diagnostic approach for ovarian cancer *Analyst* **138** 3917–26

[43] Pradhan A, Pandey P K and Singh P 2018 Overview of fluorescence spectroscopy and imaging for early cancer detection *Neurophotonics Biomed. Spectrosc.* **253** 328

[44] Chan E C Y *et al* 2009 Metabolic profiling of human colorectal cancer using high-resolution magic angle spinning nuclear magnetic resonance (HR-MAS NMR) spectroscopy and gas chromatography mass spectrometry (GC/MS) *J. Proteome Res.* **8** 352–61

[45] Smith C 1997 Colorectal cancer: radiologic diagnosis *Radiol. Clin. North Am.* **35** 439–56

[46] Yu D *et al* 2024 Comprehensive genomic profiling of small bowel adenocarcinoma by tissue and plasma biopsy *Genomics* **116** 110766

[47] Cainap C, Balacescu O, Cainap S S and Pop L A 2021 Next generation sequencing technology in lung cancer diagnosis *Biology (Basel)* **10** 1–15

[48] Li K *et al* 2024 Imaging and liquid biopsy for distinguishing true progression from pseudoprogression in gliomas, current advances and challenges *Acad. Radiol.* **31** 3366–83

[49] Sang R, Deng F, Engel A, Goldys E and Deng W 2022 Lipid-polymer nanocarrier platform enables x-ray induced photodynamic therapy against human colorectal cancer cells *Biomed. Pharmacother.* **155** 113837

[50] Salmerón-Ruiz A, Luengo Gómez D, Medina Benítez A and Láinez Ramos-Bossini A J 2024 Primary staging of rectal cancer on MRI: an updated pictorial review with focus on common pitfalls and current controversies *Eur. J. Radiol.* **175** 111417

[51] Dragsted J and Gammelgaard J 1983 Endoluminal ultrasonic scanning in the evaluation of rectal cancer: a preliminary report of 13 cases *Gastrointest. Radiol.* **8** 367–9

[52] Hamdy F C *et al* 2016 10-year outcomes after monitoring, surgery, or radiotherapy for localized prostate cancer *N. Engl. J. Med.* **375** 1415–24

[53] Avital I *et al* 2013 Evidence-based guidelines for precision risk stratification-based screening (PRSBS) for colorectal cancer: lessons learned from the us armed forces: consensus and future directions *J. Cancer* **4** 172–92

[54] Sloan-Dennison S, Laing S, Graham D and Faulds K 2021 From Raman to SESORRS: moving deeper into cancer detection and treatment monitoring *Chem. Commun.* **57** 12436–51

[55] De Oliveira Nunes L, Martin A A, Silveira L and Zampieri M 2003 FT-Raman spectroscopy study for skin cancer diagnosis *Spectroscopy* **17** 597–602

[56] Brozek-Pluska B *et al* 2012 Raman spectroscopy and imaging: applications in human breast cancer diagnosis *Analyst* **137** 3773–80

[57] Faur C I *et al* 2022 Raman spectroscopy in oral cavity and oropharyngeal cancer: a systematic review *Int. J. Oral Maxillofac. Surg.* **51** 1373–81

[58] Tahir M A, Dina N E, Cheng H, Valev V K and Zhang L 2021 Surface-enhanced Raman spectroscopy for bioanalysis and diagnosis *Nanoscale* **13** 11593–634

[59] Ravanshad R *et al* 2018 Application of nanoparticles in cancer detection by Raman scattering based techniques *Nano Rev. Exp.* **9** 1373551

[60] Wang Z *et al* 2024 Research progress in tumor diagnosis based on Raman spectroscopy *Curr. Med. Imaging Former. Curr. Med. Imaging Rev.* **20** 1–9

[61] Fenn M B *et al* 2011 Raman spectroscopy for clinical oncology *Adv. Opt. Technol.* **2011** 213783

[62] Raman C V 1923 The scattering of light by liquid and solid surfaces *Nature* **112** 281–2

[63] Hendra P J, Turner I D M, Loader E J and Stacey M 1974 The laser Raman spectra of species adsorbed on oxide surfaces. II *J. Phys. Chem.* **78** 300–4

[64] Mazaheri Tehrani A, Mohaghegh F and Materny A 2021 Coherent anti-stokes Raman scattering: basics, theoretical background, and applications *Prog. Opt. Sci. Photonics* **13** 235–54

[65] John N and George S 2017 Raman spectroscopy *Spectrosc. Methods Nanomater. Charact* **2** 95–127
[66] Fleischmann M, Hendra P J and Mcquillan A J 1974 Raman spectra of pyridine adsorbed at a silver electrode *Chem. Phys. Lett.* **26** 163–6
[67] Jeanmaire D L and van Duyne R P 1977 Surface Raman spectroelectrochemistry Part 1. Heterocyclic *J. Electroanal. Chem.* **84** 1
[68] Albrecht M G and Creighton J A 1977 Anomalously intense Raman spectra of pyridine at a silver electrode *J. Am. Chem. Soc.* **99** 5215–7
[69] Moskovits M 1978 Surface roughness and the enhanced intensity of Raman scattering by molecules adsorbed on metals *J. Chem. Phys.* **69** 4159–61
[70] Creighton J A, Blatchford C G and Albrecht M G 1979 Plasma resonance enhancement of Raman scattering by pyridine adsorbed on silver or gold sol particles of size comparable to the excitation wavelength *J. Chem. Soc. Faraday Trans. 2 Mol. Chem. Phys.* **75** 790–8
[71] Campion A, Kambhampati P, Campion A and Harris C 1998 Surface-enhanced Raman scattering *Chem. Soc. Rev.* **27** 241–50
[72] Etchegoin P G and Ru E C L 2011 Basic electromagnetic theory of SERS *Surface Enhanced Raman Spectroscopy: Analytical, Biophysical and Life Science Applications***1** ed S Schlucker (Wiley) p 37
[73] Ding S Y, You E M, Tian Z Q and Moskovits M 2017 Electromagnetic theories of surface-enhanced Raman spectroscopy *Chem. Soc. Rev.* **46** 4042–76
[74] Holze R R and Aroca 2006 Surface-enhanced vibrational spectroscopy *J. Solid State Electrochem.* **11** 335–6
[75] Xu H, Aizpurua J, Käll M and Apell P 2000 Electromagnetic contributions to single-molecule sensitivity in surface-enhanced Raman scattering *Phys. Rev. E-Stat. Physics, Plasmas, Fluids, Relat. Interdiscip. Top.* **62** 4318–24
[76] Le Ru E C and Etchegoin P G 2008 *Principles of Surface-Enhanced Raman Spectroscopy: and Related Plasmonic Effects* (Elsevier)
[77] Lombardi J R and Birke R L 2009 A unified view of surface-enhanced Raman scattering *Acc. Chem. Res.* **42** 734–42
[78] Otto A 2005 The 'chemical' (electronic) contribution to surface-enhanced Raman scattering *J. Raman Spectrosc.* **36** 497–509
[79] Otto A 2017 Charge transfer in first layer enhanced Raman scattering and surface resistance *Q. Phys. Rev.* **3** 1-14
[80] Haynes C L, Mcfarland A D and Van Duyne R P 2005 Raman spectroscopy *Anal. Chem.* **77** 338A–46A
[81] Rieder K H, Nie S and Emory S R 1994 Probing single molecules and single nanoparticles by surface-enhanced Raman scattering *Angew. Chem. Int. Ed. Engl.* **50** 1828
[82] Kneipp K *et al* 1997 Single molecule detection using surface-enhanced Raman scattering (SERS) *Phys. Rev. Lett.* **78** 1666–70
[83] Peng F *et al* 2014 Silicon nanomaterials platform for bioimaging, biosensing, and cancer therapy *Acc. Chem. Res.* **47** 612–23
[84] Liu T, Yang K and Liu Z 2020 Recent advances in functional nanomaterials for x-ray triggered cancer therapy *Prog. Nat. Sci. Mater. Int.* **30** 567–76
[85] Homola J 2008 Surface plasmon resonance sensors for detection of chemical and biological species *Chem. Rev.* **108** 462–93

[86] Dana A, Andreasen J, GrandahlHansen P, Kristensen L S, Nielsen K P and Skriver L 1985 Plasminogen activators, tissue degradation, and cancer *Adv. Cancer Res.* **44** 139–266

[87] Cao Y W C, Jin R and Mirkin C A 2002 Nanoparticles with Raman spectroscopic fingerprints for DNA and RNA detection *Science* **297** 1536–40

[88] Zong C *et al* 2018 Surface-enhanced Raman spectroscopy for bioanalysis: reliability and challenges *Chem. Rev.* **118** 4946–80

[89] Han X X, Zhao B and Ozaki Y 2009 Surface-enhanced Raman scattering for protein detection *Anal. Bioanal. Chem.* **394** 1719–27

[90] Bell S E J and Sirimuthu N M S 2006 Surface-enhanced Raman spectroscopy (SERS) for sub-micromolar detection of DNA/RNA mononucleotides *J. Am. Chem. Soc.* **128** 15580–1

[91] Bantz K C *et al* 2011 Recent progress in SERS biosensing *Phys. Chem. Chem. Phys.* **13** 11551–67

[92] Liu L, Tang Y, Dai S, Kleitz F and Qiao S Z 2016 Smart surface-enhanced Raman scattering traceable drug delivery systems *Nanoscale* **8** 12803–11

[93] Premasiri W R *et al* 2005 Characterization of the surface enhanced Raman scattering (SERS) of bacteria *J. Phys. Chem.* B **109** 312–20

[94] Qian X *et al* 2008 *In vivo* tumor targeting and spectroscopic detection with surface-enhanced Raman nanoparticle tags *Nat. Biotechnol.* **26** 83–90

[95] Antoine D *et al* 2022 Rapid, point-of-care scFv-SERS assay for femtogram level detection of SARS-CoV-2 *ACS Sens.* **7** 866–73

[96] Stuart D A, Haes A J, Yonzon C R, Hicks E M and Van Duyne R P 2005 Biological applications of localised surface plasmonic phenomenae *IEE Proc. Nanobiotechnol.* **152** 13–32

[97] Wang Y and Irudayaraj J 2013 Surface-enhanced Raman spectroscopy at single-molecule scale and its implications in biology *Philos. Trans. R. Soc. B Biol. Sci.* **368** 2012002

[98] Henzler-Wildman K and Kern D 2007 Dynamic personalities of proteins *Nature* **450** 964–72

[99] Jarvis R M and Goodacre R 2008 Characterisation and identification of bacteria using SERS *Chem. Soc. Rev.* **37** 931–6

[100] Hayazawa N *et al* 2000 Locally enhanced Raman spectroscopy with an atomic force microscope *Electrochemistry* **76** 942–9

[101] Anderson M S 2000 Locally enhanced Raman spectroscopy with an atomic force microscope *Appl. Phys. Lett.* **76** 3130–2

[102] Pettinger B, Picardi G, Schuster R and Ertl G 2000 Surface enhanced Raman spectroscopy: towards single molecule spectroscopy *Electrochem.* **68** 942–9

[103] Stockle R M, Suh Y D, Deckert V and Zenobi R 2000 Nanoscale chemical analysis by tip-enhanced Raman spectroscopy *Chem. Phys. Lett.* **318** 131–6

[104] Wessel J 1985 Surface-enhanced optical microscopy *J. Opt. Soc. Am.* B **2** 1538–41

[105] Wu D Y, Li J F, Ren B and Tian Z Q 2008 Electrochemical surface-enhanced Raman spectroscopy of nanostructures *Chem. Soc. Rev.* **37** 1025–41

[106] Pettinger B, Ren B, Picardi G, Schuster R and Ertl G 2004 Nanoscale probing of adsorbed species by tip-enhanced Raman spectroscopy *Phys. Rev. Lett.* **92** 096101

[107] Zhang R *et al* 2013 Chemical mapping of a single molecule by plasmon-enhanced Raman scattering *Nature* **498** 82–6

[108] Ding S, Zhang X, Ren B and Tian Z 2014 Surface-enhanced Raman spectroscopy (SERS): general introduction *Encyclopedia of Analytical Chemistry* (Wiley) pp 1–34

[109] Panneerselvam R *et al* 2017 Surface-enhanced Raman spectroscopy: Bottlenecks and future directions *Chem. Commun.* **54** 10–25

[110] Li J F *et al* 2010 Shell-isolated nanoparticle-enhanced Raman spectroscopy *Nature* **464** 392–5

[111] Costa M D D, Cançado L G and Jorio A 2021 Event chronology analysis of the historical development of tip-enhanced Raman spectroscopy *J. Raman Spectrosc.* **52** 587–99

[112] Pettinger B, Schambach P, Villagómez C J and Scott N 2012 Tip-enhanced raman spectroscopy: near-fields acting on a few molecules *Annu. Rev. Phys. Chem.* **63** 379–99

[113] Ding S-Y *et al* 2016 Nanostructure-based plasmon-enhanced Raman spectroscopy for surface analysis of materials *Nat. Rev. Mater.* **1** 16021

[114] Xiao L, Wang H and Schultz Z D 2016 Selective detection of RGD-integrin binding in cancer cells using tip enhanced raman scattering microscopy *Anal. Chem.* **88** 6547–53

[115] Lin Y C, Ke Z Y, Liao P H, Tseng C Y and Kong K V 2020 Reversible detection of phosphorylation and dephosphorylation by tip-enhanced Raman spectroscopy using a cyclopentadienyl ruthenium nanotag functionalized tip *Chem. Commun.* **56** 936–9

[116] Zheng C *et al* 2014 The use of Au@SiO_2 shell-isolated nanoparticle-enhanced Raman spectroscopy for human breast cancer detection *Anal. Bioanal. Chem.* **406** 5425–32

[117] Niciński K *et al* 2019 Detection of circulating tumor cells in blood by shell-isolated nanoparticle—enhanced Raman spectroscopy (SHINERS) in microfluidic device *Sci. Rep.* **9** 1–14

[118] Constantinou M, Hadjigeorgiou K and Abalde-Cela S 2022 Label-free sensing with metal nanostructure-based surface-enhanced Raman spectroscopy for cancer diagnosis *ACS Appl. Nano Mater.* **5** 12276–99

[119] Khondakar K R, Kalita P, Hickman N and Kaushik A K 2021 Raman spectroscopy/SERS based immunoassays for cancer diagnostics *Precise Diagnostics Toward Personalized Health Care* (Elsevier) pp 107–24

[120] Orendorff C J, Gole A, Sau T K and Murphy C J 2005 Surface-enhanced Raman spectroscopy of self-assembled monolayers: sandwich architecture and nanoparticle shape dependence *Anal. Chem.* **77** 3261–6

[121] Chen H Y, Lin M H, Wang C Y, Chang Y M and Gwo S 2015 Large-scale hot spot engineering for quantitative SERS at the single-molecule scale *J. Am. Chem. Soc.* **137** 13698–705

[122] Formo E V, Mahurin S M and Dai S 2010 Robust SERS substrates generated by coupling a bottom-up approach and atomic layer deposition *ACS Appl. Mater. Interfaces* **2** 1987–91

[123] Liu G L and Lee L P 2005 Nanowell surface enhanced Raman scattering arrays fabricated by soft-lithography for label-free biomolecular detections in integrated microfluidics *Appl. Phys. Lett.* **87** 074101

[124] Suresh V, Ding L, Chew A B and Yap F L 2018 Fabrication of large-area flexible SERS substrates by nanoimprint lithography *ACS Appl. Nano Mater.* **1** 886–93

[125] Liu T Y *et al* 2011 Functionalized arrays of Raman-enhancing nanoparticles for capture and culture-free analysis of bacteria in human blood *Nat. Commun.* **2** 538

[126] Shin H *et al* 2023 Single test-based diagnosis of multiple cancer types using Exosome-SERS-AI for early stage cancers *Nat. Commun.* **14** 1–10

[127] Jung H S *et al* 2021 Label-free SERS analysis of urine using a 3D-stacked AgNW-glass fiber filter sensor for the diagnosis of pancreatic cancer and prostate cancer *Anal. Chem.* **93** 3778–85

[128] Nguyen T M *et al* 2024 3D superclusters with hybrid bioinks for early detection in breast cancer *ACS Sens.* **9** 699–707
[129] Zhou Y *et al* 2023 $Ti_3C_2T_x$ MXene-facilitated non-selective trapping effect: efficient SERS detection of exosomal PD-L1 *Biosens. Bioelectron.* **237** 115493
[130] Feng S *et al* 2015 Surface-enhanced Raman spectroscopy of saliva proteins for the noninvasive differentiation of benign and malignant breast tumors *Int. J. Nanomedicine* **10** 537–47
[131] Feng S *et al* 2013 Blood plasma surface-enhanced Raman spectroscopy for non-invasive optical detection of cervical cancer *Analyst* **138** 3967–74
[132] Xie T *et al* 2023 Highly sensitive SERS detection of IL-6 in serum by Au@Fe_3O_4 nanoring-based sandwich immunoassay *Sens. Actuators B. Chem.* **375** 1–8
[133] Lin X *et al* 2017 Noninvasive detection of nasopharyngeal carcinoma based on saliva proteins using surface-enhanced Raman spectroscopy *J. Biomed. Opt.* **22** 1
[134] Printz C 2021 Female breast cancer most commonly diagnosed cancer globally *Cancer* **127** 1952–3
[135] Handy B 2009 The clinical utility of tumor markers *Lab. Med.* **40** 99–103
[136] Torre-Gutiérrez L G D *et al* 2022 Breast cancer chemotherapy treatment monitoring based on serum sample Raman spectroscopy *Lasers Med. Sci.* **37** 3649–59
[137] Liu K *et al* 2024 Robust synthesis of targeting glyco-nanoparticles for surface enhanced resonance Raman based imageguided tumor surgery *Small Sci.* **4** 200134
[138] Murali V P *et al* 2023 A clinically feasible diagnostic spectro-histology built on SERS-nanotags for multiplex detection and grading of breast cancer biomarkers *Biosens. Bioelectron.* **227** 115177
[139] Lin X *et al* 2020 Label-free liquid biopsy based on urine analysis using surface-enhanced Raman spectroscopy for noninvasive gastric and breast cancer detection *J. Raman Spectrosc.* **51** 2245–54
[140] Pastorino U *et al* 2019 Ten-year results of the Multicentric Italian Lung Detection trial demonstrate the safety and efficacy of biennial lung cancer screening *Eur. J. Cancer* **118** 142–8
[141] Lahiri A *et al* 2023 Lung cancer immunotherapy: progress, pitfalls, and promises *Mol. Cancer* **22** 1–37
[142] Yuan L *et al* 2023 Plasma extracellular vesicle phenotyping for the differentiation of early-stage lung cancer and benign lung diseases *Nanoscale Horiz.* **8** 746–58
[143] Lin C *et al* 2022 Localized plasmonic sensor for direct identifying lung and colon cancer from the blood *Biosens. Bioelectron.* **211** 114372
[144] Perumal J *et al* 2022 Machine learning assisted real-time label-free SERS diagnoses of malignant pleural effusion due to lung cancer *Biosensors* **12** 1–12
[145] Linh V T N *et al* 2024 3D plasmonic hexaplex paper sensor for label-free human saliva sensing and machine learning-assisted early-stage lung cancer screening *Biosens. Bioelectron.* **244** 115779
[146] Yang T *et al* 2014 Facile and label-free detection of lung cancer biomarker in urine by magnetically assisted surface-enhanced Raman scattering *ACS Appl. Mater. Interfaces* **6** 20985–93
[147] Zhang Z *et al* 2017 Ultrasensitive surface-enhanced Raman scattering sensor of gaseous aldehydes as biomarkers of lung cancer on dendritic Ag nanocrystals *Anal. Chem.* **89** 1416–20

[148] Paulus J 2020 Colorectal cancer colorectal cancer| 대장암 *Dbpia. Co. Kr* **66** 1–9
[149] Cîntă Pînzaru S, Andronie L M, Domsa I, Cozar O and Astilean S 2008 Bridging biomolecules with nanoparticles: surface-enhanced Raman scattering from colon carcinoma and normal tissue *J. Raman Spectrosc.* **39** 331–4
[150] Cao X *et al* 2024 LoC-SERS platform for rapid and sensitive detection of colorectal cancer protein biomarkers *Talanta* **270** 125563
[151] Yao M M *et al* 2022 Tuning the surface enhanced Raman spectroscopy performance of Au core-Ag shell nanostructure for label-free highly sensitive detection of colorectal cancer Marker *J. Alloys Compd.* **896** 163043
[152] Li M *et al* 2024 Deep learning enabled SERS identification of gaseous molecules on flexible plasmonic MOF nanowire films *ACS Sens.* **9** 979–87
[153] Canning A J *et al* 2023 miRNA probe integrated biosensor platform using bimetallic nanostars for amplification-free multiplexed detection of circulating colorectal cancer biomarkers in clinical samples *Biosens. Bioelectron.* **220** 114855
[154] Li J *et al* 2022 A duplex-specific nuclease assisted photoelectrochemical biosensor based on MoS_2@ReS_2/Ti_3C_2 hybrid for ultrasensitive detection of colorectal cancer-related piRNA-31,143 *Acta Biomater.* **149** 287–96
[155] Fousková M *et al* 2023 *In vivo* Raman spectroscopy in the diagnostics of colon cancer *Analyst* **148** 2518–26
[156] Carruba G 2007 Estrogen and prostate cancer: an eclipsed truth in an androgen-dominated scenario *J. Cell. Biochem.* **102** 899–911
[157] van Breugel S J *et al* 2023 Raman spectroscopy system for real-time diagnosis of clinically significant prostate cancer tissue *J. Biophotonics* **16** e202200334
[158] Wu K *et al* 2023 Ag NC and Ag NP/PorC film-based surface-enhanced raman spectroscopy-type immunoassay for ultrasensitive prostate-specific antigen detection *ACS Omega* **8** 18523–9
[159] Zhao J *et al* 2022 Detection of prostate cancer biomarkers via a SERS-based aptasensor *Biosens. Bioelectron.* **216** 114660
[160] Peng S *et al* 2024 Portable SERS-based lateral flow immunoassay strips with self-calibration for detection of a prostate cancer biomarker *Sens. Actuators B Chem.* **401** 135012
[161] Zhao J *et al* 2023 SERS-based biosensor for detection of f-PSA%: Implications for the diagnosis of prostate cancer *Talanta* **261** 124654
[162] Ge H *et al* 2024 Label-free SERS detection of prostate cancer based on multi-layer perceptron surrogate model method *Spectrochim. Acta-A Mol. Biomol. Spectrosc.* **304** 123407
[163] Chai A W Y, Lim K P and Cheong S C 2020 Translational genomics and recent advances in oral squamous cell carcinoma *Semin. Cancer Biol.* **61** 71–83
[164] Sasahira T and Kirita T 2018 Hallmarks of cancer-related newly prognostic factors of oral squamous cell carcinoma *Int. J. Mol. Sci.* **19** 2413
[165] Sciubba J J 2001 Oral cancer. The importance of early diagnosis and treatment *Am. J. Clin. Dermatol.* **2** 239–51
[166] Abati S, Bramati C, Bondi S, Lissoni A and Trimarchi M 2020 Oral cancer and precancer: a narrative review on the relevance of early diagnosis *Int. J. Environ. Res. Public Health* **17** 1–14
[167] Han S *et al* 2019 Nanoparticle-based assay for detection of S100P mRNA using surface-enhanced Raman spectroscopy *J. Biomed. Opt.* **24** 1

[168] Amber A, Nawaz H, Bhatti H N and Mushtaq Z 2023 Surface-enhanced Raman spectroscopy for the characterization of different anatomical subtypes of oral cavity cancer *Photodiagnosis Photodyn. Ther.* **42** 103607

[169] Farnesi E *et al* 2023 Label-free SERS and MD analysis of biomarkers for rapid point-of-care sensors detecting head and neck Cancer and infections *Sensors (Basel)* **23** 8915

[170] Farooq A, Wood C D, Ladbury J E and Evans S D 2024 On-chip Raman spectroscopy of live single cells for the staging of oesophageal adenocarcinoma progression *Sci. Rep.* **14** 1761

[171] Faur C I *et al* 2023 A new detection method of oral and oropharyngeal squamous cell carcinoma based on multivariat analysis of surface enhanced Raman spectra of salivary exosomes *J. Pers. Med.* **13** 762

[172] Li S X *et al* 2014 Potential of cancer screening with serum surface-enhanced Raman spectroscopy and a support vector machine *Laser Phys. Lett.* **11** 065603

[173] Feng S *et al* 2014 Saliva analysis combining membrane protein purification with surface-enhanced Raman spectroscopy for nasopharyngeal cancer detection *Appl. Phys. Lett.* **104** 073702

[174] Li X, Yang T, Li S, Zhang S and Jin L 2015 Discrimination of rectal cancer through human serum using surface-enhanced Raman spectroscopy *Appl. Phys. B Lasers Opt.* **119** 393–8

[175] Connolly J M *et al* 2016 Non-invasive and label-free detection of oral squamous cell carcinoma using saliva surface-enhanced Raman spectroscopy and multivariate analysis *Nanomed. Nanotechnol. Biol. Med.* **12** 1593–601

[176] Xiao R *et al* 2016 Non-invasive detection of hepatocellular carcinoma serum metabolic profile through surface-enhanced Raman spectroscopy *Nanomed. Nanotechnol. Biol. Med.* **12** 2475–84

[177] Qiao X *et al* 2018 Selective surface enhanced Raman scattering for quantitative detection of lung cancer biomarkers in superparticle@MOF structure *Adv. Mater.* **30** 1702275

[178] Chen Y *et al* 2018 Salivary analysis based on surface enhanced Raman scattering sensors distinguishes early and advanced gastric cancer patients from healthy persons *J. Biomed. Nanotechnol.* **14** 1773–84

[179] Banaei N *et al* 2019 Machine learning algorithms enhance the specificity of cancer biomarker detection using SERS-based immunoassays in microfluidic chips *RSC Adv.* **9** 1859–68

[180] Buhas B A *et al* 2023 High-accuracy renal cell carcinoma discrimination through label-free SERS of blood serum and multivariate analysis *Biosensors* **13** 813

[181] Hwang I J *et al* 2024 Confined growth of Ag nanogap shells emitting stable Raman label signals for SERS liquid biopsy of pancreatic cancer *Biosens. Bioelectron.* **248** 115948

[182] Lee S *et al* 2024 Early-stage diagnosis of bladder cancer using surface-enhanced Raman spectroscopy combined with machine learning algorithms in a rat model *Biosens. Bioelectron.* **246**

[183] Hajab H *et al* 2024 Surface-enhanced Raman spectroscopy of the filtrate portions of the blood serum samples of breast cancer patients obtained by using 30 kDa filtration device *Spectrochim. Acta-A Mol. Biomol. Spectrosc.* **311** 1–11

[184] Fălămaş A, Rotaru H and Hedeşiu M 2020 Surface-enhanced Raman spectroscopy (SERS) investigations of saliva for oral cancer diagnosis *Lasers Med. Sci.* **35** 1393–401

[185] Chen S *et al* 2019 Identifying non-muscle-invasive and muscle-invasive bladder cancer based on blood serum surface-enhanced Raman spectroscopy *Biomed. Opt. Express* **10** 3533

[186] Panikar S S *et al* 2020 Anti-fouling SERS-based immunosensor for point-of-care detection of the B7–H6 tumor biomarker in cervical cancer patient serum *Anal. Chim. Acta* **1138** 110–22

[187] Srajer J, Schwaighofer A and Nowak C 2013 Surface-enhanced Raman spectroscopy for biomedical diagnostics and imaging *Biomed. Spectrosc. Imaging* **2** 51–71

[188] Chakraborty A, Ghosh A and Barui A 2020 Advances in surface-enhanced Raman spectroscopy for cancer diagnosis and staging *J. Raman Spectrosc.* **51** 7–36

[189] Huang X, El-Sayed I H, Qian W and El-Sayed M A 2006 Cancer cell imaging and photothermal therapy in the near-infrared region by using gold nanorods *J. Am. Chem. Soc.* **128** 2115–20

[190] Feng J *et al* 2017 Bioconjugation of gold nanobipyramids for SERS detection and targeted photothermal therapy in breast cancer *ACS Biomater. Sci. Eng.* **3** 608–18

[191] Parimi D S, Kumar J, Panneerselvam R, T S and Suresh A K 2024 Sustainable golden nanoflowers grafted food-waste derived biotemplate for the direct SERS-detection of carcinogenic herbicides from agro-farms *Mater. Today Chem.* **36** 101985

[192] Li Q *et al* 2013 High surface-enhanced raman scattering performance of individual gold nanoflowers and their application in live cell imaging *Small* **9** 927–32

[193] Potara M *et al* 2017 Carboplatin-loaded, Raman-encoded, chitosan-coated silver nanotriangles as multimodal traceable nanotherapeutic delivery systems and pH reporters inside human ovarian cancer cells *ACS Appl. Mater. Interfaces* **9** 32565–76

[194] Hu F, Zhang Y, Chen G, Li C and Wang Q 2015 Double-walled Au nanocage/SiO_2 nanorattles: integrating SERS imaging, drug delivery and photothermal therapy *Small* **11** 985–93

[195] Panikkanvalappil S R, Hira S M, Mahmoud M A and El-Sayed M A 2014 Unraveling the biomolecular snapshots of mitosis in healthy and cancer cells using plasmonically-enhanced raman spectroscopy *J. Am. Chem. Soc.* **136** 15961–8

[196] Shao D *et al* 2016 Janus silver-mesoporous silica nanocarriers for SERS traceable and pH-sensitive drug delivery in cancer therapy *ACS Appl. Mater. Interfaces* **8** 4303–8

[197] Kim Y K *et al* 2015 One-pot synthesis of multifunctional Au@Graphene oxide nanocolloid core@shell nanoparticles for raman bioimaging, photothermal, and photodynamic therapy *Small* **11** 2527–35

[198] Zhang W, Wang Y, Sun X, Wang W and Chen L 2014 Mesoporous titania based yolk-shell nanoparticles as multifunctional theranostic platforms for SERS imaging and chemo-photothermal treatment *Nanoscale* **6** 14514–22

[199] Torres-Herrero B *et al* 2023 Remote activation of enzyme nanohybrids for cancer prodrug therapy controlled by magnetic heating *ACS Nano* **17** 12358–73

[200] Wu L A, Li W E and Chen Y F 2017 DNA-assisted assembly of plasmonic core-satellite nanostructures for surface-enhanced Raman spectroscopy (SERS) *IEEE 12th Int. Conf. Nano/Micro Eng. Mol. Syst. NEMS 2017* 2017 206–9

[201] Kuzminova A, Procházka M and Kylián O 2021 Gas-phase synthesis of mesoporous films of Ag/C:H:N:O core-satellite nanoparticles for surface-enhanced Raman spectroscopy *Mater. Lett.* **305** 130797

[202] Cho S H, Baek K M and Jung Y S 2020 Scalable nanofabrication of plasmonic nanostructures for trace-amount molecular sensing based on surface-enhanced raman spectroscopy (SERS) *Smart Sensors and Systems* (Springer) pp 71–92

[203] Sha M Y, Xu H, Natan M J and Cromer R 2008 Surface-enhanced Raman scattering tags for rapid and homogeneous detection of circulating tumor cells in the presence of human whole blood *J. Am. Chem. Soc.* **130** 17214–5

[204] Wu P and Cai C 2015 Synthesis of magnetic Fe3O4–Au hybrids for sensitive SERS detection of cancer cells at low abundance *J. Mater. Chem.* B **3** 4487–95

[205] Jermyn M *et al* 2017 Highly accurate detection of cancer *in situ* with intraoperative, label-free, multimodal optical spectroscopy *Cancer Res.* **77** 3942–50

[206] Hobro A J and Lendl B 2009 Stand-off Raman spectroscopy *TrAC-Trends Anal. Chem.* **28** 1235–42

[207] Sparén A and Svensson O 2016 Transmission Raman: methods and applications *Encyclopedia Spectroscopy and Spectrometry* (Academic) pp 469–74

[208] Orlando A *et al* 2021 A comprehensive review on Raman spectroscopy applications *Chemosensors* **9** 1–28

[209] Kerssens M M, Matousek P, Rogers K and Stone N 2010 Towards a safe non-invasive method for evaluating the carbonate substitution levels of hydroxyapatite (HAP) in micro-calcifications found in breast tissue *Analyst* **135** 3156–61

[210] Li H *et al* 2021 Raman microspectroscopic investigation and classification of breast cancer pathological characteristics *Molecules* **26** 921

[211] Eshraghi-Arani M and Dehghani-Bidgoli Z 2021 Raman spectroscopy-based breast cancer detection using self constructing neural networks *Iran. J. Med. Phys.* **18** 89–95

[212] Desroches J *et al* 2018 A new method using Raman spectroscopy for *in vivo* targeted brain cancer tissue biopsy *Sci. Rep.* **8** 1792

[213] Santos F, Wolthuis R, Koljenovic S, Almeida R M and Puppels G J 2005 Fiber-optic probes for *in vivo* Raman spectroscopy in the highwavenumber region *Anal. Chem.* **77** 6747–52

[214] Mohs A M *et al* 2010 Hand-held spectroscopic device for *in vivo* and intraoperative tumor detection : contrast enhancement, detection sensitivity, and tissue penetration *Anal. Chem.* **82** 9058–65

[215] Ren W and Irudayaraj J 2021 Surface-enhanced Raman spectroscopy for cancer characterization *Principles and Clinical Diagnostic Applications of Surface-Enhanced Raman Spectroscopy* (Elsevier) ch 10 pp 373–93

[216] Zhang Y, Zhao S, Zheng J and He L 2017 Surface-enhanced Raman spectroscopy (SERS) combined techniques for high-performance detection and characterization *TrAC-Trends Anal. Chem.* **90** 1–13

[217] Blanco-Formoso M and Alvarez-Puebla R A 2020 Cancer diagnosis through sers and other related techniques *Int. J. Mol. Sci.* **21** 2253

[218] Shen K *et al* 2024 A magnetically embedded pump-free LoC-SERS device based on enzyme-mediated cascade reaction for gastric cancer-related D-amino acids detection *Sens. Actuators B Chem.* **409** 135615

[219] Fan M *et al* 2024 LC-MS/MS-assisted label-free SERS blood analysis by self-position plasmonic platform for tumor screening *Chem. Eng. J.* **483** 149348

[220] Ryu J *et al* 2024 Quantification of putative ovarian cancer serum protein biomarkers using a multiplexed targeted mass spectrometry assay *Clin. Proteomics* **21** 1–20

[221] Wu L, Dias A and Diéguez L 2022 Surface enhanced Raman spectroscopy for tumor nucleic acid: towards cancer diagnosis and precision medicine *Biosens. Bioelectron.* **204** 114075

[222] Kang Z *et al* 2023 Early screening of cervical cancer based on tissue Raman spectroscopy combined with deep learning algorithms *Photodiagnosis Photodyn. Ther.* **42** 103557
[223] Cao D *et al* 2023 Diagnosis and staging of cervical cancer using label-free surface-enhanced Raman spectroscopy and BWRPCA-TLNN model *Vib. Spectrosc.* **128** 103587
[224] Cheng N *et al* 2024 Serum analysis based on SERS combined with 2D convolutional neural network and Gramian angular field for breast cancer screening *Spectrochim. Acta A Mol. Biomol. Spectrosc.* **312** 124054

Chapter 7

Optical biopsy and chemometrics for skin cancer diagnostics

Yulia A Khristoforova, Ivan A Bratchenko, Lyudmila A Bratchenko, Irina A Matveeva, Alexandr A Moryatov, Sergey V Kozlov, Oleg I Kaganov, Andrey E Orlov and Valery P Zakharov

7.1 Introduction

Skin cancer is one of the most common type of cancers with an increasing prevalence worldwide. Melanoma is much less common type but it responsible for the most deaths of all skin cancers. GLOBOCAN estimated 325 000 persons diagnosed as having melanoma, and approximately 57 000 persons died of the disease in 2020 [1]. The data published in by Arnold *et al* [2] estimated the global burden from melanoma to increase to 510 000 new cases and 96 000 deaths by 2040. Moreover, although the risk of melanoma generally increases with age, melanoma is becoming more common among younger adults [2]. Early detection of any tumor and adequate therapy and/or surgery is the best strategy in successful patient treatment.

For many years, classification of skin tumors started from a naked eye examination and was complemented with dermoscopic investigation of suspicious tissues [3]. However, deep and precise analysis of tumor morphology and other important clinical features could only be analyzed by a qualified specialist with extensive experience in tumors classification [4]. Today, 'optical biopsy' [5] is one of several promising methods being utilized to detect tumors based on their spectral features caused by the comparative presence of different chemical components. Various optical modalities including terahertz spectroscopy [6], ultraviolet and visible fluorescence spectroscopy [7], Raman spectroscopy (RS) [8, 9], diffuse reflectance spectroscopy [10] demonstrated a possibility to diagnose cancer, including rare tumors and tumors with atypical clinical features [11, 12]. In recent years, RS has been increasingly used to investigate biological tissues and fluids for diagnostic tasks, particularly for skin cancer detection.

doi:10.1088/978-0-7503-5949-8ch7

RS is a well-known spectroscopic technique based on inelastic scattering of light when interacting with molecular bonds of tissues' chemical elements. RS spectrum of a tissue is a superposition of the signals caused by the contribution of the active molecules of the components presented in the tissue. The intensity of the RS peaks for a particular molecule is directly proportional to the concentration of that molecule within a tissue. Therefore, a Raman spectrum is an intrinsic molecular fingerprint of the sample, revealing detailed information about DNA, protein, and lipid content as well as macromolecular conformations, which can be extracted from the measured spectra, which makes RS an outstanding approach for precise detection of malignant and benign tissues [13]. It is important to note that, in addition to the Raman shift, the scattered light contains an audio frequency (AF) signal received after interaction with the tissues. The spectral properties of the AF signal depend on the presence of endogenous or native fluorophores in the tissues [14]. Therefore, combined analysis of RS and AF spectral features can improve optical diagnostic performance due to expansion of spectral markers characterization of biochemical changes during tumor growth.

The use of chemometrics methods has become widespread for Raman data analysis, which has been clearly reflected in a large number of manuscripts in the last few years [15, 16]. The combination of RS and the chemometrics methods provides an opportunity to build statistical models for recognizing concentrations or group information on specimens using their spectral features. Numerous research papers demonstrate analysis of Raman data using principal component analysis (PCA) [17], projection on the latent structures (PLS) [8, 18, 19], hierarchical cluster analysis (HCA) [20], support vector machine (SVM) [21], and convolution neural network (CNN) [22], etc. In particularly, this chapter presents use of advanced statistical methods (PLS-DA, CNN, the multivariate curve resolution alternating least squares (MCR-ALS)) for skin tumor identification based on Raman and AF spectral features.

This chapter presents the results and performance of the PLS-DA [8] and CNN [22] classifiers for the analysis of 'optical biopsy' data for malignant skin tumors detection, particularly for melanoma. In addition, we estimated the prognostic possibility of combining the individual patient factors with the results of optical biopsy when detecting skin cancer and the possibility of differentiating skin tumors by separate biochemical components defined using the MCR-ALS method.

7.2 Raman portable device and studied patients cohort

We developed a portable RS system equipped with a commercially available Raman probe [23]. The stimulation of the collected spectra was performed by a laser module (LuxxMaster LML-785.0RB-04, PD-LD) with the central wavelength of 785 nm. The handheld Raman probe (RPB785, InPhotonics) is able to focus the exciting radiation as well as collect and filter the scattered radiation. The collected signal was decomposed into a spectrum using a portable spectrometer (QE65Pro, Ocean optics). Spectra registration was carried out in the 780–1000 nm region with the spectral resolution of 0.2 nm. All *in vivo* spectra measurements were performed with the signal-accumulation time of 60 s and the detector cooling down to−15 °C. The Raman probe is positioned directly over the tissue sample at a distance of 7–8 mm. The averaged diameter of the irradiated tissue area was about 3.5 mm. The laser power density on the skin was about 0.3 W cm^{-2} and did not caused any damage to the skin or discomfort in patients.

Due to a low efficiency of utilized detector in 920–1000 nm area, the analysis of the spectral data was carried out in 803–914 nm range that corresponds to Raman shift of 300–1800 cm^{-1}. The raw spectral data were centered, smoothed by Savitsky-Golay filter, and normalized by using the standard deviation of a standard normal variate method (SNV). Data centering decreases the model rank by one and is applicable in uniform model cases. The SNV method subtracts the mean value from each spectrum and divides each signal value by the standard deviation of the whole spectrum. The SNV method is used for levelling the experimental data dispersion.

It should be noted that application of the proposed portable setup hardly allows extracting the Raman peaks in the 300–1200 cm^{-1} region because of the low signal-to-noise ratio (SNR). In this spectral region, the melanin AF overlaps a weak Raman signal [24] and mainly the AF skin features may be analyzed. In the 1200–1800 cm^{-1} range a smaller AF contribution is observed, which makes it possible to extract tissue Raman peaks in the registered signal. The SNR for the extraction of Raman bands in the 1200–1800 cm^{-1} wavenumber region with the proposed portable system was about 3. After preprocessing, in the analyzed spectral range 803–914 nm (or 300–1800 cm^{-1}) each of the obtained joint Raman and AF spectra is a discrete set of 515 intensity values.

All analyzed experimental data were collected from May 2017 to December 2019 at *in vivo* clinical settings at Samara Regional Clinical Oncology Dispensary. The protocols of the *in vivo* tissue diagnostics were approved by the ethical committee of Samara State Medical University (Samara Region, Samara, Russia, protocol No 132, 29 May 2013), the clinical studies fall within *The Code of Ethics of a Doctor of Russia*, approved at the *4th Conference of the Russian Medical Association*, and within the *World Medical Association Declaration of Helsinki*. The patients involved in *in vivo* experiments examined by general practioners in local Volga Region clinics and directed to Samara Regional Clinical Oncology Dispensary with suspected skin cancer. Experimental spectral cohort of skin cancer sized of 617 samples of skin tumors from 615 patients including various pigmented and non-pigmented skin diseases was achieved using developed portable setup [23] in *in vivo* clinical setting. Each patient was examined by a specialized oncologist both in local clinics and in specialized Oncology Dispensary. The oncologist made a provisional diagnosis of the studied skin neoplasm on the basis of visual examination. After the examination of the oncologist, we utilized the portable RS system for the registration of neoplasms spectra. The final (ground truth) diagnosis for each tested lesion was defined on the basis of histopathology. The final spectral dataset analyzed in this study consisted of 204 malignant neoplasms (70 malignant melanomas (MM), 122 basal cell carcinomas (BCC), 12 squamous cell carcinomas (SCC)) and 413 benign neoplasms (26 dermatofibromas (DF), 62 papillomas (PP), 40 hemangiomas (HE), 113 seborrheic keratosis (SK), 170 nevi (NE), 1 cutaneous horn and 1 benign tumor of epidermal appendage). The detailed distribution of human skin lesions, including information on tumor locations, patients, etc, can be found elsewhere.

The diagnostic performance of the proposed RS system was evaluated according to different tasks or dichotomous groupings based on clinical relevance. These tasks included:

1. Discrimination of malignant (MM, BCC and SCC) versus benign (DF, PP, HE, SK, NE, cutaneous horn, benign tumor of epidermal appendage) neoplasms;
2. Discrimination of MM versus benign pigmented skin neoplasms (NE + SK);
3. Discrimination of MM versus SK.

The AF of skin tissues stimulated by 785 nm laser is a non-linear decreasing function, whereas the Raman signal is a set of separate bands, combing a number of narrow sub-bands merged into a wider peak. Due to a complex biochemical composition of skin tissues, the precise determination of exact chromophores is quite complicated and for skin tissue classification. Nevertheless, to interpret the observed bands in the recorded skin Raman spectra, we were guided by the known peak locations of the isolated functional groups [25–27]. Thus, the recorded skin Raman spectra have fingerprint bands within the range of 1200–1800 cm^{-1} with the following possible associations: Amide III (collagen, elastin) at 1230 cm^{-1}, Amide III, stretching of C–N, in-plane bending of N–H in collagen, elastin at 1275 cm^{-1}, a CH3CH2 wagging mode in collagen at 1335 cm^{-1}, a CH_2 scissoring mode associated with lipids at 1445 cm^{-1}, in-plane stretching of the aromatic rings in melanin at 1570 cm^{-1}, and a C = C stretching mode in lipids at 1665 cm^{-1} [25–27]. AF spectra are visually distinctive for pigmented and non-pigmented tissues, but visual analysis is not sufficient to separate benign and malignant neoplasms.

7.3 Partial least squares discriminant analysis of *in vivo* skin Raman spectra

7.3.1 Statistical analysis

We applied a multivariate PLS-DA to find AF shape features and Raman sub-bands that could be useful for skin tissues classification for different spectroscopic cases:

1. The whole registered spectral dataset (containing AF and Raman signals in 300–1800 cm^{-1} region) was analyzed (referred to as 'Full' task);
2. Only the AF part (300–1200 cm^{-1} region) of the spectral dataset was analyzed ('AF');
3. Only the Raman part (1200–1800 cm^{-1} region) of the spectral dataset was analyzed ('Raman');
4. Joint analysis of AF and Raman parts was performed (results were combined with logistic regression implementation) ('Raman + AF').

The PLS-DA is able to construct a regression model to identify spectra for the neoplasm classes based on the significant spectral differences. The stability of the obtained classification PLS-DA models was checked by means of 10-fold cross-validation. The number of principal components (PCs) for PLS-DA models was chosen by the criterion of the local minimum of the root mean square error (RMSE) of the performed 10-fold cross-validation. Despite that, the increase of PCs number leads to the minimization of RMSE and increase in accuracy of the classification model, RMSE in cross-validation starts varying in comparison with RMSE for the obtained model, and one should only use a number of first PCs that do not cause RMSE variations during the cross-validation process. To build a statistical model for all classification tasks we utilized from 1 to 4 PCs in different models.

In addition, we calculated the variable importance in projection (VIP) scores for all constructed PLS-DA models (figure 7.1). VIP is a weighted sum of PC loadings and solely highlights the importance of the variables (discrete values of spectral intensities) for predicting the reliability of the model [28]. The higher the VIP score value the more important the corresponding variable is in the PLS model. In our work, the VIP scores are able to find the informative bands of the neoplasm spectra in regression specification to classify different tumor types. Figure 7.1 shows that the VIPs are a mix of Raman and AF properties. In malignant versus benign neoplasms Raman narrow bands in the 1125–1185, 1440–1470, and 1640–1680 cm^{-1} regions, the 'AF' VIPs utilize data based on the curvature of wide AF bands. In the MM versus pigmented (NE + SK) and MM versus SK models, narrow low-intensity Raman bands are masked with a wide high-intensity AF curve.

7.3.2 Classification model

The results of skin tissues classification for three diagnostic tasks (malignant versus benign; MM versus NE + SK and MM versus SK) are presented in table 7.1 for the separate and joint Raman and AF analyses of skin neoplasms and for the 'Full' spectra analysis. Figure 7.2 demonstrates ROC curves (b, d, f) for the constructed models and box-plots (a, c, e) for differentiating of malignant versus benign neoplasms (a, b), MM versus Pigmented (NE + SK), (c) MM versus SK using analysis of full 300–1800 cm^{-1} region spectral range for 1 spectroscopic cases. ROC curves and box-plots for the other spectroscopic tasks can be found elsewhere [8].

The 'Raman + AF' classifier demonstrates best performance for the MM versus SK task and for the Malignant versus Benign neoplasms separation. However, there is no significant difference for the obtained ROC AUCs for Raman + AF' and 'Raman' classifiers (for all considered diagnostic tasks $p > 0.1$). For the MM versus NE + SK task, the best performance is demonstrated by the 'Full' spectra classifier; however, its difference from the 'Raman + AF' classifier is not statistically relevant ($p > 0.3$), as well as from 'Raman' classifier ($p > 0.07$). Our subsequent discussion will be focused on 'Raman + AF' classifier description.

The better discrimination models demonstrate higher ROC AUC values, and it is reasonable to compare ROC AUCs of the constructed classification models. In the case of Malignant (MM, BCC, SCC; $n = 204$) versus benign (DF, PP, HE, SK, NE, cutaneous horn, benign tumor of epidermal appendage; $n = 413$) neoplasms classification, the highest ROC AUC is 0.75 (0.71–0.79, 95% CI) and is obtained for Raman

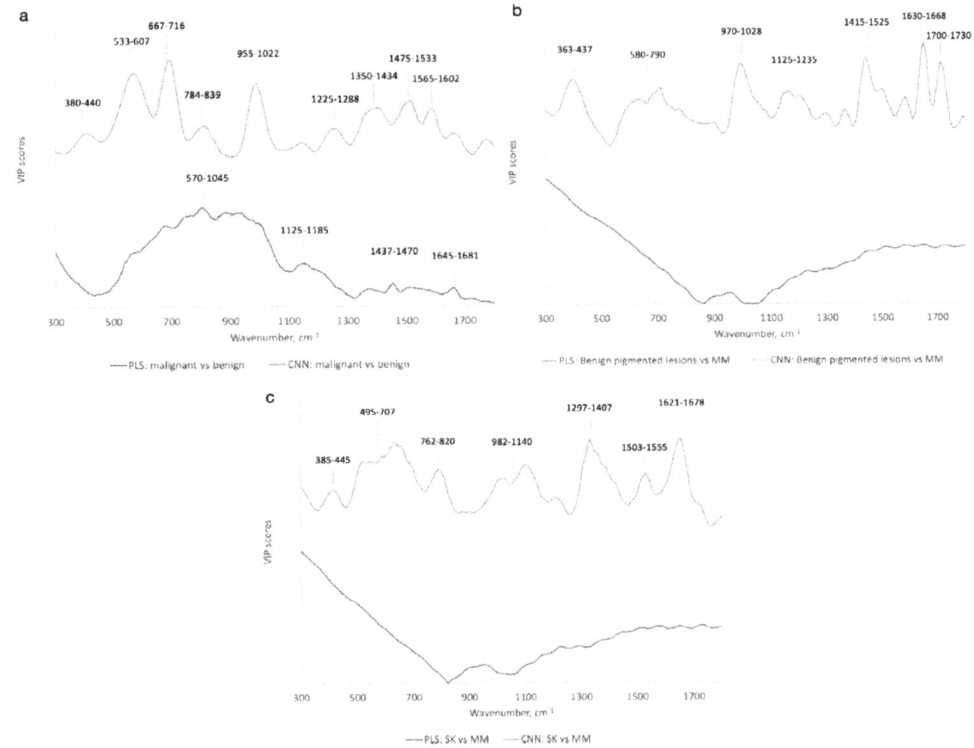

Figure 7.1. VIPs for different classification models using PLS-DA and CNN analysis: (a) Malignant versus Benign, (b) MM versus pigmented (NE + SK), (c) MM versus SK; MM–malignant melanoma, NE–nevus, SK—seborrheic keratosis. Reprinted from [22], Copyright (2022), with permission from Elsevier.

Table 7.1. Skin tissue classification for three diagnostic tasks: (1) Malignant (MM, BCC, SCC) versus Benign (DF, PP, HE, SK, NE, cutaneous horn, benign tumor of epidermal appendage); (2) MM versus NE + SK; 3) and MM versus SK.

Classification model	PLS-DA	
Malignant (204) versus benign (413)	Full	0.60 (0.56–0.65)
	RS	0.75 (0.71–0.79)
	AF	0.62 (0.57–0.67)
	Joint AF + RS	0.75 (0.71–0.79)
MM ($n = 70$) versus Ne + SK ($n = 283$)	Full	0.69 (0.63–0.76)
	RS	0.61 (0.53–0.69)
	AF	0.66 (0.59–0.74)
	Joint AF + RS	0.66 (0.59–0.74)
MM (70) versus SK (113)	Full	0.80 (0.73–0.86)
	RS	0.75 (0.67–0.83)
	AF	0.80 (0.73–0.87)
	Joint AF + RS	0.81 (0.74–0.87)

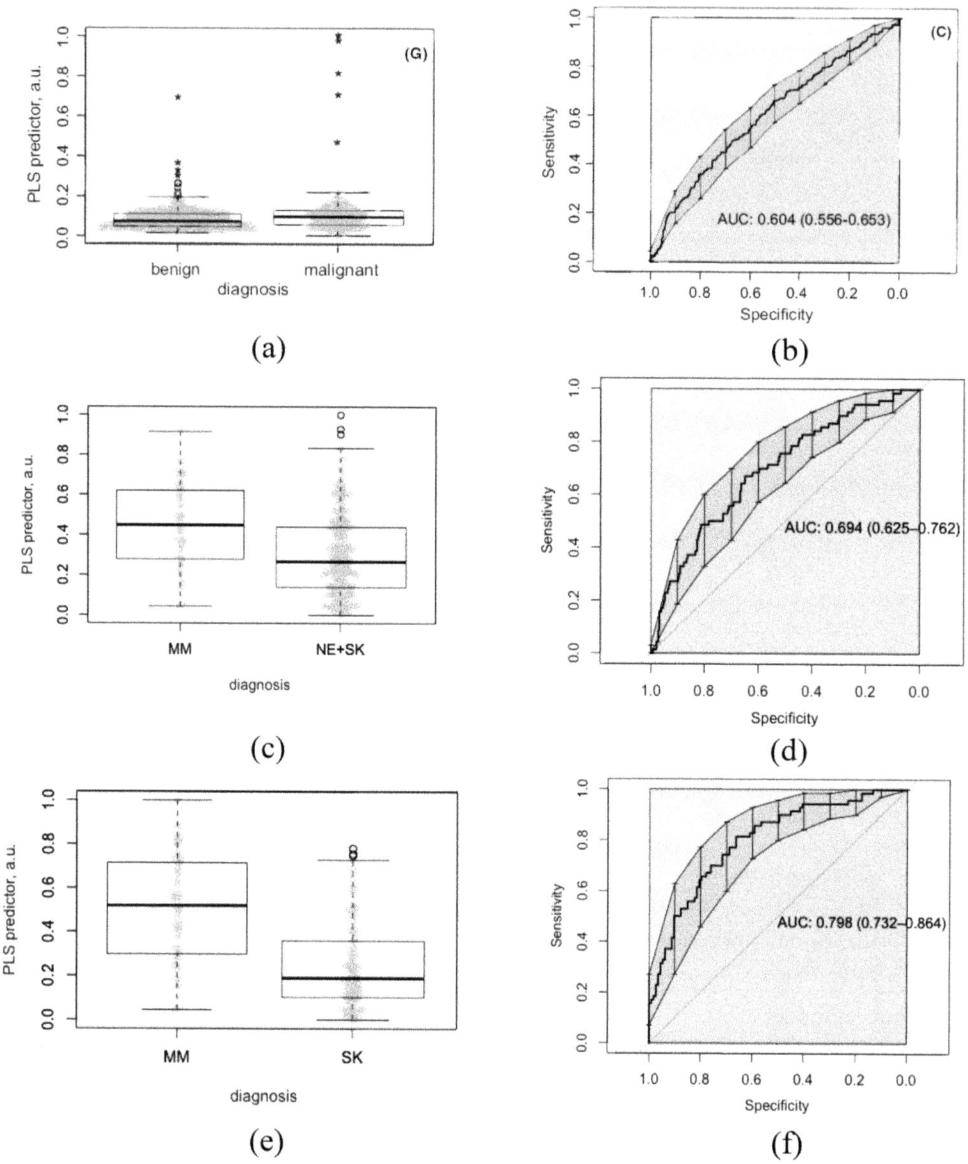

Figure 7.2. Neoplasms classification based on PLS-DA analysis of full 300–1800 cm^{-1} spectral range: (a, c, e) box-plots for obtained PLS predictors, circles (o) are values over 1.5 times the interquartile range, stars (×) are values over 3 times the interquartile range; (b, d, f) ROC curves and 95% CIs are derived from the respective posterior probabilities. Reprinted from [8], Copyright (2021), with permission from John Wiley & Sons Ltd.

spectra analysis. The combination of Raman and AF features based on logistic regression shows the same ROC AUC, while full spectra analysis provides only 0.60 (0.56–0.65, 95% CI) ROC AUC. Only 'AF' analysis demonstrates 0.62 (0.57–0.67, 95% CI) ROC AUC. The best separation of MM ($n = 70$) versus NE + SK ($n = 283$) is possible with 'AF' and 'Full' spectra analysis, demonstrating 0.66 (0.59–0.74, 95% CI) and 0.69 (0.63–0.76, 95% CI) ROC AUCs, respectively. 'Raman' analysis shows only 0.61 (0.53–0.69, 95% CI) ROC AUC, 'Raman + AF' analysis shows 0.66 (0.59–0.74, 95% CI) ROC AUC. In the case of MM ($n = 70$) versus SK ($n = 113$) classification, the highest ROC AUC of 0.81 (0.74–0.87, 95% CI) is obtained for the joint 'Raman + AF' analysis; separately, 'Raman' and 'AF' analyses demonstrate ROC AUCs of 0.75 (0.67–0.83, 95% CI) and 0.80 (0.73–0.87, 95% CI), respectively. 'Full' analysis shows 0.80 (0.73–0.86, 95% CI) ROC AUC.

7.3.3 Summary

The analysis of the obtained results shows that the joint Raman and AF study of skin tissues optical features provides the best performance in skin neoplasms classification, which is due to simultaneous analysis of Raman and AF tissue features. The lowest performance was obtained for the classification of MM and pigmented lesions (NE + SK). This result is caused by the high AF rate in the registered spectra caused by melanin masked low-intensity Raman peaks [23, 24, 29].

Important to note, that according to the achieved ROC AUCs all four considered spectroscopic tasks (Raman, AF, Full and Raman + AF) demonstrate statistically insignificant changes ($p > 0.2$) for MM versus NE + SK and for MM versus SK classification tasks. At the same time, for Malignant versus Benign neoplasms classification task Raman classifier shows higher performance than AF classifier (changes are statistically significant, $p < 0.01$), while Raman + AF classifier shows equal results to the Raman classifier. Such results may be explained by AF dominance in the collected signal. Strong AF signal masks weak Raman peaks and spectra analysis is difficult, especially for pigmented lesions. Thus, further studies are required to accurately establish the best way of skin noisy spectra analysis with low-cost Raman devices.

The proposed approach provides a capability to classify skin neoplasms with a mean accuracy higher than the accuracy of GPs and trainees, and with a comparable or less accuracy of trained dermatologists and experts. However, it is quite complicated to draw some exact conclusions as discussed studies are based on different populations, different devices, and different data and models. Further studies may include incorporating patients' demographics [30, 31] into the analysis or applying networks for extracting more useful contribution-specific information [32].

7.4 Combination of spectral data and patients' risk factors for classification of *in vivo* skin tumor spectra

Different personal factors may be potential prerequisites for developing skin cancer. The risk of melanoma generally increases with age and incidence is greater among older populations [2, 33]. The National Cancer Institute has reported [34, 35] that melanoma is more common in men than women and more frequent among whites in comparison with other races or ethnicities. High risk can also be associated with personal patient's and family history [36, 37]. Therefore, incorporating patient-specific information can improve the accuracy of disease identification based on clinical studies.

7.4.1 Statistical analysis

We estimated the prognostic possibility of combining individual patient factors with the results of optical biopsy for detecting skin cancer by chemometrics [31]. The 803–914 nm spectral region corresponding to the 300–1800 cm^{-1} wavenumber region in terms of Raman spectroscopy was also analyzed. The PLS-DA method was applied to build a regression model between the analyzed tumor predictors and tumor types. Stability of the PLS-DA classification was checked by means of 10-fold cross-validation. The number of latent variables (LVs) for the PLS-DA models was chosen according to the minimum of the RMSE in the 10-fold cross-validation. To determine the differentiation accuracy of the tumor analysis, the PLS predictors were calculated as numeric values of tumor diagnosis in the built regression model.

At the initial appointment, the oncologist collected the patient history and potential risk factors for skin cancer growth by survey: gender (G), age (A), tumor localization (L), family history (FH), personal history (PH), sun exposure (SE), size (S), and occupational hazards (OH). All the collected demographic indicators were defined by the patient survey. However, due to different reasons, for some patients, the set of collected risk factors was not full. Only gender, age, and localization factors were received for all the 617 skin neoplasm spectra. Therefore, we considered two spectra datasets:

(I) the spectral data of all 617 skin neoplasms with only three indicators: (G), (A), (L);

(II) the spectral data of only 481 out of the 617 skin neoplasms with all eight indicators: (G), (A), (L), (FH), (PH), (SE), (S), (OH).

All the risk factors were digitized:

G: 1—male; 2—female;

A: 1—under 29, 2–30 to 39, 3—from 40 to 49, 4—from 50 to 59, 5—from 60 to 69, 6—over 70;

L: 1—head and neck, 2—trunk, 3—upper limb, 4—lower limb;

FH: 0—no malignant diseases in close relatives (); 1—close relatives' malignant diseases, 2—close relatives' skin cancer disease;

PH: 0—the patient had no serious disease; 1—the patient had a different disease; 2—the patient had a malignant disease;

SE: 0—the patient avoids suntan; 1—the patient gets suntan without sunburns; 2—the patient often has sunburns;

S: 1—from 0 to 5 mm; 2—from 6 to 20 mm; 3—21 mm;

OH: 0—no occupational hazards; 1—occupational hazards due to the skin contact with chemicals (e.g., work with petroleum products, on chemical plants, etc).

The digitization of the patient factors was performed by the specialized oncologists of Samara Regional Clinical Oncology Dispensary.

7.4.2 Spectral data and three demographic factors

In this way, each skin tumor was presented as 518 tumor predictors including 515 spectral parameters, respectively, representing discrete intensity values after pre-processing and three risk factor parameters (age, gender, and localization) for PLS analysis.

We built three classification models: (1) malignant (n = 204) versus benign (n = 413) neoplasms (2) MM (n = 70) versus benign pigmented (Ne and SK, n = 283), (3) MM (n = 70) versus SK (n = 113). The ROC AUCs of the skin tumors diagnosis by PLS-DA analysis for all classification models are gathered in table 7.2. The significance of patient's data for type of cancer growth was estimated when all factors were combined with the spectral data, and when each factor was added separately.

As one may see, the combination of spectral data and patient risk factors was significant for some classification tasks. Statistical improvement was achieved for the classification of 204 malignant tumors and 413 benign tumors, from 0.610 to 0.818 ROC AUC, $p = 2 \times 10^{-11}$, when spectral data in the 300–1800 cm^{-1} range were combined with three individual patient factors. In addition, patient demographics, gender, age, and tumor localization, were statistically significant for detecting malignant tumor type when each factor was added separately. 70 MMs and 283 benign pigmented skin neoplasms were differentiated with a statistical improvement from 0.709 to 0.825, $p = 0.02$ when the three risk factors were simultaneously added to the spectral data. However, these factors were insignificant when separately adding.

7.4.3 Spectral data and eight demographic and patients' risk factors

When eight patients' risk factors were included in model each skin tumor was presented as 523 discrete predictors (515 spectral parameters and eight patients factors such gender, age, localization, family history, personal history, sun exposure, size, and occupational hazards). We considered the same classification models. The ROC AUCs of the skin tumors diagnosis by PLS-DA analysis for all classification models can be found in table 7.2.

We achieved the following results. The classification of malignant (n = 157) versus benign (n = 324) neoplasms using the PLS analysis was performed with the 0.610 (0.556–0.663) ROC AUC on the basis of only the spectral data and with the 0.789 (0.746–0.832) ROC AUC when supplying the spectral data with eight risk factors. For this set, age is also the most important risk factor. MMs (n = 49) were differentiated from the benign pigmented neoplasms (n = 221) with the 0.789 (0.718–0.861) ROC AUC using only the Raman and AF spectral data, and the 0.849 (0.785–0.914) ROC AUC when combining the spectral and the risk factors variables. However, in this case, there were no significant differences ($p = 0.14$) between the ROC AUCs obtained for the models with the eight risk factors and without those. When analyzing MMs (n = 49) versus SKs (n = 90), the discrimination model showed the 0.820 (0.748–0.892) ROC AUC that was obtained by

Table 7.2. Results of PLS-DA models [31]. Reprinted under the CC BY 4.0 license from [31].

Model	ROC AUC
I.1 Malignant (n = 204) versus Benign (n = 413), cohort with 3 risk factors	
Only spectral data (800–914 nm)	0.600 (0.567–0.652)
Spectral data with gender	0.691 (0.647–0.736), $p = 0.008$
Spectral data with age	0.804 (0.767–0.840), $p = 9 \times 10^{-9}$
Spectral data with localization	0.759 (0.718–0.800), $p = 3 \times 10^{-6}$
Spectral data with all risk factors	0.818 (0.778–0.841), $p = 2 \times 10^{-11}$
II.1 Malignant (n = 157) versus Benign (n = 324), cohort with 8 risk factors	
Only spectral data (800–914 nm)	0.610 (0.556–0.663)
Spectral data with gender	0.707 (0.658–0.756), $p = 0.006$
Spectral data with age	0.718 (0.671–0.766), $p = 0.002$
Spectral data with localization	0.680 (0.628–0.732), $p = 0.035$
Spectral data with family history	0.625 (0.570–0.677), $p = 0.35$
Spectral data with personal history	0.609 (0.556–0.663), without improvement
Spectral data with sun exposure	0.609 (0.555–0.663), without improvement
Spectral data with size	0.689 (0.639–0.738), $p = 0.02$
Spectral data with occupational hazards	0.616 (0.563–0.669), $p = 0.43$
Spectral data with all risk factors	0.789 (0.746–0.832), $p = 5 \times 10^{-7}$
I.2 MM (n = 70) versus Ne + SK (n = 282), cohort with 3 risk factors, n = 351	
Only spectral data (800–914 nm)	0.690 (0.630–0.761)
Spectral data with gender	0.751 (0.685–0.818), $p = 0.2$
Spectral data with age	0.771 (0.706–0.837), $p = 0.1$
Spectral data with localization	0.772 (0.709–0.835), $p = 0.1$
Spectral data with all risk factors	0.825 (0.766–0.884), $p = 0.02$
II.2 MM (n = 49) versus Ne + SK (n = 172) (cohort with 8 risk factors, n = 221)	
Only spectral data (800–914 nm)	0.789 (0.718–0.861)
Spectral data with gender	0.801 (0.729–0.873), $p = 0.4$
Spectral data with age	0.808 (0.734–0.881), $p = 0.37$
Spectral data with localization	0.804 (0.737–0.871), $p = 0.4$
Spectral data with family history	0.796 (0.726–0.866), $p = 0.45$
Spectral data with personal history	0.744 (0.668–0.819), without improvement
Spectral data with sun exposure	0.798 (0.725–0.870), $p = 0.44$
Spectral data with size	0.806 (0.736–0.876), $p = 0.38$
Spectral data with occupational hazards	0.788 (0.714–0.861), without improvement
Spectral data with all risk factors	0.849 (0.785–0.914), $p = 0.14$
I.3 MM (n = 70) versus SK (n = 113) (cohort with 3 risk factors, n = 182)	
Only spectral data (800–914 nm)	0.791 (0.728–0.859)
Spectral data with gender	0.791 (0.722–0.859), without improvement
Spectral data with age	0.791 (0.723–0.859), without improvement
Spectral data with localization	0.841 (0.783–0.900), $p = 0.15$
Spectral data with all risk factors	0.844 (0.786–0.902), $p = 0.15$

(*Continued*)

Table 7.2. (*Continued*)

Model	ROC AUC
II.3 MM (n = 49) versus SK (n = 90) (cohort with 8 risk factors, n = 139)	
Only spectral data (800–914 nm)	0.814 (0.740–0.888)
Spectral data with gender	0.815 (0.741–0.889), $p = 0.49$
Spectral data with age	0.815 (0.740–0.889), $p = 0.49$
Spectral data with localization	0.851 (0.784–0.918), $p = 0.25$
Spectral data with family history	0.816 (0.743–0.889), $p = 0.48$
Spectral data with personal history	0.815 (0.742–0.889), $p = 0.49$
Spectral data with sun exposure	0.815 (0.741–0.889), $p = 0.49$
Spectral data with size	0.860 (0.795–0.925), $p = 0.19$
Spectral data with occupational hazards	0.815 (0.740–0.889), $p = 0.49$
Spectral data with all risk factors	0.820 (0.748–0.892), $p = 0.46$

combining the spectral and the eight risk factors, while the analysis of only the spectral data was performed with the 0.814 (0.740–0.888) ROC AUC.

7.4.4 Summary

Our results show that among all risk factors, patient demographics such as gender, age, and tumor localization are statistically significant in detecting a skin tumor type due to their univocal definition, in contrast to the behavior factors data that were collected by staff or patients and might, therefore, lack accuracy. For some of the classification tasks, it was found that the combination of spectral data and patient risk factors could be significant. Specific total trends for each skin tumor type are observed for patient age, gender, and tumor localization. However, these demographic features did not allow us to discriminate different tumor types, especially pigmented tumors within an individual demographic group, therefore distinguishing skin tumors with similar demographics was possible using the Raman and AF spectral data only.

Diagnostic performance when combining the patient demographic data with the optical data was evaluated in several works [30, 38, 39]. In [30], Zhao *et al* were investigated whether incorporating such patient demographics as gender, skin type, localization, and age into Raman spectral analysis can improve the diagnostic performance for malignant skin cancer. The authors reported that ROC AUC improved significantly from 0.913 (0.892–0.933) to 0.934 (0.917–0.952) ($p < 0.05$) after combining only the Raman data with all the demographics using the PLS analysis to differentiate the malignant and benign skin lesions. In comparison with the study by Zhao *et al* [30], in our work we analyzed a larger set of risk factors for cancer growth including not only the demographics but the patient lifestyle and behavior factors as well. We similarly found that combining all the risk factors with the spectral data can perform better in discriminating the malignant and benign tumors and increase the ROC AUC from 0.600 to 0.818 with the three factors and from 0.610 to 0.789 with the eight factors. We increased the ROC AUCs by 30%–36% taking into account the patient risk factors while in the study by Zeng *et al* [30], the improvement was only by 2%. Probably, this greater improvement of the malignant skin cancer identification is a result of a different SNR of the spectral data. Our spectral data were recorded with a lower SNR (approximately 3) that results in a low accuracy of detecting malignant neoplasms by only the Raman and AF spectra (0.600 and 0.610 ROC AUC in models I.1 and II.1) and in a significant improvement when the patient factors were added. In [30], the authors used a highly sensitive spectroscopic system that allowed them to obtain a high ROC AUC 0.913 using only the Raman spectral data.

7.5 Convolutional neural networks for the analysis of *in vivo* Raman skin spectra

7.5.1 CNN architecture

Neural networks for analysis of Raman spectra are a very promising tool to obtain a more precise skin cancer diagnosis. We applied CNNs for the analysis of spectral data of skin tumors [22]. The analysis of the spectral data was performed for joint RS and AF implementation and the same diagnostic tasks that were considered in the previous sections.

The choice of the CNN architecture for recognition of current spectral dataset of skin neoplasms consisted of consecutive stages. At the first stage, the verified CNN configurations and advanced deep learning practice based on CNN were analyzed. Analyzing the published results has shown that the following CNN configurations are characterized by the prospects for recognition of Raman spectra: simple sequential CNNs [40], CNNs containing the inception module [41], CNNs with residual connections [42], ensembled CNNs [43], CNNs based on a combination of convolutional layers with recurrent layers [44]. It should be noted that for Raman spectra recognition, recurrent neural networks can be used not only in combination with CNN, but also as an independent model. For instance, Yu *et al* [45] demonstrated the application of the LSTM-based recurrent network to analyze a Raman dataset in the task of marine pathogens classification. Utilization of long short-term memory (LSTM)-based recurrent networks has also been demonstrated for recognition and classification of SERS spectra of nine clinically important *Staphylococcus* species [40] and for recognition of generating synthetic Raman data in the cancer tissue classification problem [46]. One of the features of utilizing artificial neural networks is the need for an empirical choice of the network topology and optimization of hyperparameters for the solved task. Therefore, empirical optimization of the topology and hyperparameters was then performed. Thus, we chose network topology as a combination of a residual one-dimensional convolutional base, a recurrent layer, and a fully connected classification level. The residual one-dimensional convolutional base is a directed acyclic graph with two branches, one of which implements the residual connection, the other is a sequential combination of the convolutional layer, the pooling layer, the convolutional layer, and the pooling layer. Convolutional layers learn filter maps for different types of patterns in the input. The pooling layers extract the most prominent structures. The residual connection [47] is implemented using the convolution of the input tensor with the convolution window equal to 1 for linear reduction of the dimension. The residual one-dimensional convolutional base is followed by a recurrent layer characterized by 64-dimensionality of the output space, the fraction of the units to drop for the linear transformation equals 0.1. The *binary_crossentropy* loss function is used as a feedback signal for training the weight tensors. The CNN is trained using the *adamax* algorithm. The number of epochs was determined by the local minimum of the loss function during cross-validation. We utilized 110 epochs in a malignant versus benign model, 70 epochs in MM versus NE + SK model, and 75 epochs in MM versus SK model. In order to avoid a 'black box' classification, model explanation and evaluating the variables contribution to the constructed model are required. In the current work, an algorithm of calculating permutation-based variable importance was used. The permutation-based method for assessing variable importance in the constructed model is used in traditional machine learning; the perspective of its application and its adaptation for analyzing deep learning models are described in references [48–50]. Figure 7.3 demonstrates a schematic diagram of the proposed approach for analyzing the Raman spectral dataset and corresponding structural features using the proposed CNN.

Each dataset consisted of 617 samples of skin tumors and was divided into a training set (80% of spectral dataset) and a test set (20% of spectral dataset). The 10-fold cross-validation was used to check the stability of each classification model, malignant versus benign neoplasms classification, MM versus Ne + SK, and MM versus SK.

7.5.2 Classification models

Table 7.3 demonstrates the achieved performance for the classification models based on the PLS-DA and CNN implementation. The application of CNN leads to the

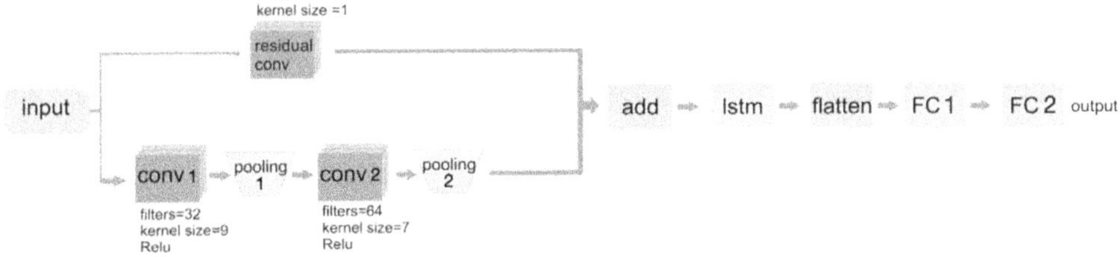

Figure 7.3. Schematic diagram of the architecture of one-dimensional CNN for the recognition of Raman spectra and classification of skin tissues where: **input** is an input layer with output shape (912, 1); **conv1** is a one-dimensional convolutional layer with padding = 'same' and output shape (912, 32); **pooling1** is an average pooling layer with pool_size = 4, strides = 4 and output shape (228, 32); **conv2** is a one-dimensional convolutional layer with padding = 'same' and output shape (228, 64); **pooling2** is an average pooling layer with pool_size = 4, strides = 4 and output shape (57, 64); **residual conv** is a one-dimensional convolutional layer with strides = 16 and output shape (57, 64); **add** is a layer that adds residual tensor and convolutional base, output shape (57, 64); **lstm** is a recurrent layer; **flatten** is a flatten layer; **FC1** is a fully connected layer with units = 128 and *Relu* activation function; **FC2** is a fully connected layer with units = 1 and *sigmoid* activation function. Reprinted from [22], copyright (2022), with permission from Elsevier. All rights reserved.

Table 7.3. Skin tissue classification for three diagnostic tasks: (1) malignant (MM, BCC, SCC) versus benign (DF, PP, HE, SK, NE, cutaneous horn, benign tumor of epidermal appendage); (2) MM versus NE + SK; (3) and MM versus SK—with PLS-DA, and CNN classifiers.

Classification model	PLS-DA (spectral data)	PLS-DA (spectral and patients' data)	CNN
Malignant (204) versus benign (413)	0.75 (0.71–0.79)	0.818 (0.778–0.841)	0.96 (0.94–0.97)
MM (n = 70) versus Ne + SK (n = 283)	66 (0.59–0.74)	0.825 (0.766–0.884)	0.90 (0.85–0.94)
MM (70) versus SK (113)	0.81 (0.74–0.87)	0.844 (0.786–0.902)	0.92 (0.87–0.97)

overall increase in skin malignant and benign tumors classifications. The achieved improvement in ROC AUC for CNN is significant ($p < 0.01$) in comparison to the PLS-DA implementation for all the three discussed tasks. For discriminating malignant and benign neoplasms, the achieved ROC AUC with CNN implementation is as high as 0.96 (0.94–0.97; 95% CI). For the two other dichotomy classification tasks, the ROC AUCs are slightly lower.

Figure 7.1 demonstrates VIPs for all constructed PLS-DA and CNN models. Figure 7.1 shows that in the case of PLS-DA, the VIPs utilize the data from narrow bands in the 1125–1185, 1437–1470, and 1645–1681 cm^{-1} regions (related to the Raman spectra), while in the low-wavelength region (300–1000 cm^{-1}), the PLS-DA captures only AF features. The PLS-DA VIPs utilize the data based on the curvature of wide AF bands in the analyzed spectra. The VIPs of mixed Raman and AF spectra analyzed in this study are a combination of Raman and AF properties where the narrow low-intensity Raman bands are masked with wide high-intensity AF peaks. For the analysis of pigmented lesions (MM versus pigmented benign and MM versus SK), strong AF dominates weak Raman bands and the PLS-DA analysis utilizes mostly wide AF features. The CNN VIPs also highlight the most informative bands that provide the best performance for the obtained classifier. One can see that CNN utilizes more Raman bands in the analysis in comparison to PLS-DA. For malignant versus benign neoplasms, the differentiation CNN not only uses information from the bands in the 1000–1800 cm^{-1} region, but also information from the bands in the 380–1000 cm^{-1} region. To distinguish between MM and pigmented lesions, the CNN utilizes the exact Raman bands instead of wide AF information. The PLS-DA VIPs highlight the most informative Raman bands near 1450 and 1650 cm^{-1} and primarily use information from the AF region near 470–1050 cm^{-1} for malignant and benign neoplasms discrimination. To distinguish between MM and pigmented lesions (NE + SK), the PLS-DA utilizes the bands near 1300 and 1650 cm^{-1}, and near 570, 720, and 1000 cm^{-1} for MM and SK discrimination. However, in the case of the MM and SK discrimination, the mentioned bands are strongly affected by a high AF signal.

7.5.3 Summary

In recent decades the application of CNN in cancer detection and screening have been widely increased as there is a need to analyze complex biomedical data. Such applications included analysis of cancer images [51], nodules malignancy assessment [52], prediction of cancer type based on gene expression [53], prediction of cancer survival [54] and many others applications [38, 55–58]. Analysis of the recent publications dedicated to CNN application in cancer detection and classification showed an opportunity to significantly increase the accuracy of performed analysis in comparison to standard statistical methods. Thus, it is not surprising, that in the case of Raman spectra analysis CNN may outperform standard approaches as PLS-DA. CNN is able to catch hidden in the complex information (as mixed Raman and AF spectra) signs of specific target groups, and utilize such data in precise classification of different groups (cancer types in the considered task). At the same time, special attention should be paid to the analysis of the obtained data during groups classification to avoid overestimation of the models and avoid utilization of noises in the models. In the case of PLS-DA application such important information may be found in VIP distributions, as VIPs represent weighted sum of PCs. In the current study, shape of the VIPs totally depends on the composition of Raman bands and AF peaks in the registered spectral database, and therefore we are sure, that the constructed classification models do not utilize random noises. In the case of CNN implementation, we utilize a well-known approach based on VIPs estimations using a model-specific approach [41]. Such an approach helped us to achieve better results in comparison to PLS-DA, as VIP analysis in CNN is able to highlight very weak Raman bands masked by huge AF signal. Once again the VIP shapes demonstrate (figure 7.1), that what is utilized in the CNN-based classification model data is based only on specific spectral bands, and does not contain random noises. Thus, the obtained results of skin tissues CNN classification based on Raman spectra analysis are solid and stable, and may be applied in future clinical applications. In summation, according to the obtained results, the discussed portable Raman systems in combination with CNN analysis can be applied for skin neoplasm detection to improve the accuracy of provisional and clinical diagnosis.

7.6 Multivariate curve resolution alternating least squares analysis of *in vivo* skin Raman spectra

It is known that Raman spectra contain an extremely large amount of information on all the chemical substances that can be found in skin. Many components of skin tissue that are accepted as biomarkers have similar peak positions in Raman spectra and overlap the spectrum of other substances such as the extracellular matrix, etc. Moreover, in addition to differences caused by the disease development, there are also some within-group differences associated with comorbidities and skin phenotypes. It is also important to understand that the quality of the Raman spectra recorded using portable Raman probes is usually slightly lower than the spectra recorded using a Raman microscope [8, 23]. For example, we used a portable spectroscopic system to record Raman spectra, with a SNR equal to 3. Therefore, the spectra may also contain a signal associated with the optical system.

In our study to analyze the low SNR Raman spectra of skin, we propose using the MCR-ALS method. The MCR-ALS method is widely used to reconstruct concentration profiles in chemical analysis [59, 60]. The main advantage of MCR analysis, in a fully unsupervised mode with the unknown basis, is its ability to physically interpret the components into which the original Raman spectra are divided. As a result of this analysis, we obtain the spectra of the substances constituting the sample and their contribution to the Raman spectrum.

We aimed to study of the possibilities of the MCR-ALS method for analyzing skin tissues *in vivo*. In a clinical setting, high-quality recording of Raman spectra can be difficult due to a large patient flow and the limited time available for patient examination. SNR is determined by multiple factors, including the laser power, the detector cooling temperature, and the signal-accumulation time. It was revealed that there is a linear relationship between SNR and temperature (see [61]). Although it is possible to increase the SNR due to the strong cooling of the detector, the portability will be lost. Raman microscopy is usually used to investigate thin sections of tissues, but if we investigate tissues *in vivo*, it is expensive and, in most cases, inefficient to use Raman microscopy. Therefore, it can be assumed that the skin Raman spectra subjected to analysis by the MCR-ALS method will have a rather low SNR. We take into account the fact that the Raman spectra of some skin tissue components also have similar peaks and bands, for example, collagen, elastin, and keratin [27, 62–64]. Nevertheless, we believe that it is possible to distinguish groups of components, for example, proteins, the moisturizing factor, and pigments (melanin), since some of the Raman peaks of the selected groups are located in different spectral bands. In addition, we investigated the possibilities of using the spectral profiles obtained by MCR-ALS analysis to classify skin tissues.

For this analysis we used the spectral cohort of skin cancer described above (in section 7.2), however, we additionally added normal spectra of the same patients involved in this *in vivo* study. Also, not all skin tumor types were considered by MCR-ALS. In total, 1000 spectra were analyzed: 540 of normal skin, 113 of SK, 122 of BCC, 67 of MM, and 158 of PN. The spectra were preprocessed with baseline removal with asymmetric least squares (lambda $= 6$, $p = 0.1$, number of iterations $= 10$) to analyze only Raman components and smoothing by Savitzky–Golay method (derivative order $= 0$, window width $= 15$, polynomial order $= 1$). The skin tumor spectra were cut in the range from 860–920 nm, which corresponds to 1114–1874 cm^{-1}.

7.6.1 Multivariate curve resolution alternating least squares analysis

In this study, we use the MCR-ALS method to analyze the Raman spectra of skin tissue and distinguish the disease markers. MCR is a group of methods which can be used to solve the curve resolution problem in spectroscopy, and ALS is an algorithm that is used for the MCR basic bilinear model.

The MCR problem can be defined as follows. Suppose we have a mixture of A components. Every individual component is usually called a 'pure component'. Every pure component has a spectrum, which can be represented as a column vector s_i with size J, which is a number of values in each spectrum (corresponding to the number of wavelengths or wavenumbers).

If we mix the components into one mixture and take a spectrum of this mixture, the spectrum will be just a linear combination of the spectra of the pure components [65]. This can be written as follows:

$$d = c_1 s_1^T + c_2 s_2^T + \cdots + c_A s_A^T, \tag{7.1}$$

where d is a vector of spectral values representing the spectrum of the mixture (J); c_1, c_2, …, c_A are concentrations of the pure components in the mixture; and s_1, s_2, …, s_A are the spectra of the pure components.

The equation can be written in a more compact form:

$$D = CS^T, \tag{7.2}$$

where C is a matrix of concentrations of the pure components in the mixture, and S is a matrix of the spectra of the pure components.

The task of the MCR methods is to get C and S by knowing D. This is not a trivial task, as the expression above does not have a unique solution. For example, one of the solutions is what the PCA gives; however, the scores do not correspond to the real concentration values nor do the loadings represent the spectra of the pure components. In fact, it is impossible to obtain C and S precisely; what we obtain is a sort of estimate, and we can rewrite the equation as:

$$D = CS^T + E, \tag{7.3}$$

where E is the error matrix [65].

The main advantage of MCR analysis is the ability to physically interpret the components into which the original Raman spectra are divided. As a result of the analysis, we obtain the spectra of the substances constituting the sample and their contribution to the Raman spectrum. Its contribution, in fact, is directly related to the real concentrations of the substances. Among the limitations of the MCR method is the difficulty of unmixing substances with similar Raman spectra, when the substance does not contain unique Raman peaks in the spectrum [65]. In addition, the research problem is to choose the optimal number of components into which the spectra will be unmixed. It may depend on both the study objective and the characteristics of the Raman spectra.

It should be specially noted that MCR analysis could be sensitive to noise in the analyzed Raman spectra. In practical application, the efficiency of evaluating the component concentration in a test sample can decrease due to the fact that the spectra contain a noise signal caused by the optical system or the fluorescence signal.

Previously, we studied the possibility of applying the MCR-ALS method to the analysis of Raman spectra of proteinogenic amino acid mixtures [66] and the effect of noise in Raman spectra on the analysis result [67]. Our studies demonstrate the possibility of unmixing several spectrally similar components of one complex mixture under noisy conditions. Using the MCR-ALS method makes it possible to successfully estimate the amino acid concentrations in a mixture, even when the Raman spectra have a low SNR (from 3 to 5).

For unmixing the spectra, we used the MCR-ALS GUI v4c by András Gorzsás [68]. To analyze experimental skin Raman spectra, we utilized the MCR-ALS method, and in this case we do not know the exact number of substances contained in the skin sample. Feng *et al* [27] report that eight components captured the skin constituents as measured in *in vivo* human skin cancers. However, this also depends on the characteristics of the Raman spectra. Therefore, it should be investigated how many components it is necessary to obtain in the original Raman spectra for an optimal result. This can be undertaken based on *a priori* knowledge or by analyzing the dataset using singular value decomposition (SVD) [68]. Figure 7.4 shows the numerical results of the singular value decomposition for set of raw Raman spectra and set of preprocessed Raman spectra. The number of components is usually selected, after which a large drop in eigenvalues is observed or the eigenvalues approximate 0. In both cases, figure 7.4 displays a gradual decrease with no abrupt drop in eigenvalues. Thus, at first glance, the number of components for a set of raw Raman spectra can reasonably be assumed to be 2 (3 is already close to 0 on the SVD plot). The number of components for a set of preprocessed spectra can reasonably be assumed to be 5–6 (7 is already close to 0 on the SVD plot). That is, in our case, preprocessing increases the number of reconstructed components (see figure 7.4). However, it is further shown that the choice of the number of components according to the SVD results does not allow the MCR analysis to reconstruct diagnostically useful spectral profiles (see section 7.3.1). Therefore, we chose the number of components based on *a priori* knowledge and other considerations.

The estimation of the initial values was performed using a SIMPLISMA-based algorithm with a default value of 10% allowed noise [70].

As constraints, we used a default spectrum equal-length closure constraint (this is the most common closure constraint for general spectroscopic data and means an equal spectral-area normalization for the MCR-ALS algorithm to avoid possible

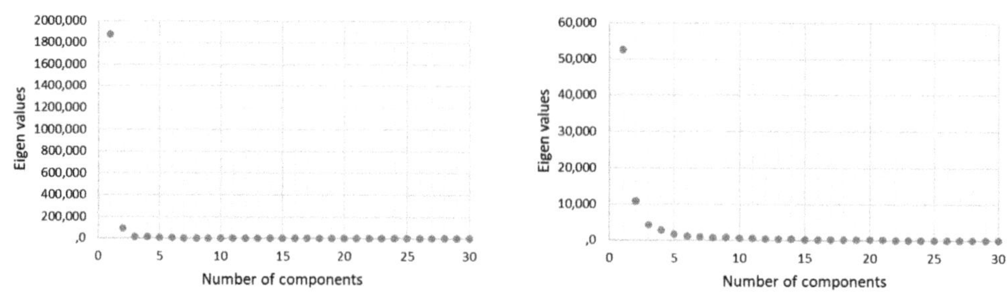

(a) (b)

Figure 7.4. Determining the number of components by singular value decomposition: (a) set of raw Raman spectra, (b) set of preprocessed Raman spectra. Reprinted under the CC BY 4.0 license from [69].

scale indeterminacies) and a non-negativity constraint in both the spectrum and the concentration profiles, which is also hard-coded in the GUI with no user control. It is implemented as a mild constraint, using a fast non-negative least squares algorithm [68]. In the case of using the spectrum basis in section 7.3.3 (which is described below), we also used equality constraints for spectra profiles. Equality constraints allow the user to fix values in the spectral profiles, such as the spectrum of a known compound present in the dataset [68].

The maximum number of iterations to be performed, if convergence or divergence does not happen before, was set to 150. The convergence criterion (the percentage of change in the standard deviation of residuals between two consecutive iterations) was set to 0.1 (default setting). In other words, the convergence is achieved when the change in the standard deviation of the residuals is lower than or equal to 0.1% between two consecutive iterations. After selecting the number of components, setting the constraints and the end conditions for the modeling, the MCR-ALS algorithm can be started. After initial estimation is given for C, it is optimized iteratively using the ALS algorithm until the convergence condition is met and the maximum number of iterations is reached [68].

In section 7.6.2, the preprocessed Raman spectra were studied: 540 spectra of normal skin, 113 of K, 122 of BCC, 67 of MM, and 158 of PN. The spectra of normal skin were divided into a different number of components from 4 to 30, and the spectra of the diseases into 5 components.

In section 7.6.3, we also investigate 540 spectra of normal skin, 113 of K, 122 of BCC, 67 of MM, and 158 of PN. However, there is one important difference between sections 6.2 and 6.3. In section 7.6.2, only matrix D is known, while matrices C and S^T remain undefined. In section 7.6.3 we also define matrix S^T.

In other words, in section 7.6.2. we only know the matrix of the original Raman spectra, that is, the matrix of mixtures, and the matrices of concentrations of the components and the spectra of the components are not known. In section 7.6.3, in addition to the matrix of mixtures, we also know the matrix of the spectra of the components; only the matrix of the concentrations of these components remains unknown. In this case, the matrix of the spectra of the components is called a 'basis' or 'basic spectra'.

The fact is that in the case of MCR-ALS analysis, without using a basis we cannot unambiguously determine into which specific components the Raman spectra are divided (for example, to which specific substance each selected component corresponds). Using a basis, we can solve this problem. In this case, the set of components into which the Raman spectra are divided remains fixed and uniquely determined. As a result, we can unambiguously determine what the concentrations of the components in the tissue sample are. The disadvantage of this approach is the fact that we often do not know what components the tissue sample consists of, so it is not possible to set the basis in advance.

We solve this problem in the following way. First, we subject the Raman spectra to MCR-ALS analysis without using a basis (see section 7.6.2). In section 7.6.3, as a basis, we use several spectra obtained in section 7.6.2, that, in our opinion, most accurately represent the contribution of some skin components. In addition to the fixed bases, we set the possibility of using four additional bases, which are identified in advance. In other words, the Raman spectra were unmixed into eight components, four of which were strictly defined.

Spectra equality is used to fix spectral profiles. For all the components that are to be constrained, the row contains numbers (i.e., spectral intensities at each wavenumber); for unconstrained components, the row contains NaN values (see [68]).

7.6.2 Unmixing preprocessed *in vivo* Raman spectra

As described earlier, we conducted the MCR-ALS analysis of 1000 preprocessed *in vivo* Raman spectra: 540 of normal skin, 113 of K, 122 of BCC, 67 of MM, and 158 of PN. The spectra of normal skin were divided into a different number of components from 4 to 30, and the disease spectra into 5 components.

Spectra analysis revealed that with a large number of components into which the Raman spectra are unmixed, MCR-ALS reconstructs single peaks, and with a decrease in the components, these peaks are combined into more complex spectra. Below we describe only some of the spectra, which, in our opinion, are most similar to the Raman spectra of the components that make up the skin tissue (figure 7.5(A–D)).

Component 1 (figure 7.5(A)) corresponds to the contribution of the optical system. A similar component representing the contribution of optic filter is shown in references [69]. The contribution of microscope optics in Raman spectra was highlighted in [71], where the authors applied an non-nativ matrix factorization (NNMF) algorithm to the *in vivo* Raman spectra of upper epidermis. It seems quite logical that in [71] this component was one of the last obtained, and in our study, the first. The reason for this is that we used a spectroscopic setup with a low SNR instead of a Raman microscope.

The ability to identify the parasitic signal associated with the contribution of the optical system can potentially be used in preprocessing the recorded Raman signals. In the spectrum of component 2 (figure 7.5(B)), the peaks at 1174 and 1230 cm^{-1} correspond to the natural moisturizing factor of the skin [71]. The peaks at 1390 and 1520 cm^{-1} are the linear stretching of the C–C bonds within the rings and the in-plane stretching of the aromatic rings of melanin [27, 71, 72]. The area from 1650 to 1800 cm^{-1} is due to C = C and C = O stretching and corresponds to skin lipids. In general, the most intense regions in these spectra are the melanin regions, so the second component can be considered predominantly melanin. A similar shape of the spectrum was obtained in [71], where melanin exhibits broad Raman bands in the 1200–1700 cm^{-1} range with two local maxima at ≈1370 and 1580 cm^{-1}.

In the spectrum of component 3 (figure 7.5(C)), one can see four peaks. The peak at 1150 cm^{-1} corresponds to the contribution of the natural moisturizing factor, and that at 1280 cm^{-1} to amide III and urocanic acid [71, 73]. The most pronounced peak at 1450 cm^{-1} corresponds to the C–H bending proteins and may be contributed by keratin, collagen, and elastin [27]. In addition, the peak at 1450 cm^{-1} may also correspond to the contribution of urocanic acid [71]. The peak at 1660 cm^{-1} is the amide I of proteins and may be contributed by collagen [62, 74]. In other words, component 3 represents the contribution of various proteins of the skin tissue and,

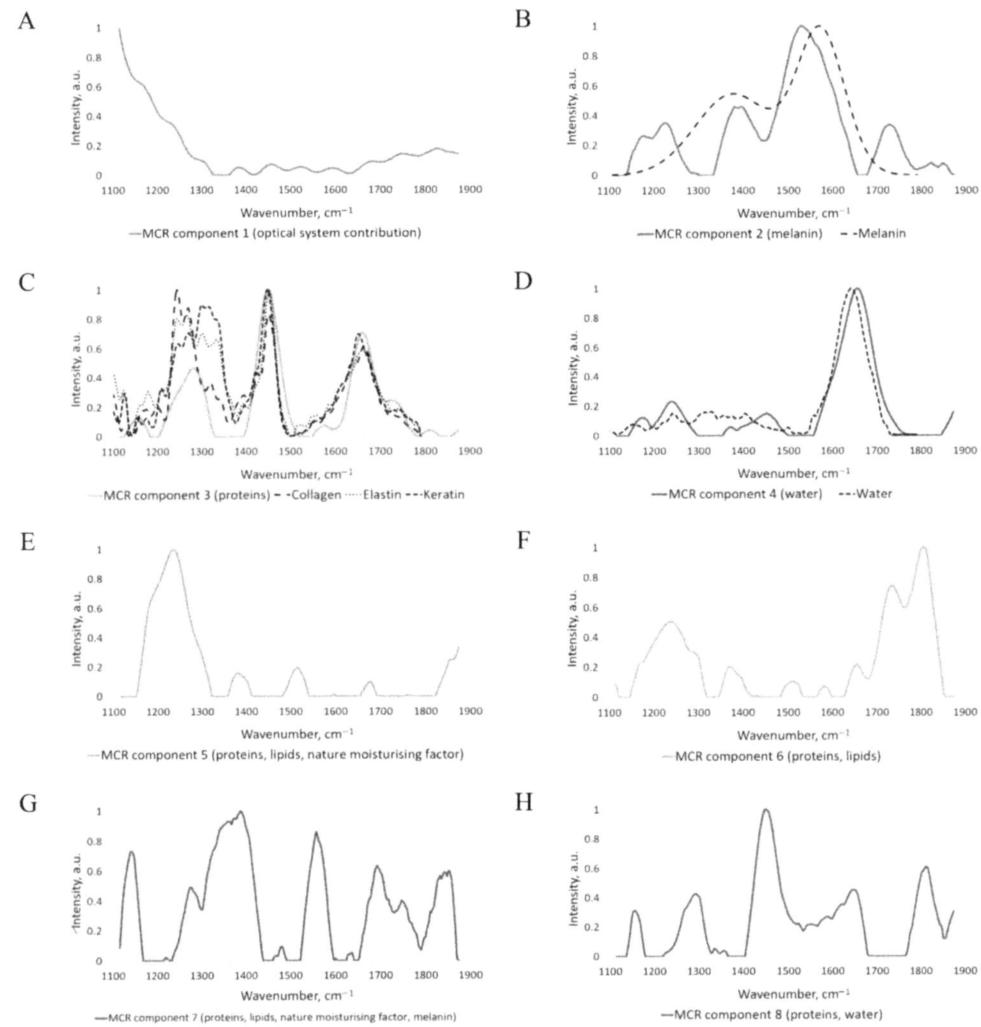

Figure 7.5. Raman spectra obtained by MCR-ALS analysis of the *in vivo* Raman spectra of skin (solid lines denote the spectra obtained in our study, dashed lines, the spectra obtained in [27]): (A) component 1 (optical system contribution), (B) component 2 (melanin), (C) component 3 (proteins), (D) component 4 (water), (E) component 5 (proteins, lipids, nature moisturizing factor), (F) component 6 (proteins, lipids), (G) component 7 (proteins, lipids, nature moisturizing factor, melanin), (H) component 8 (proteins, water). Reprinted under the CC BY 4.0 license from [69].

possibly, of the natural moisturizing factor, including urocanic acid. Moreover, the contribution of collagen is so high that the peaks at 1450 and 1660 cm^{-1} are visible even when the raw Raman spectra of skin with fluorescence are decomposed (see section 7.3.1). Comparison with the results obtained by Feng *et al* shows the similarity of this spectrum with the spectra of collagen, elastin, and keratin in the range from 1400 to 1800 cm^{-1}. Thus, in [27] we can also see the peaks corresponding to amide III (1269 cm^{-1}), to CH bending proteins (1450 cm^{-1}), and C–O amide I vibration (1665 cm^{-1}). Nevertheless, Feng *et al* were able to distinguish the spectra of collagen, elastin, and keratin separately, while we obtained only the spectrum of their mixture.

In the spectrum of component 4 (figure 7.5(D)), the most intense peak is at 1650 cm^{-1} and corresponds to water. Comparison with the results by Feng *et al* [27] shows that the spectra match almost completely.

The other components reconstructed as a result of the MCR-ALS analysis [69] apparently correspond to the contribution not of a specific skin component or related substances, but of a group of components. This may be attributed to superposition of peaks and bands, which prevents the MCR-ALS method from working correctly.

It is important to understand that the reason for the superposition of peaks and bands is not only the nature of these substances. The quality of the equipment used also plays a great role. The overlapping of spectral peaks and bands occurs in the presence of intense noise, i.e., in the Raman spectra with a low SNR.

Feng *et al* used Raman microscopy to record the spectra and identified eight different components [27]. Yakimov *et al* also used Raman microscopy but applied an NNMF algorithm instead of MCR-ALS and identified ten different components [71]. In our case, using a portable conventional Raman spectroscopy setup, we managed to explicitly reconstruct four components, whereas the rest of the components represent the contribution of several completely different groups of substances. Nevertheless, we can use the four spectra of components obtained as a basis and evaluate their concentration in the skin Raman spectra.

In section 7.6.3, we also investigate 540 spectra of normal skin, 113 of K, 122 of BCC, 67 of MM, and 158 of PN. However, there is one important difference between sections 3.2 and 3.3. In section 7.6.2, only matrix D is known, while matrices C and S^T remain undefined, whereas in section 7.6.3 we also define matrix S^T.

In other words, in section 7.6.2. we only know the matrix of the original Raman spectra, that is, the matrix of mixtures, while the matrices of concentrations of the components and the spectra of the components remain unknown. In section 7.6.3, in addition to the matrix of mixtures, we also know the matrix of the spectra of the components; only the matrix of the concentrations of these components remains unknown. In this case, the matrix of the spectra of the components is called a basis or basic spectra.

7.6.3 The contribution of individual components to the Raman spectra of various diseases

As described in section 7.6.2, we also investigated 1000 preprocessed *in vivo* Raman spectra: 540 of normal skin, 113 of K, 122 of BCC, 67 of MM, and 158 of PN. The only difference is that we used the MCR-ALS method with a basis that contained four fixed spectra (see figure 7.5(A–D)). MCR-ALS is performed with 99.4893% explained variation and 6.711% lack of fit (these indicators are detailed in [70]). As a result, we obtained four additional Raman spectra. These spectra are presented in figure 7.4(E–H). The concentrations of the components were rendered using box-plot diagrams. They are presented in [69] (see Supplementary figure 7.S4). As one can see [69] (see Supplementary figure 7.S4), components 1, 3, and 4 (proteins, water, and optical contribution; see figure 7.5(A, C, D)) are expressed almost identically in the spectra of all diseases. The most striking differences are seen in the example of component 2 (figure 7.5(B)). As we mentioned earlier, component 2 presumably represents the contribution of melanin. The concentrations of component 2 are high in K, MM, and PN, and low in normal skin and BCC. It is well-known that, on average, the content of melanin in K, MM, and PN is higher than in normal skin [27].

Among the box-plots of additional components (figure 7.5(E–H)), the box-plots of components 5 and 7 (figure 7.5(E, G)) should be distinguished. As can be seen in Supplementary figure 7.S4, component 5 is less pronounced in K and BCC and is more pronounced in PN and MM. Referring to the spectrum of this component (figure 7.5(E)), a band from 1150 to 1320 cm^{-1} of amide III can be distinguished. This spectrum may correspond to the contribution of lipids and natural moisturizing factor [61, 71, 74]. Besides this, in the spectra of components 5 and 6 (figure 7.5(E, F)) we see an intense peak at 1240 cm^{-1} that corresponds to the contribution of proteins. If we compare components 3, 5, and 6 with the spectra of collagen, elastin, and keratin, it can be noted that components 5 and 6 somehow complement the spectrum of component 3 in the range from 1150 to 1320 cm^{-1}. The contribution of proteins might have been distributed among these components. Component 7 (figure 7.5(G)) is most pronounced only in BCC, and its contribution is extremely insignificant in the Raman spectra of other diseases. We can note peaks at 1144 cm^{-1} (natural moisturizing factor); 1275 and 1750 cm^{-1} (lipids); 1355, 1386, and 1559 cm^{-1} (melanin); and 1694 cm^{-1} (collagen) [27, 71]. In the spectrum of component 8 (figure 7.5(H)) one can see intense peaks at 1450 and 1650 cm^{-1}, which suggests that this is also part of the total contribution of proteins and water. The spectrum of component 6 (figure 7.5(F)) shows an intense band at 1700–1850 cm^{-1}, which may correspond to the contribution of lipids [27].

Thus, components 2–4 represent the contribution of certain substances or groups of substances (e.g., proteins), whereas components 5–8 represent the contribution of several completely different groups of substances with a set of overlapping peaks, which leads to their ratio redistribution in different diseases.

The limitation of this study lies in the fact that we cannot compare the concentration values of skin components (i.e., the values of the contribution of the reconstructed spectra to the total Raman spectrum) with their true values. We can only indirectly confirm general patterns, noting, for example, an increased average level of melanin in pigmented neoplasms.

Furthermore, taking into account the obtained concentrations [69] (see Supplementary figure 7.S4), we applied the binary logistic regression for two cases:

- malignant neoplasms versus benign neoplasms;
- malignant melanoma (MM) versus pigmented neoplasms (K + PN).

Using the results of the binary logistic regression we obtained box-plot diagrams and ROC curves of the predicted values (see figure 7.6).

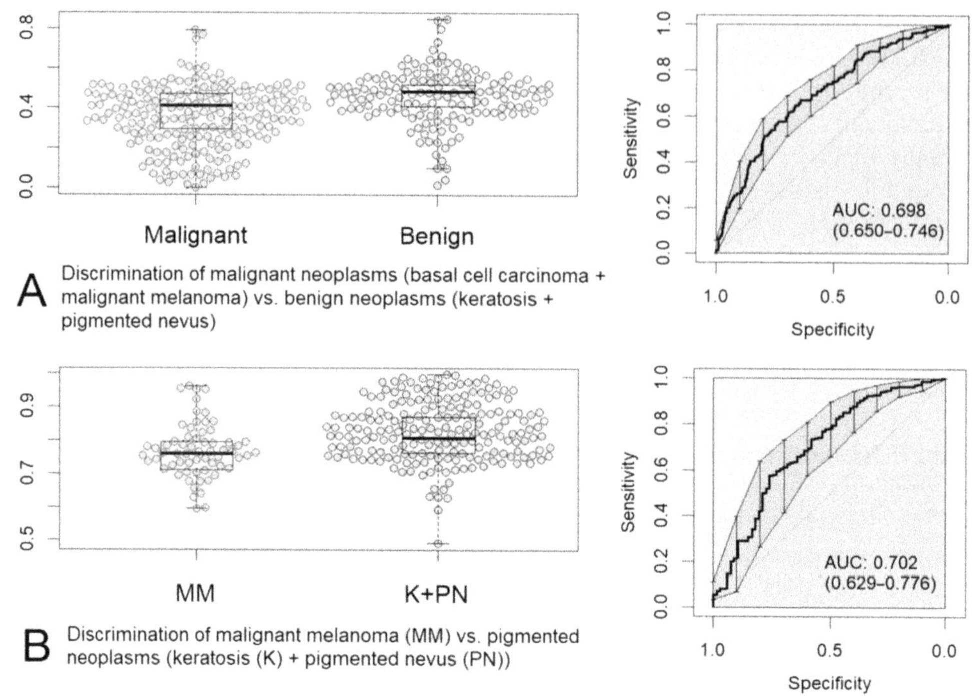

Figure 7.6. Box-plot diagrams and ROC curves of predicted values obtained as a result of logistic regression: (A) malignant neoplasms (basal cell carcinoma + malignant melanoma) versus benign neoplasms (keratosis + pigmented nevus), (B) malignant melanoma (MM) versus pigmented neoplasms (keratosis + pigmented nevus). Reprinted under the CC BY 4.0 license from [69]).

In the case of malignant (MM, BCC; $n = 189$) versus benign (K, PN; $n = 271$) neoplasm classification, the ROC AUC is 0.698 (0.650–0.746, 95% CI), and in the case of MM ($n = 67$) versus pigmented neoplasms ($n = 271$) classification, the ROC AUC is 0.702 (0.629–0.776, 95% CI).

In [8], the data were processed by means of regression analysis using PLS-DA, and the AUCs of similar classification models were 0.75 (0.71–0.79) and 0.61 (0.53–0.69), respectively. Thus, we can conclude that PLS-DA (applied to Raman spectra, as is described in [8]) and MCR-ALS analysis followed by binary logistic regression produce nearly the same results.

We applied the PLS-DA for two cases:

- malignant neoplasms versus benign neoplasms;
- malignant melanoma (MM) versus pigmented neoplasms (K + PN).

The box-plot diagrams and ROC curves of the predicted values are presented in figure 7.7.

In the case of malignant (MM, BCC; $n = 189$) versus benign (K, PN; $n = 271$) neoplasm classification, the ROC AUC is 0.632 (0.581–0.683, 95% CI), whereas in the case of MM ($n = 67$) versus pigmented neoplasms ($n = 271$) classification, the ROC AUC is 0.658 (0.583–0.733, 95% CI). Thus, we can conclude that PLS-DA

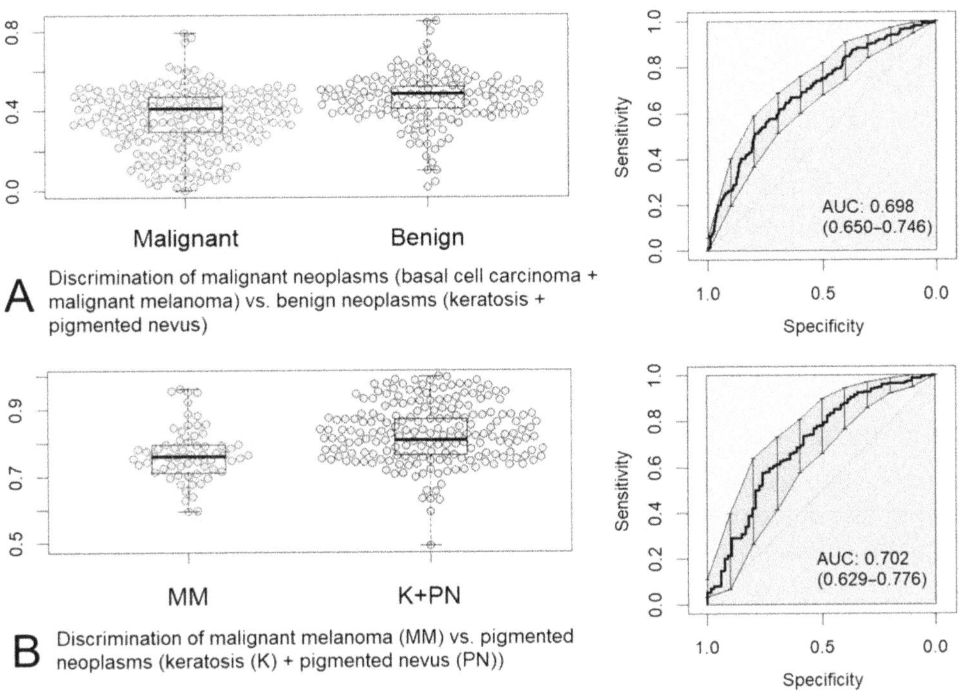

Figure 7.7. Box-plot diagrams and ROC curves of the predicted values obtained as a result of PLS-DA: (A) malignant neoplasms (basal cell carcinoma + malignant melanoma) versus benign neoplasms (keratosis + pigmented nevus), (B) malignant melanoma (MM) versus pigmented neoplasms (keratosis + pigmented nevus). Reprinted under the CC BY 4.0 license from [69]).

applied to the profiles of the component concentrations gives approximately the same result as the logistic regression (figure 7.7).

7.6.4 Summary

The results obtained in this study demonstrate the possibility of unmixing several spectrally similar components using MCR-ALS analysis even under noisy conditions of the recorded Raman spectra. This gives grounds to talk about a possible effective use of the MCR-ALS method in portable devices for diagnosing neoplasms, when the speed and ease of use of the device are more important than its high spectral resolution.

Moreover, in addition to our initial problem of analyzing the Raman spectra in order to classify them, we were also able to use the MCR-ALS method to identify the parasitic signal associated with the contribution of the optical system. In other words, the method can be used as part of the Raman setup software to correct the setup bias. Eliminating the influence of optical equipment can be extremely useful in multicenter and transnational research, when completely different equipment with different technical characteristics is used to record Raman spectra.

Unmixing such spectrally similar components as different proteins or lipids is still a challenge. In this study, we were unable to unmix them into separate components. The use of more localized measurement equipment for recording Raman spectra, for example, a Raman microscope, could make it possible to achieve better results.

Another limitation of this study is the fact that we do not have an approved and confirmed method for determining the composition of the skin *in vivo*. We can only evaluate the MCR-ALS method using the classification models.

Nevertheless, despite some limitations of the method, we have obtained a satisfactory classification result for some diseases. We plan to devote our future research to supplementing our methodology with other methods for analyzing Raman spectra, such as using neural networks.

7.7 Conclusions

In summation, according to the obtained results, the discussed portable Raman systems in combination with advanced statistical analysis can be applied for skin neoplasm detection to improve the accuracy of provisional and clinical diagnosis. The performance of CNN-based tumor classification with the proposed portable Raman device allowed us to achieve the better performance that is comparable to the accuracy of the Raman devices with deeply-cooled detectors. The accuracy of automatic analysis with the proposed CNN-based approach is higher than the accuracy provided by GPs and trainees, and is comparable or higher with respect to the accuracy of trained dermatologists. The increased accuracy of CNN implementation is a result of a more precise (compared to PLS-DA) accounting of low-intensity Raman bands in the intense AF background. The classification performance can be further improved by adding complementary information to the analysis such as patients' demographics or by analysis of spectral active components extracted by MCR-ALS. It is important to note that the proposed approach may be combined with other optical techniques, such as dermoscopy-based systems, for more precise tumors detection. Proposed Raman systems complemented with CNN can be tested for their ability to detect rare forms of skin cancer such as amelanotic melanoma [12], dermatofibrosarcoma [11], other illness (track diabetes [75, 76], find kidney disorders [19], or coronary heart disease [77]), and to find tumors in other organs. The proposed system should be evaluated in large-scale multicenter trials to prove its applicability in clinical settings. Note, that the latest studies demonstrated that portable RS systems may compete with deeply-cooled RS systems in the detection of specific components in tissues [78], so the application of portable RS setups maybe very effective in some clinical applications.

Acknowledgments

This work was partly supported by the Russian Science Foundation under Grant No. 21–75–10097 (https://rscf.ru/project/21-75-10097/) and also performed within the framework of the strategic project 'Development of the high-tech sector of the economy 'Information technologies in healthcare' of the development program of Samara State Medical University until 2030.

Conflict of interest statement

The authors declare no conflict of interest.

References

[1] Sung H, Ferlay J, Siegel R L, Laversanne M, Soerjomataram I, Jemal A and Bray F 2021 Global cancer statistics 2020: Globocan estimates of incidence and mortality worldwide for 36 cancers in 185 countries *CA Cancer J. Clin.* **71** 209–49

[2] Arnold M, Singh D and Laversanne M 2022 Global Burden of Cutaneous Melanoma in 2020 and Projections to 2040 *JAMA Dermatol.* **158** 495–503

[3] Argenziano G *et al* 2016 Dermoscopy improves accuracy of primary care physicians to triage lesions suggestive of skin cancer *J. Clin. Oncol.* **24** 1877–82

[4] Anderson A M, Matsumoto M, Saul M I, Secret A M and Ferris L K 2018 Accuracy of skin cancer diagnosis by physician assistants compared with dermatologists in a large health care system *JAMA Dermatol* **154** 569–573

[5] Alfano R R and Pu Y 2013 Optical biopsy for cancer detection in H Jelinkova *Laser For Medical Applications* (Cambridge: Woodhead Publishing Limited) pp 325–67

[6] Zaytsev K I, Kudrin K G, Karasik V E, Reshetov I V and Yurchenko S O 2015 In vivo terahertz spectroscopy of pigmentary skin nevi: pilot study of non-invasive early diagnosis of dysplasia *Appl. Phys. Lett.* **106** 053702

[7] Borisova E *et al* 2020 Multispectral fluorescence detection of pigmented cutaneous tumours *Proceedings of the Third Int. Conf. Biophotonics* 11585 1158504

[8] Bratchenko I A, Bratchenko L A, Moryatov A A, Khristoforova Y A, Arte-myev D N, Myakinin O O, Orlov A E, Kozlov S V and Zakharov V P 2021 In vivo diagnosis of skin cancer with a portable Raman spectroscopic device *Exp. Dermatol.* **30** 652–63

[9] Cordero E, Latka I, Matthäus C, Schie I W and Popp J 2018 In-vivo Raman spectroscopy: from basics to applications *J. Biomed. Opt.* **23** 071210

[10] Colas V, Blondel W, Khairallah G, Daul C and Amouroux M 2021 Proposal for a skin layer-wise decomposition model of spatially-resolved diffuse reflectance spectra based on maximum depth photon distributions: a numerical study *Photonics* **8** 444

[11] Bratchenko L A, Khristoforova Y A, Moryatov A A and Bratchenko I A 2021 Raman spectroscopy based diagnosis of dermatofibrosarcoma protuberans: case report *Photodiagnosis Photodyn. Ther.* **35** 102351

[12] Bratchenko I A, Khristoforova Y A, Bratchenko L A, Moryatov A A, Kozlov S V, Borisova E G and Zakharov V P 2021 Optical biopsy of amelanotic melanoma with Raman and autofluorescence spectra stimulated by 785 nm laser excitation *J. Biomed. Photon. Eng.* **7** 020308

[13] Bashkatov A N, Zakharov V P, Bucharskaya A B, Borisova E G, Khristoforova Y A, Genina E A and Tuchin V V 2020 Malignant tissue optical properties *Multimodal Optical Diagnostics of Cancer* ed V V Tuchin, J Popp and V Zakharov (Springer International Publishing) pp 3–106

[14] Vo-Dinh T and Cullum B 2003 Fluorescence spectroscopy for biomedical diagnostics *Biomedical Photonics Handbook* ed T Vo-Dinh (Boca Raton: CRC Press) pp 739–88

[15] Geladi P 2003 Chemometrics in spectroscopy. Part 1. Classical chemometrics *Spectrochim. Acta B.* **58** 767–82

[16] Ralbovsky N M and Lednev I K 2019 Raman spectroscopy and chemometrics: a potential universal method for diagnosing cancer *Spectrochim. Acta* A **219** 463–87

[17] Zhu Y, Liu S, Li M, Liu W, Wei Z, Zhao L and Ma Y 2022 Preparation of an AgNPs@ Polydimethylsiloxane (PDMS) multi-hole filter membrane chip for the rapid identification of food-borne pathogens by surface-enhanced Raman spectroscopy *Spectrochim. Acta* A **267** 120456

[18] Gao S, Lin Y, Zhao X, Gao J, Xie S, Gong W and Lin J 2022 Label-free surface enhanced Raman spectroscopy analysis of blood serum via coffee ring effect for accurate diagnosis of cancers *Spectrochim. Acta* A **267** 120605

[19] Bratchenko L A, Bratchenko I A, Khristoforova Y A, Artemyev D N, Konovalova D Y, Lebedev P A and Zakharov V P 2021 Raman spectroscopy of human skin for kidney failure detection *J. Biophotonics* **14** e202000360

[20] Arslan A H, Ciloglu F U, Yilmaz U, Simsek E and Aydin O 2022 Discrimination of waterborne pathogens, Cryptosporidium parvum oocysts and bacteria using surface-enhanced Raman spectroscopy coupled with principal component analysis and hierarchical clustering *Spectrochim. Acta* A **267** 120475

[21] Ryzhikova E, Ralbovsky N M, Sikirzhytski V, Kazakov O, Halamkova L, Quinn J and Lednev I K 2021 Raman spectroscopy and machine learning for biomedical applications: Alzheimer's disease diagnosis based on the analysis of cerebrospinal fluid *Spectrochim. Acta* A **248** 119188 …

[22] Bratchenko I A, Bratchenko L A, Khristoforova Y A, Moryatov A A, Kozlov S V and Zakharov V P 2022 Classification of skin cancer using convolutional neural networks analysis of Raman spectra *Comput. Methods Programs Biomed.* **219** 106755

[23] Khristoforova Y A, Bratchenko I A, Myakinin O O, Artemyev D N, Mory-atov A A, Orlov A E, Kozlov S V and Zakharov V P 2019 Portable spectroscopic system for *in vivo* skin neoplasms diagnostics by Raman and autofluorescence analysis *J. Biophotonics* **12** e20180 040 0

[24] Mahadevan-Jansen A and Richards-Kortum R 1996 Raman spectroscopy for the detection of cancers and precancers *J. Biomed. Opt.* **1** 31

[25] Bashkatov A N, Zakharov V P, Bucharskay, A B, Borisova E G, Khristoforova Y A, Genina E A and Tuchin V V 2020 Malignant tissue optical properties *Multimodal Optical Diagnostics of Cancer* (Cham: Springer) pp 3–106

[26] Movasaghi Z, Rehman S and Rehman I U 2007 Raman spectroscopy of biological tissues *Appl. Spectrosc. Rev.* **42** 493

[27] Feng X, Moy A J, Nguyen H T M, Zhang J, Fox M C, Sebastian K R, Reichenberg J S, Markey M K and Tunnell J W 2017 Raman active components of skin cancer *Biomed. Opt. Express* **8** 2835

[28] Chong I G and Jun C H 2005 Performance of some variable selection methods when multicollinearity is present *Chemom. Intell. Lab. Syst.* **78** 103–12

[29] Wang S, Zhao J, Lui H *et al* 2012 *In vivo* near-infrared autofluorescence imaging of pigmented skin lesions: methods, technical improvements and preliminary clinical results *Skin Res. Technol.* **19** 20–6

[30] Zhao J, Zeng H, Kalia S and Lui H 2019 Incorporating patient demographics into Raman spectroscopy algorithm improves *in vivo* skin cancer diagnostic specificity *Transl. Biophoton.* **1** e20190 0 016

[31] Khristofova Y *et al* 2022 Combination of optical biopsy with patient data for improvement of skin tumor identification *Diagnostics (Basel)* **12** 2503

[32] Arnaout R, Curran L, Zhao Y, Levine J C, Chinn E and Moon-Grady A J 2021 An ensemble of neural networks provides expert-level prenatal detection of complex congenital heart disease *Nat. Med.* **27** 882–91

[33] Risk factors and cancer, global cancer observatory global cancer observatory https://gco.iarc.fr/da-458tabases.php. (accessed 28 October 2021)

[34] National Cancer Institute. Cancer stat facts: Melanoma of the skin https://seer.cancer.gov/statfacts/html/melan.html (accessed 28 October 2021)

[35] American Cancer Society. Risk factors for melanoma skin cancer https://cancer.org/cancer/melanomaskin-cancer/causes-risks-prevention/risk-factors.html (accessed 28 October 2021)

[36] Diseati L, Scheinfeldt L B, Kasper R S, Zhaoyang R, Gharani N, Schmidlen T J, Gordon E S, Sessions C K, Delaney S K, Jarvis J P *et al* 2015 Common genetic risk for melanoma encourages preventive behavior change *J. Pers. Med.* **5** 36–49

[37] Gordon R 2013 Skin cancer: an overview of epidemiology and risk factors *Semin. Oncol. Nurs.* **29** 160–9

[38] Pacheco A G and Krohling R A 2020 The impact of patient clinical information on automated skin cancer detection *Comput. Biol. Med.* **116** 103545

[39] Kharazmi P, Kalia S, Lui H, Wang Z J and Lee T K 2018 A feature fusion system for basal cell carcinoma detection through datadriven feature learning and patient profile *Ski. Res. Technol.* **24** 256–64

[40] Tang J-W, Liu Q-H, Yin X-C, Pan Y-C, Wen P-B, Liu X, Kang X-X, Gu B, Zhu Z-B and Wang L 2021 Comparative analysis of machine learning algorithms on surface enhanced Raman spectra of clinical staphylococcus species *Front. Microbiol.* **12** 696921

[41] Hu J, Zou Y, Sun B, Yu X, Shang Z, Huang J, Jin S and Liang P 2022 Raman spectrum classification based on transfer learning by a convolutional neural network: application to pesticide detection *Spectrochim. Acta* A **265** 120366

[42] Ho C-S, Jean N, Hogan C A, Blackmon L, Jeffrey S S, Holodniy M, Banaei N, Saleh A A E, Ermon S and Dionne J 2019 Rapid identification of pathogenic bacteria using Raman spectroscopy and deep learning *Nat. Commun.* **10** 4927

[43] Yan H, Yu M, Xia J, Zhu L, Zhang T, Zhu Z and Sun G 2020 Diverse region-based CNN for tongue squamous cell carcinoma classification with raman spectroscopy *IEEE Access* **8** 127313–28

[44] Wang P *et al* 2021 Discrimination of blood species using Raman spectroscopy combined with a recurrent neural network *OSA Contin.* **4** 672

[45] Yu S, Li X, Lu W, Li H, Fu Y V and Liu F 2021 Analysis of Raman spectra by using deep learning methods in the identification of marine pathogens *Anal. Chem.* **93** 11089–98

[46] Wu M, Wang S, Pan S, Terentis A C, Strasswimmer J and Zhu X 2021 Deep learning data augmentation for Raman spectroscopy cancer tissue classification *Sci. Rep.* **11** 1

[47] He K, Zhang X, Ren S and Sun J 2016 Deep residual learning for image recognition *Proc. of the IEEE Conf. on Computer Vision and Pattern Recognition* 770–8

[48] Date Y and Kikuchi J 2018 Application of a deep neural network to metabolomics studies and its performance in determining important variables *Anal. Chem.* **90** 1805–10

[49] Lagerquist M A R, Gagne D J, Jergensen G E, Elmore K L, Homeyer C R and Smith T 2019 Making the black box more transparent: understanding the physical implications of machine learning *Bull. Amer. Meteor. Soc.* **100** 2175–99

[50] Yang J-B, Shen K-Q, Ong C-J and Li X-P 2009 Feature selection for MLP neural network: the use of random permutation of probabilistic outputs *IEEE Trans. Neural Netw.* **20** 1911–1922
[51] Hoar D, Lee P Q, Guida A, Patterson S, Bowen C V, Merrimen J, Wang C, Rendon R, Beyea S D and Clarke S E 2021 Combined transfer learning and test-time augmentation improves convolutional neural network-based semantic segmentation of prostate cancer from multi-parametric MR images *Comput. Methods Programs Biomed.* **210** 106375
[52] Bonavita I, Rafael-Palou X, Ceresa M, Piella G, Ribas V and Ballester M A G 2020 Integration of convolutional neural networks for pulmonary nodule malignancy assessment in a lung cancer classification pipeline *Comput. Methods Programs Biomed.* **185** 105172
[53] Mostavi M, Chiu Y-C, Huang Y and Chen Y 2020 Convolutional neural network models for cancer type prediction based on gene expression *BMC Med. Genomics* **13** 44
[54] Guillermo L-G, Jerez J M, Franco L and Veredas F J 2020 Transfer learning with convolutional neural networks for cancer survival prediction using gene-expression data *PLoS One* **15** e0230536
[55] Ding S, Wu Z, Zheng Y, Liu Z, Yang X, Yang X, Yuan G and Xie J 2021 Deep attention branch networks for skin lesion classification *Comput. Methods Programs Biomed.* **212** 106447
[56] Goyal M, Knackstedt T, Yan S and Hassanpour S 2020 Artificial intelligence-based image classification methods for diagnosis of skin cancer: challenges and opportunities *Comput. Biol. Med.* **127** 104065
[57] Alfed N and Khelifi F 2017 Bagged textural and color features for melanoma skin cancer detection in dermoscopic and standard images *Expert Syst. Appl.* **90** 101–10
[58] Kothari R *et al* 2021 Raman spectroscopy and artificial intelligence to predict the Bayesian probability of breast cancer *Sci. Rep.* **11** 6482
[59] Garrido M, Rius F X and Larrechi M S 2008 Multivariate curve resolution–alternating least squares (MCR-ALS) applied to spectroscopic data from monitoring chemical reactions processes *Anal. Bioanal. Chem.* **390** 2059–66
[60] de Juan A and Tauler R 2021 Multivariate curve resolution: 50 years addressing the mixture analysis problem—a review *Anal. Chim. Acta* **1145** 59–78
[61] Desroches J *et al* 2015 Characterization of a Raman spectroscopy probe system for intraoperative brain tissue classification *Biomed. Opt. Express* **6** 2380–97
[62] Kuhar N, Sil S, Verma T and Umapathy S 2018 Challenges in application of Raman spectroscopy to biology and materials *RSC Adv.* **8** 25888–908
[63] Khalid M, Bora T, Ghaithi A A, Thukral S and Dutta J 2018 Raman spectroscopy detects changes in bone mineral quality and collagen cross-linkage in staphylococcus infected human bone *Sci. Rep.* **8** 9417
[64] Nguyen H T, Zhang Y, Moy A J, Feng X, Sebastian K R, Reichenberg J S, Fox M C, Markey M K and Tunnell J W 2021 Characterization of *ex vivo* nonmelanoma skin tissue using Raman spectroscopy *Photonics* **8** 282
[65] Felten J, Hall H, Jaumot J, Tauler R, De Juan A and Gorzsás A 2015 Vibrational spectroscopic image analysis of biological mate-rial using multivariate curve resolution–alternating least squares (MCR-ALS) *Nat. Protoc.* **10** 217–40
[66] Matveeva I A, Myakinin O O, Khristoforova Y A, Bratchenko I A, Tupikova E N and Zakharov V P 2020 Possibilities for de-composing Raman spectra of amino acids mixture by Multivariate Curve Resolution (MCR) analysis *Fourth International Conference on Terahertz*

and Microwave Radiation: Generation, Detection, and Applications (Tomsk, Russia) Vol. 11582 pp 299–306

[67] Matveeva I A, Bratchenko L A, Myakinin O O, Tupikova E N and Zakharov V P 2021 The effect of noise in Raman spectra on the reconstruction of the concentration of amino acids in the mixture by multivariate curve resolution (MCR) analysis *J. Biomed. Photonics Eng.* **7** 020309

[68] Gorzsás A 2017 *MCR-ALS GUI V4c, Open-Source MATLAB Script from the Vibrational Spectroscopy Core Facility* (Umeå, Sweden: Umeå University)

[69] Matveeva I, Bratchenko I, Khristoforova Y, Bratchenko L, Moryatov A, Kozlov S, Kaganov O and Zakharov V 2022 Multivariate curve resolution alternating least squares analysis of *in vivo* skin Raman spectra *Sensors* **22** 9588

[70] Ruckebusch C 2016 *Resolving Spectral Mixtures: With Applications from Ultrafast Time-Resolved Spectroscopy to Super-Resolution Imaging* (Amsterdam: Elsevier)

[71] Yakimov B P, Venets A V, Schleusener J, Fadeev V V, Lademann J, Shirshin E A and Darvin M E 2021 Blind source separation of molecular components of the human skin *in vivo*: non-negative matrix factorization of Raman microspectroscopy data *Analyst* **146** 3185–96

[72] Huang Z, Lui H, Chen M X, Alajlan A, McLean D I and Zeng H 2004 Raman spectroscopy of *in vivo* cutaneous melanin *J. Biomed. Opt.* **9** 1198–205

[73] Duraipandian S, Mo J, Zheng W and Huang Z 2014 Near-infrared Raman spectroscopy for assessing biochemical changes of cervical tissue associated with precarcinogenic transformation *Analyst* **139** 5379–86

[74] Bankapur A, Zachariah E, Chidangil S, Valiathan M and Mathur D 2010 Raman tweezers spectroscopy of live, single red and white blood cells *PLoS One* **5** e10427

[75] Guevara E, Torres-Galván J C, Ramírez-Elías M G, Luevano-Contreras C and González F J 2018 Use of Raman spectroscopy to screen diabetes mellitus with machine learning tools *Biomed. Opt. Express* **9** 4998–5010

[76] Paolillo F R, Mattos V S, de Oliveira A O, Guimarães F E G, Bagnato V S and de Castro Neto J C 2019 Noninvasive assessments of skin glycated proteins by fluorescence and Raman techniques in diabetics and nondiabetics *J. Biophotonics* **12** e201800162

[77] Yu P E 2022 Hemoglobin heme conformation in patients with different oxygen saturation values *J. Biomed. Photonics Eng.* **8** 40505

[78] Fales A M, Ilev I K and Pfefer T J 2021 Evaluation of standardized performance test methods for biomedical Raman spectroscopy *J. Biomed. Opt.* **27** 074705

Chapter 8

Hyperspectral imaging and histology with Raman spectroscopy

Tim McNamara and Bryan Hennelly

8.1 Introduction

Raman spectroscopy enables detailed visualization of molecular compositions, providing a 'fingerprint' by which materials can be identified, a capability that is of growing interest in medical diagnostics. Hyperspectral imaging and histology with Raman spectroscopy represent important recent advancements in the medical and scientific communities, offering an innovative approach to the molecular analysis of tissues. The Raman spectrum at each point in the image can be recorded with micrometre resolution using a variety of different modalities, producing a three dimensional dataset, where the third dimension is the Raman wavenumber. Raman spectroscopy is non-destructive and label-free, thereby allowing for the recording of hyperspectral information without altering the samples properties. This chapter introduces the various techniques and methodologies involved in hyperspectral Raman imaging, focussing particularly on their application in histological studies.

One of the most transformative applications of this technology is virtual staining, a non-invasive method that mimics traditional chemical staining processes used in histology. Virtual staining does not require the physical application of dyes to tissue samples, preserving the original specimens while providing essential information about tissue morphology and pathology. This technique is finding important application in clinical settings, particularly during surgical procedures, where it facilitates rapid intra-surgical pathological diagnostics. By allowing pathologists and surgeons to visualize and assess histopathological details in real-time, virtual staining significantly enhances the decision-making process during surgeries, potentially improving patient outcomes by enabling more precise and timely interventions.

Furthermore, the integration of machine learning with hyperspectral Raman imaging opens new avenues for automated tissue classification and diagnosis.

doi:10.1088/978-0-7503-5949-8ch8

Machine learning algorithms can analyze complex hyperspectral data to identify patterns that may not be immediately visible to the human eye, even to the trained pathologist, thereby providing an additional layer of diagnostic insight. This capability is especially valuable in scenarios where rapid and accurate tissue analysis is critical, such as during tumour resection surgeries.

This chapter is structured to provide a comprehensive overview of various Raman spectroscopy techniques, including spontaneous Raman, stimulated Raman spectroscopy (SRS), and coherent anti-Stokes Raman scattering (CARS). Each section will detail the specific contributions of these techniques to hyperspectral imaging, discuss their practical applications, and explore the future potential of integrating these approaches with advanced computational methods for enhanced diagnostic accuracy. There is a particular emphasis on SRS owing to its high-speed and its recently proven application for real-time virtual staining and tissue classification.

We begin in the next section with a review of the various opto-electronic modalities for recording and processing a hyperspectral image. This is followed by a series of sections that review stimulated Raman histology, whereby the Raman hyperspectral image can be processed to produce an H&E-like stained image for pathological interpretation or machine learning based classification. We conclude with a section that offers a vision of the future of this exciting area of research.

8.2 Recording a hyperspectral Raman image

8.2.1 Overview

In this section, we briefly review the state of the art in recording a hyperspectral Raman image, which is the precursor to Raman histology. We begin with a review of spontaneous Raman systems that employ a line-scanning approach. Spontaneous Raman spectroscopy remains the gold standard in the field in the sense that all of the coherent Raman systems attempt to produce the same information with higher speed, but none can match it in terms of quantitative accuracy. Next we will review the SRS system which is the basis for most of the research that is reviewed in this chapter. SRS is very high-speed but it is typically used to record only one or two Raman wavenumbers. Finally, we will review two alternative coherent Raman methods, which although not as fast as SRS, can provide broadband spectra.

8.2.2 Spontaneous Raman scattering

Hyperspectral imaging with spontaneous Raman is not as commonly applied as SRS, but it has seen growing interest in recent years. Raman spectroscopy is a phenomenon whereby incident light interacts with molecular vibrations, resulting in scattered light with shifted wavelengths. This effect provides a unique spectral fingerprint for each molecule across the full spectral window, typically encompassing 400 cm^{-1}–3500 cm^{-1}, and is primarily limited by the ability of the recording equipment rather than the signal generated. The setup for spontaneous Raman is comparably simple compared to other methods, typically requiring a single laser source that is focused on a sample. The Raman scattered light is separate from the laser using a longpass filter and is directed to a spectrograph where the spectral intensity is measured. The method can easily be coupled with a microscope by focussing the laser through the microscope objective and collecting the back-scattered photons via the same objective. This approach, termed 'epi-Raman' is the most common and requires a dichoric beamsplitter to separate the laser and Raman photons since the input laster and output photons share the same path into and out of the objective. A confocal aperture is commonly included in the setup to enable 3D resolution as well as reducing the impact of laser induced luminescence from the glass substrate, which can be mitigated using background subtraction algorithms [12]. This architecture is adopted by many commercial Raman instrument companies including Horiba.

Typically, recording a single spectrum from a biological sample requires an acquisition time in the order of 1 s. This is because, despite its high spectral resolution and relatively simple setup, spontaneous Raman is an inherently weak process with fewer than 1 in 1e^6 photons being Raman scattered. This means that typical hyperspectral imaging, whereby the sample is point-scanned through the laser focus, becomes prohibitively time consuming. Nevertheless, because of the attractiveness of confocal Raman in terms of spectra some authors have advanced the approach toward 150 ms acquisition times, which is made possible with singular value decomposition (SVD) denoising [13].

In recent years, reducing the total time required for recording spontaneous Raman spectra has been a goal of many researchers, employing novel processing methods such as optical setups that allow for parallelized acquisition. Figure 8.1(a)

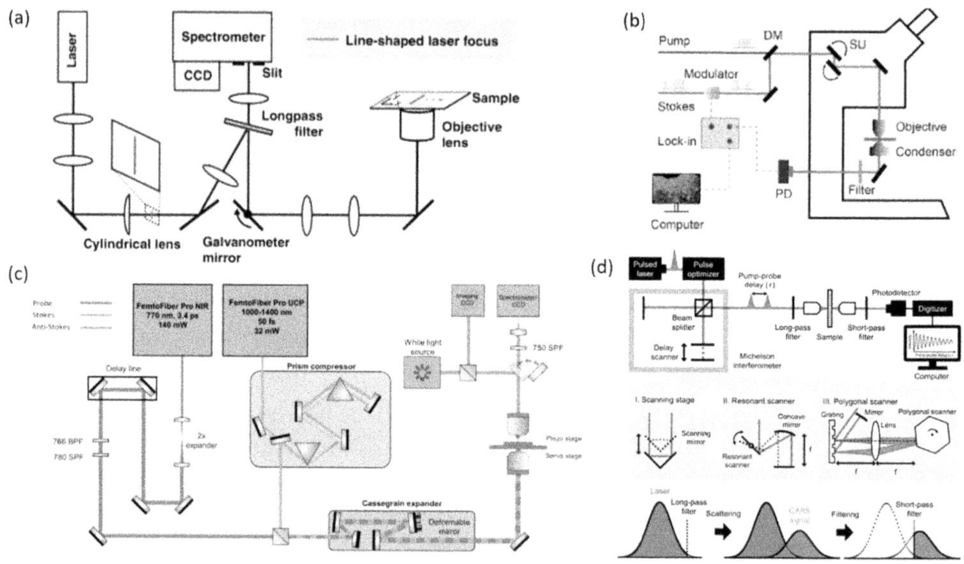

Figure 8.1. Diagram of the optical setup for the various Raman hyperspectral imaging modalities using (a) line-scanning spontaneous Raman (reprinted from [7], copyright 2016, with permission from Elsevier Ltd, all rights reserved); (b) stimulated Raman Spectroscopy point scanning (reprinted with permission from [11], copyright 2024, American Chemical Society); (c) broadband coherent anti-Stokes Raman Spectroscopy (reproduced from [8] CC BY 4.0); (d) Fourier transform Coherent anti-Stokes Raman Spectroscopy (reproduced from [9] CC BY 4.0).

is one such example developed by Fujita *et al* in [7]. This system, similar to the Renishaw commercial Raman instruments, projects a laser line at the sample plane that is focused by a cylindrical lens combined with the microscope objective. Raman scattering occurs in the sample at all points along this line. The back-scattered photons are imaged to the line that is the spectrograph slit. A galvo mirror is placed in the system such that the illuminating line can be scanned accross the sample, while the back-scattered light will also be incident on the static spectrograph slit. Although this line-scanning approach affords less depth resolution than confocal Raman, it has the significant advantage of enabling parallel Raman spectra recorded all along the line and therefore represents the state of the art for hyperspectral Raman imaging with full band. One limitation of this approach is the stronger background signal from glass, when compared with confocal. For this reason line-scanning often requries the use of quartz or expensive Raman grade CaF_2 substrates [14].

Also worth mentioning is reference [15] in which the same research group have proposed an even higher-speed line-scanning Raman system for hyperspectral imaging. Although this method is limited to the CH-band, it facilitates hyperspectral imaging at a speed that is comparative to broadband CARS (BCARS), reviewed below. This technique employs multiple line illuminations for sample scanning, significantly improving the throughput compared single-line scanning. This system utilizes a powerful continuous-wave laser and a multi-slit detection setup to scan the sample in parallel, reducing the overall scan time to approximately 10 min per megapixel. A bandpass filter narrows the detected spectral range to focus on specific Raman bands while filtering out 'unwanted' fingerprint regions. Additionally, the system incorporates a custom-built confocal slit array, enhancing signal clarity and reducing noise. Importantly, SVD is applied to the spectral data for noise reduction and signal enhancement, making this approach highly effective for rapid and precise biomedical imaging and diagnostics.

8.2.3 Stimulated Raman spectroscopy

SRS is the core technology behind many advancements in virtual staining and disease classification methodologies discussed in this review chapter. Since its innovation by the Xie group a decade ago [16], SRS has gained widespread adoption due to its exceptionally fast acquisition speeds and enhanced signal clarity compared to traditional Raman techniques. SRS differs from spontaneous Raman spectroscopy by utilizing two synchronized laser beams—a pump and a Stokes beam—to induce and amplify molecular vibrations within the sample. This enhancement is achieved through a nonlinear interaction process, where the energy difference between the two beams matches the vibrational energy of the sample's molecular bonds, and the basic system used for hyperspectral imaging is shown in figure 8.1(b), which is taken from [10].

Unlike the inherently weak inelastic scattering of spontaneous Raman, SRS amplifies the Raman signal, significantly enhancing detection sensitivity and speed. This makes it ideal for rapid and detailed molecular imaging. The implementation of SRS involves critical optical components including a pulse laser system to generate the necessary beam properties, acousto-optic modulators (AOMs) to precisely control beam frequencies, and lock-in amplifiers (LIAs) to detect the subtle changes in intensity resulting from the Raman effect.

One of the most significant milestones achieved by the Xie group in the development of SRS was the successful suppression of non-resonant background (NRB) noise, a pervasive challenge in traditional Raman techniques. Another key innovation from the Xie group that propelled the use of SRS was the development of high-speed tuning systems for the pump laser making use of fibre lasers and optical parametric oscillators (OPOs), allowing rapid and precise adjustments across different Raman shifts to scan multiple molecular bonds efficiently. These adjustments typically require sequential tuning to cover a broad spectral range, traditionally increasing the recording time. However, recent advancements have sought to circumvent this limitation by using broadband SRS techniques that can capture multiple wavenumbers simultaneously, thus speeding up the data acquisition process without sacrificing spectral information [17]. This approach, though more complex optically, reduces the need for multiple sequential acquisitions and integrates advanced optical modulation and signal detection strategies to manage the increased data throughput effectively.

8.2.4 Broadband coherent anti-Stokes Raman spectroscopy

BCARS offers a significant advancement in the field of hyperspectral Raman imaging by providing full-spectrum Raman images without the need for the wavelength scanning required in SRS. This technique, which is depicted in figure 8.1(c), [18] utilizes a unique laser configuration that allows for the simultaneous probing of the entire biologically-relevant Raman spectrum, ranging from 500 cm^{-1} to 3500 cm^{-1}. Unlike SRS, which enhances specific Raman lines by tuning the pump and Stokes beams to match molecular vibrations, BCARS generates a broadband spectrum in a single acquisition. This is achieved through the use of a supercontinuum source combined with a narrowband probe. The broadband nature of the light source in BCARS accesses a wide range of Raman shifts simultaneously, enabling the capture of comprehensive chemical information across the full fingerprint and CH-stretch regions in a single shot.

One of the primary advantages of BCARS is its ability to provide detailed chemical maps of samples without the need for sequential tuning, which is a time-consuming aspect of SRS. However, BCARS systems typically face challenges with NRB noise, which can obscure the weaker Raman signals and distort the spectral data. Advanced numerical methods, such as the Kramers–Kronig transform or most recently using deep learning methods, [19, 20] are employed to numerically remove NRB-induced distortions and retrieve the Raman-like spectrum from the raw BCARS data.

The acquisition time for BCARS, at approximately 3 milliseconds per spectrum, positions it between the ultra-fast SRS and the slower spontaneous Raman spectroscopy. This makes BCARS an ideal candidate for applications that benefit from rapid imaging but require more comprehensive spectral information than SRS can provide. For example, BCARS can be used to scan wide areas of tissue to provide a full spectral map within several minutes, which is significantly faster than spontaneous Raman but with a richer dataset than SRS. Furthermore, BCARS can complement SRS in a hybrid imaging approach, where SRS is used for initial rapid screening to identify regions of interest with potential pathological significance. Subsequently, these targeted areas can be examined in greater detail using BCARS to obtain comprehensive biochemical information. This complementary use of both technologies leverages the speed of SRS for screening and the spectral breadth of BCARS for detailed analysis, potentially providing a powerful toolset for biomedical research and diagnostic applications.

8.2.5 Fourier transform coherent anti-Stokes Raman spectroscopy (FT-CARS)

For the sake of completeness we also briefly review FT-CARS as another possible method for hyperspectral Raman imaging, which has received some attention for its ability to acquire broadband Raman spectra at extraordinarily high speeds. As illustrated in figure 8.1(d), the basic principle in FT-CARS is to split a femtosecond pulse laser beam into two paths to create a pump and a probe beam. These beams interact in a sample through a Michelson interferometer setup where one arm is fixed and the other includes a rapidly scanning delay line. This configuration generates a CARS signal whose frequency components are down-converted into a range that can be rapidly read by conventional photodetectors. The technique's capability to rapidly scan the delay line allows it to perform spectroscopic measurements much faster than traditional methods, reaching acquisition rates of up to 50 000 spectra per second [21]. In figure 8.1(d), the delay scan is implemented using a polygonal mirror array in its Fourier plane, which, through its rotation, scans the delay line at high speeds. This setup enables a rapid succession of Raman spectra over a wide range of Raman shifts, making FT-CARS highly suitable for very high-speed spectral recording. Another advantage is that the NRB, a problem in BCARS, is mitigated by the FT recording process.

Despite these technological advancements, the application of FT-CARS in biological sampling poses specific challenges, and has yet to be fully tested to the same level as SRS or BCARS. The rapid scanning required by FT-CARS (such as the polygonal mirror array in the figure), while beneficial for speed, might simply be too fast to record useful broadband spectra from a biological sample, which are inherently weak scatterers. Biological samples often exhibit lower Raman scattering efficiencies, which means that the high-speed capabilities of FT-CARS might not translate directly to practical speeds when imaging biological tissues. The faster the scan, the lower the signal-to-noise ratio tends to be, unless compensated by high laser powers or advanced noise-reduction technologies (such as the use of LIAs in SRS). This could necessitate slower scanning to accumulate sufficient signal, balancing the inherent advantages of the method's speed

In table 8.1 a comparison of the various hyperspectral Raman modalities is provided for bioimaging.

Table 8.1. Comparison of Raman hyperspectral modalities.

Acquisition mode	Effective per-pixel dwell time	Spectral resolution	Bandwidth (cm^{-1})
Point scan Raman	150 ms* [13]	1–10 cm^{-1}	400–4000
Line scan Raman	24 ms* [7]	1–10 cm^{-1}	400–4000
Multi-line scan Raman	617 μs* [15]	3–5 cm^{-1}	2800–3200
32-channel SRS	40 μs [17]	10 cm^{-1}[22]	2800–3200
Dual-channel SRS	10 μs [2]	10 cm^{-1}	10–20
BCARS	3 ms*	10–30 cm^{-1}[23]	400–4000

*Dwell times achieved using SVD denoising.

8.2.6 Preprocessing

Preprocessing in hyperspectral Raman imaging is a necessary first step before any virtual staining or classification algorithms. This step ensures the accuracy and relevance of the spectral data obtained from various Raman spectroscopy modalities. Each method comes with its own set of challenges and requirements that dictate the necessary preprocessing steps. In spontaneous Raman spectroscopy, preprocessing involves wavenumber calibration [24] to align spectral features accurately with their true positions. Intensity calibration is required to ensure that the response from the spectrometer is consistent across different wavelengths from one instrument to another. Cosmic ray removal is necessary for hyperspectral imaging, this is best done by comparing a given spectra with other recorded spectra in the dataset to indemnify and replace data affected by cosmic rays [25]. Background subtraction is another critical step, particularly to remove signals arising from the substrate or medium, which can obscure or distort the Raman signal; glass in particular can be problematic but it can be effectively removed using a least squares regression method [12]. Additionally, baseline removal is employed to correct for distortions due to autofluorescence or other broad spectral features, often using techniques like polynomial fitting or rolling ball algorithms [12]. For SRS, preprocessing may include spectral phasing to correct phase shifts in the signal, ensuring proper alignment of spectral peaks. Additionally, signal enhancement techniques, such as lock-in amplification, are utilized to bolster the weak Raman signal against a dominant NRB, which is a common challenge in SRS. While BCARS preprocessing must also correct wavenumber calibration for spectral accuracy, the most significant step is the removal of non-resonant background (NRB) noise, often using methods like the Kramers–Kronig transform or, more recently, deep learning methods [19, 20]. This step is crucial as NRB can significantly obscure or distort the actual Raman signal in the collected spectra. Intensity calibration is trivial in BCARS. FT-CARS primarily involves transforming time-domain signals into the frequency domain to extract Raman spectra using a discrete Fourier transform. Across all these modalities, SVD is a powerful tool used for denoising hyperspectral datasets. SVD works by decomposing the dataset into singular vectors and values, which can be truncated to minimize noise while preserving the essential structure of the data.

8.3 Virtual staining with procedural approaches

8.3.1 Overview

We use the term procedural approach to refer to the identification of a small subset of wavenumber information that can be directly related to the molecular bonds associated with clinical H&E staining, which are then used to 'virtually stain' a hyperspectral stimulated Raman image such that is has the same appearance as an H&E image. The goal here is to make use of the label-free molecular information provided by real-time stimulated Raman in order to produce histopathology images that are equivalent to an image that could be obtained by chemical staining. This procedural approach is not probabilistic as for the case of generative deep learning methods. It provides a direct chemical link between the label-free imaging and the labelled imaging by exploiting the chemistry involved in chemical staining. The primary source of information for procedural generation of H&E images the procedural methods reviewed below are the CH_2 (found in cell bodies) and CH_3 (in cell nuclei) chemical bonds, relating directly to the 2845 cm^{-1} and 2930 cm^{-1} wavenumbers. These bonds are found in abundance in cell bodies and cell nuclei. Where the 2930 cm^{-1} region has stronger responses to nucleic acids and similar contributions as the 2845 cm^{-1} from lipids and proteins, by subtracting the 2845 cm^{-1} from the 2930 cm^{-1} image the contribution from proteins and lipids is weakened thereby enhancing the contrast for nucleic acid specific peaks.

Two research groups have made significant contributions to this area in recent years, both of which have spun out start-up companies to commercialize their technologies towards real-time histopathology imaging in surgery to assist with identifying diseased tissue and tumour margins. The Xie group, which pioneered the development of SRS, have developed a high-speed low-noise SRS bioimaging system that can be tuned to 2845 and 2930 cm^{-1} and two wavenumber images can be recorded sequentially [1, 26–28]. This hyperspectral dataset is then subject to a bespoke image processing algorithm to produce an H&E-like image. The Rigneault group at the university of Marseilles make use of a customized SRS system capable of recording the two wavenumbers simultaneously (via a phase) and the resultant hyperspectral image is subject to a pseudo-automated image processing routine that can be tuned to produce convincing H&E-like images [2, 29–31]. This group also makes use of the second harmonic generation (SHG) signal that can also be generated by the same system, in order to further enhance the quality of their virtual staining.

8.3.2 Stimulated Raman histology—The Xie Group [1]

The Xie group were the first to develop low-noise stimulated Raman scattering (SRS) bioimaging systems in 2008, [27] pioneering a technique that significantly improved the sensitivity and speed of label-free imaging for biological applications. They went on to commercialize this breakthrough through the company Invenio

Imaging. A key innovation by the Xie group was the use of a fibre laser system for SRS imaging, which provided a more stable, compact, and user-friendly light source compared to traditional laser setups. This innovation allowed for better noise suppression and enhanced signal quality, particularly in live-cell and tissue imaging, by stabilizing the power and phase of the laser output. Combined with their methods to minimize the NRB, the fibre laser-based SRS system became a practical and powerful tool for real-time, high-contrast imaging in biomedical research and clinical diagnostics.

SRS images are captured at 2845 cm^{-1} and 2930 cm^{-1} using the portable setup shown in figure 8.2(a) relating to information from the CH_2 and CH_3 chemical bonds, respectively. In figure 8.2(b) virtually stained SRH images are compared with corresponding H&E images for low-grade and anaplastic brain tissue sample; the MRI image on the left indicates the region from which this tissue was been excised. Brain surgery is a particularly suitable application for real-time SRH due to the need to carefully and accurately identify tumour margins during surgery. A key component in the SRH system is the image processing method that takes as input the two wavenumber images and produces as output a convincing virtually stained H&E-like image. This image processing method is illustrated in figures 8.2 (c)–(i). The 2845 cm^{-1} (CH_2) and 2930 cm^{-1} (CH_3) recordings are shown in figures 8.2(c) and (d). The data from each recording is placed in a separate channel of a two-channel image. A blurred version of the two-channel image is generated by performing a Gaussian blur, the initial unblurred image is then divided by the blurred image to remove artefacts in either acquisition or tissue preparation producing a new denoised two-channel image. A nucleic index is generated by subtracting the channels of the new denoised two-channel image (corresponding to CH_3–CH_2) shown in figure 8.2(e). The next step is to create an RGB image using these two channels. A simple example of creating an RGB image from the nucleic map and the denoised 2845 cm^{-1} image is shown in figure 8.2(f) where in this case the two channels are mapped to a blue scale and a green scale, respectively. Creating a convincing virtual H&E image requires a more nuanced approach in mapping to the RGB colours. The virtual H&E image is generated by taking each channel independently and mapping these to two different RGB colour schemes, followed by combining the two RGB images. The 2845 cm^{-1} CH_2 image pixel intensity is linearly related to a white to pink colour scale. Separately, the CH_2–CH_3 image pixel intensity is linearly mapped to a white to purple colour scale. The combined RGB image is shown in figure 8.2(g) and compared with the real H&E image in figure 8.2(h). Each of these images contains 1024×1024 pixels. Given the high-speed of data aquisition for SRH, it is possible to scan the slide capturing a large grid and generating mosaic image of a wide field of tissue as shown in figure 8.2(i).

The Xie group has utilized this method in a variety of studies [32–36] demonstrating the ability of stimulated Raman histology to be used as a diagnostic tool both by histopathologists by providing real-time H&E images in surgery as well and in conjunction with computational methods for automated diagnosis.

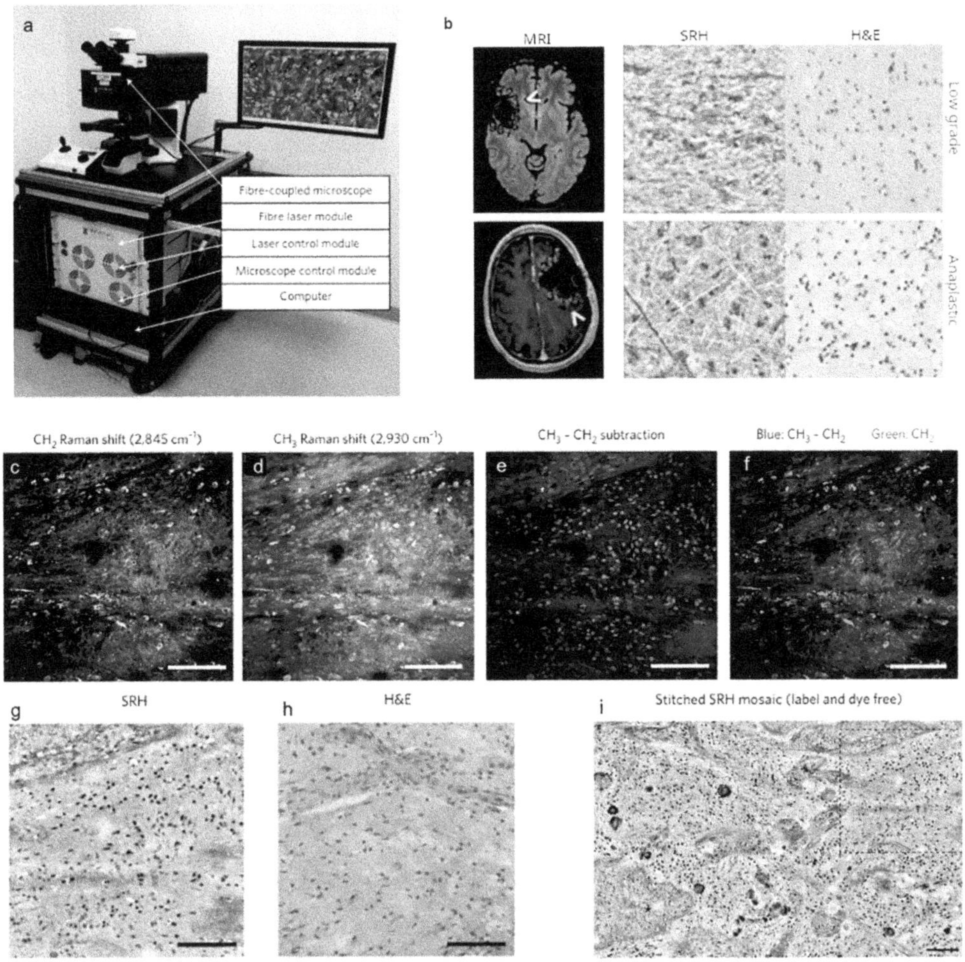

Figure 8.2. (a) Invenio Imaging SRS system In operating room; (b) MRI of recurrent oligodendroglioma and glioblastoma side by side with comparison of virtually stained SRH and true H&E images. The remaining image parts relate to the virtual staining method: (c,d) Individual wavenumber rasters of 2845 cm^{-1} and 2930 cm^{-1} relating to CH_2 and CH_3, respectively; (e) subtraction of these two images. (f) False colour composite where the blue band is the CH_2–CH_3 and green the CH_2. (g) The false colour composite image is input to a look-up table to produce the virtually stained SRH image; (h) True H&E stained image for comparison. (i) The system records a grid of NxN images which are then stitched together to form a large mosaic SRH image. (a), (c) and (d) reprinted by permission from Springer Nature Customer Service Centre GmbH: Springer Nature, Nature Biomedical Engineering, [1], copyright 2017. (b) Reproduced from [32] CC BY 4.0.

8.3.3 Virtual hematoxylin, eosin and saffron colouring—the Rigneault group [2]

Separately, the Rigneault group has also focused on SRH using a bespoke stimulated Raman system and using more complex image processing methods [2, 29, 31]. The key methods for virtual staining proposed by the Rigneault group are shown in figure 8.3 below. This includes a novel optical system, as shown in

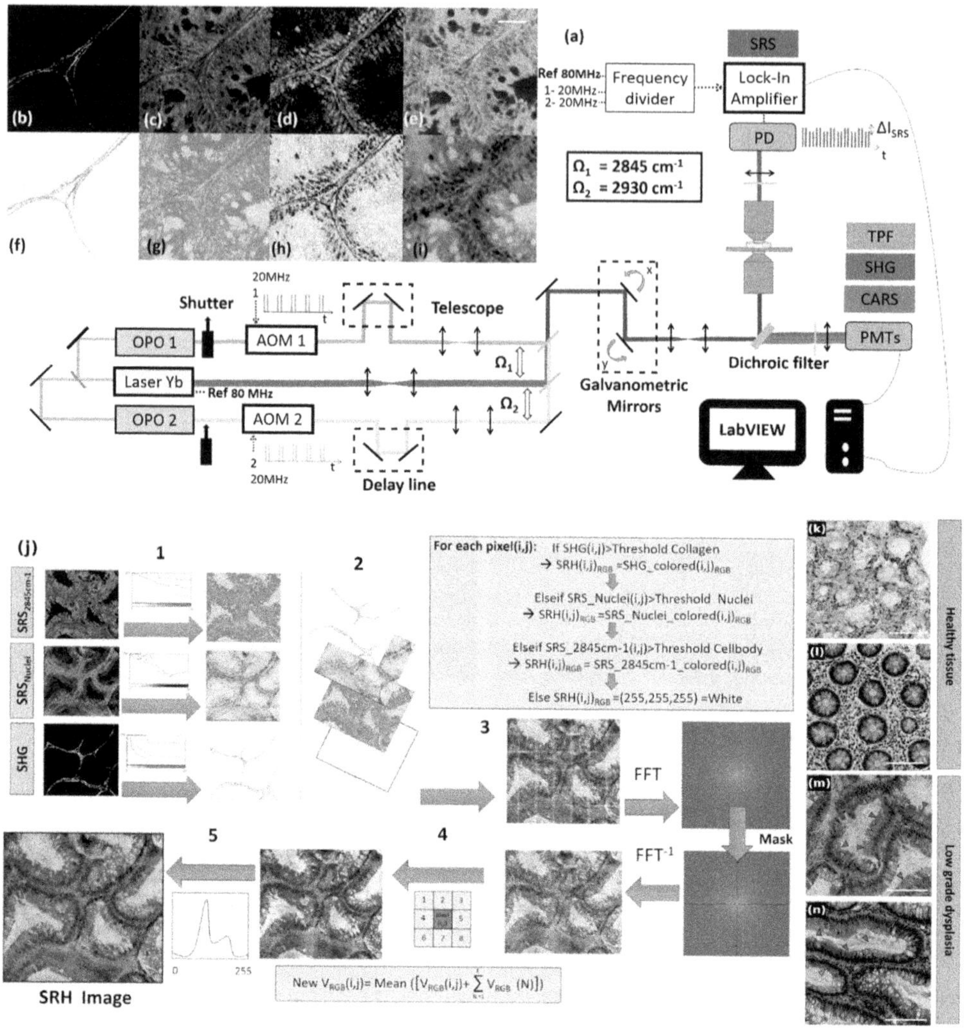

Figure 8.3. [2] (a) Optical diagram of FM-SRS, TPEF/CARS and SHG capable system. (b–d) Grayscale images relating to SHG, 2845 cm^{-1} and (2930 cm^{-1}–2845 cm^{-1}). (e) A simple histologically relevant visualization of collagen, lipids/proteins and nuclei by combining the three greyscale images previously mentioned as the channels in an RGB image. (f–h) Colour images generated from the previously described grayscale images, mapped to orange (collagen), pink and violet (lipids/proteins and nuclei). (i) A virtual HES image generated by hierarchically superimposing the three coloured images described previously. (j, 1–5) Illustration of the algorithm used to generate a large virtually stained HES image; see text for further details. This figure has been reproduced from figures 1–3 [2] CC BY 4.0.

figure 8.3(a), which combines multiple imaging modalities, including both stimulated Raman and SHG in their virtual staining method. The SRS setup uses a mode-locked ytterbium (Yb) fibre laser operating at 1031 nm as a Stokes beam. Two OPOs are tuned to different wavelengths (797.3 nm and 792.2 nm) to probe the CH_2 and CH_3 vibrations making use of the same two wavenumbers used by the Xie group.

These beams are recombined and scanned across tissue samples to create high-resolution images. There are, however, a number of advancements over the methods used by the Xie group. Firstly, the authors introduce a method called frequency-modulated SRS (FM-SRS); whereas traditional SRS requires the two wavenumbers (2845 cm^{-1} for CH_2 and 2930 cm^{-1} for CH_3) images to be recorded sequentially and the difference to be calculated, FM-SRS enables the difference to be recorded directly using a single-channel lock-in amplifier, thereby speeding up the process. This is achieved by setting a 180° phase between AOM_1 and AOM_2 shown in the figure. As well as speed, another advantage of this approach is lower noise. Noise can accumulate during the separate sequential imaging processes, therefore the capturing of two wavenumber signals in a single acquisition may reduce noise by minimizing time between measurements and reducing the likelihood of noise interference from external factors or sample movement. In using the FM-SRS modality it is possible to simultaneously record a CARS signal, TPEF, SHG and SRS, the latter two being utilized for virtual staining.

The algorithm demonstrated in figure 8.3(j) illustrates the virtual staining algorithm in λ-switch mode, as described in [2], and will be discussed in that context in the next paragraph. Figure 8.3(b–i) show the virtual hematoxylin, eosin and saffron (HES) staining method being applied to standard λ-switch SRS in which the 2845 cm^{-1} and 2930 cm^{-1} are recorded sequentially by alternating between OPO 1 and OPO 2. Figure 8.3(b) shows the SHG image, which is particularly useful for visualizing non-centrosymmetric and highly ordered molecular arrangements such as those found in collagen [37]. Figure 8.3(c) shows the 2845 cm^{-1} a signal in the CH_2 region relating to proteins/lipids. Finally figure 8.3(d) shows the subtraction: 2930 cm^{-1}–2845 cm^{-1}. Figure 8.3(e) demonstrates a false colour composite built by combining these three greyscale images into a standard RGB image. Figure 8.3(f–g) illustrates the colour layers generated by applying colour maps to the greyscale images (b,c,d): orange for the SHG, pink for the 2845 cm^{-1} (CH_2) and dark blue for the 2930 cm^{-1}–2845 cm^{-1} (nucleic map). A virtually stained patch is the combination of these images, as shown in figure 8.3(i). The method for producing a full-scale virtual label-free HES-like image is described below. (k) Shows a virtually stained healthy tissue, contrasted with (l) which is a true HES stained image. (m) Similarly shows a virtual HES image of low-grade dysplasia contrasted with with (n) a true HES image.

In order for the methods to be clinically relevant, it is necessary to produce wide-field virtually stained images for the clinician. This is achieved by recording and processing a grid of smaller virtually stained images, followed by stitching these images together into a large mosaic. However, this approach can result in discontinuities at the borders and to mitigate this problem further image processing is required. The full pipeline is illustrated in figure 8.3(j). Starting with Step 1, where a colour gradient from white to a targeted colour is generated: orange to mimic a saffron dye for collagen, pink to mimic eosin, and dark blue to mimic hematoxylin. In Step 2, we see the hierarchically exclusive composition of the colour maps applied to each individual pixel. For each channel, there is a user-adjustable threshold, of the form K times the mean of the given channel with the constraint $0 < K < 2$. The user may adjust the value of K to increase or decrease sensitivity of the given channel. Should the pixel value be above a defined threshold, the colour corresponding to the channel will be set. If the pixel is not accepted by the first threshold it will go on to the next. Should none of the channel's values be accepted by the corresponding thresholds the pixel will default to white. This sequence of steps is applied to each of the smaller images, and the results are stitched accordingly. Step 3 is the stitching step. This involves a filter in the spatial frequency domain, whereby the discrete Fourier transform (DFT) of the image is calculated using an FFT algorithm, followed by multiplication with a cross-hair mask and an inverse DFT. This process helps to remove obvious linear discontinuities between neighbouring 100 μm^2 images. Step 4 involves a standard box blur being applied to smooth the image and a final user guided colour correction may be applied via histogram to better match a standard HES image in Step 5.

Figure 8.3(k) shows a virtual HES image of a healthy tissue sample contrasted with figure 8.3(l) a ground truth image from a similar region. Similarly, figure 8.3(m) shows a virtual HES image of a low-grade dysplasia contrasted with figure 8.3(n), the corresponding ground truth physically stained image. In both cases the virtually generated label-free images bear a convincing similarity to their labelled counterparts, albeit with some subtle variations in colour intensity and contrast. Variations of these types can be effectively addressed using methods of style transfer and deep learning, which are reviewed in the next section.

8.4 Virtual staining with style transfer

8.4.1 Overview

In the previous section we reviewed methods for mapping from a stimulated Raman label-free image to an image that is visually similar to a labelled H&E or HES histological image using procedural algorithms that map from specific Raman wavenumbers to various colour maps. While these methods are advantageous in terms of computational time as well as the existence of a clear chemical link between the label and label-free images, there is, however, the disadvantage of variable results in terms of subtle variations in colour intensity and contrast when comparing the label-free and labelled images. This can be mitigated to an extent using manual tuning of the procedural algorithms. To better address these issues, deep learning based image-to-image translation methods have been investigated, which can be collectively described as style transfer methods. Style transfer [38] is a field within machine learning involving the algorithmic manipulation of an image's semantic content to embody the stylistic characteristics of another. While many style transfer techniques originated in image synthesis and have traditionally been associated with artistic, design, and entertainment applications, their utility has expanded into the realm of data augmentation and analysis. Notably, in the domain of histology, researchers have begun to leverage style transfer methodologies to transform between a variety of sensing modalities, such as bright-field microscopy with staining agents. Raman spectroscopy is no exception to this, and novel approaches hold significant promise for enhancing data interpretability and potentially uncovering new insights within histological studies.

Early style transfer networks utilized a dual loss function based on minimizing (1) the difference between extracted features of a given input image with a newly generated image, and (2) the differences in the co-occurrences of feature matrices from the generated image to the target style image [39]. While there were significant successes with this methodology, it often led to local artefacts that detracted from the verisimilitude of the generated images. Adversarial approaches quickly emerged that were less prone to this issue in the form of generator-adversary network (GAN) architectures. In the GAN architecture a generator would produce novel images and place it within a collection of original images, i.e. a set of true images and generated images. The generator architecture works in tandem with a discriminator architecture; The loss applied to the generator is based on how well the discriminator is fooled into misclassifying the generated image as a true image. The end result is a greater emphasis on global contexts within an image. Unfortunately these GAN networks even in the context of style transfer were more likely to hallucinate features locally in order to maintain the global context. In an attempt to maintain the increased global context and simultaneously bolster local accuracy the cycle consistent GAN architecture emerged [40]. The core idea in the CycleGAN architecture is to devise a two-way transfer between domains with dual-generators and discriminators where a mapping is only successful if it can translate from domain A to domain B, and independently be translated from domain B back to domain A in such a way that the image $Ax_i \mapsto Bx_i$ and $Bx_i \mapsto Ax_i$. Recently, these methods have been applied to produce virtual staining using SRS (and other forms of nonlinear spectroscopy) images, and these contributions are described in the subsequent sections. While the procedural methods explored earlier have no need of co-registered label-free and matching labelled data, traditional generative deep learning methods often do have this requirement. One of the significant advantages of the CycleGAN is its potential to circumvent this need by utilizing the full cyclical mapping from the original domain to the transformed and back to original. The total differences between the original image and its regenerated counterpart provide reasonable ground truth, ensuring no information necessary to reproduce itself was lost while translating the image style between the two domains.

8.4.2 Computational tissue staining—the Blocklitz group [3]

In their work on computational tissue staining, the Blocklitz group were the first to transfer nonlinear microscopy (NLM) images to histopathologically stained H&E images in an unsupervised manner. They contrasted the semi-supervised conditional GAN (CondGAN) model with the unsupervised cycle consistent conditional GAN (CycleCGAN) model to explore the potential for label-free style transfer methods with nonlinear microscopy.

Initially, a series of NLM images are recorded where signals relating to CARS, TPEF and SHG are used to generate a false colour composite by setting each as the channels in an RGB image. An example of these images is seen in figure 8.4(A) and

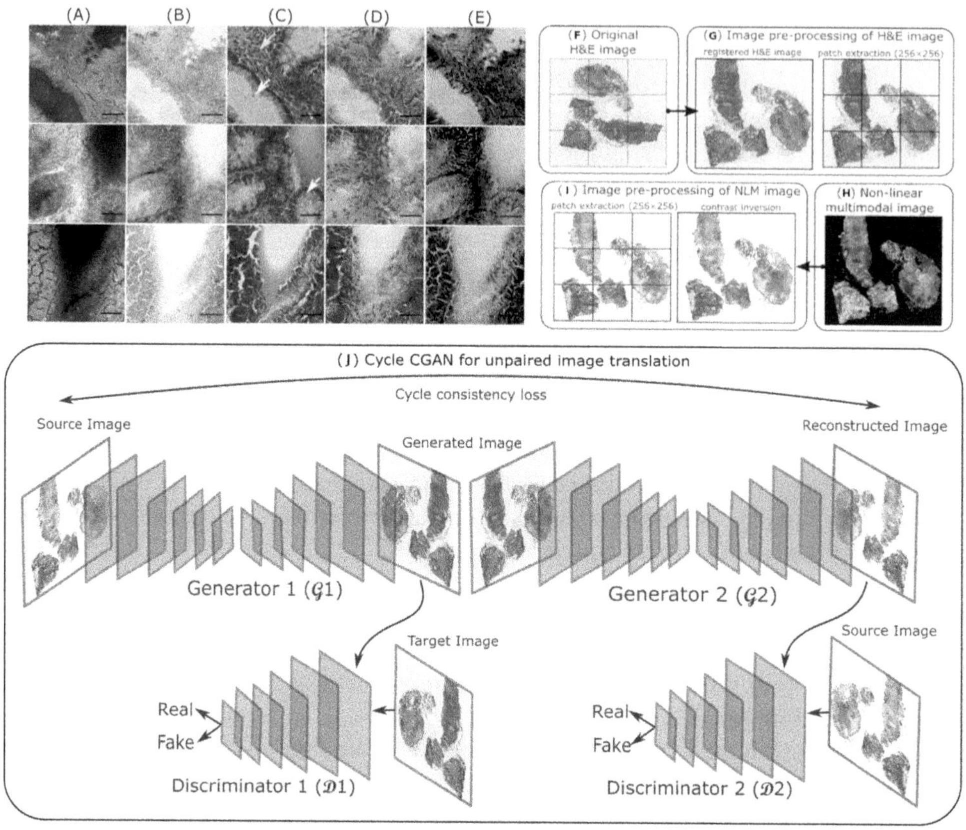

Figure 8.4. (A) False colour composites relating the CARS,TPEF and SHG to RGB channels. (B) Inverted false colour composites to better match an H&E colour distribution. (C) True H&E images recorded via bright-field microscopy. (D) Virtual H&E stain generated via conditional GAN and (E) virtual H&E generated via CycleGAN. (F-H) Illustration of the preprocessing steps undertaken. (F) Shows the raw H&E input image. (G) Illustrates the image registration to NLM data and 256×256 patch extraction. (H) The initial false colour composite of CARS, TPEF and SHG before contrast inversion. (J) Illustrates the conditional GAN architecture. (K) Illustrates the CycleGAN architecture figure Reproduced from figures 2 and 3 in [3] CC BY 4.0.

(H). In order to aid the training using colour styles close to that of an H&E style, these false colour composites are inverted, moving from red and green hues, to purples, and blues. Ground truth images of H&E stains are also recorded via bright-field microscopy, examples of which can be seen in figure 8.4(C). The inverted false colour composite images are passed through both a CondGAN and a CycleGAN where H&E-resembling virtually stained images are produced. Examples of this can be seen in figure 8.4 (D) for the conditional GAN and (E) for the CycleGAN. As is visually apparent between the images generated by both networks, they achieve comparable results despite the lack of paired images for the CycleGAN.

Before discussing the networks themselves we will briefly discuss the preprocessing methods as shown in figure 8.4(F–H) The images were prepared such that both inputs should match in terms of both pixel count and pixel size. The NLM images were recorded with a pixel size of 0.227 μm^2, and the bright-field microscopy images 0.219 μm^2. The H&E images were registered to align with the NLM data, an example of this translation can be seen in figure 8.4(F–G). Non-overlapping image patches of pixel count 256 × 256 were extracted from both datasets as shown in figure 8.4(G) for H&E and figure 8.4(I) for NLM images. The inversion of the false colour composites discussed earlier is implemented before patch extraction in order to better match the initial input image to the expected colour distribution of the histopathologically stained H&E image.

The CondGAN, while taking significantly less time to train, requires strongly supervised input data with images that share spatial dimensions, resolution and are co-registered to one another. As shown in equation (8.1) and figure 8.4(J) there are two sources of loss in the CondGAN, the conditional loss and the discriminator loss.

$$L_{\text{Generator}} = \underbrace{\lambda MAE(z_{\text{generated}}, z_{\text{target}})}_{\text{Conditional Loss}} + \underbrace{(1 - D(z_{\text{generated}}))}_{\text{Discriminator Loss}} \tag{8.1}$$

$$L_{\text{Discriminator}} = \underbrace{D(z_{\text{generated}})^2}_{\text{Generated input mislabelled}} + \underbrace{(1 - D(z_{\text{target}}))^2}_{\text{Real input mislabelled}} \tag{8.2}$$

The conditional loss is given by the mean absolute error between the image generated and the known paired target image for the given input. This is followed by the inversion of the discriminator loss. This is because the discriminator component of the generator loss is determined by how frequently the generator fools the discriminator. The architectures used for the generator and discriminator were selected from the available literature. In the case of the discriminator it was based on the PatchGAN architecture first proposed by Isola *et al* [41]. The generator was inspired by the U-NET model, an autoencoder with skip connections between encoder and decoder layers of corresponding dimensions [42].

The Blocklitz group compared this CondGAN with CycleCGAN, the latter having the significant advantage of not requiring directly paired data. This can be described by the loss function given in equation (8.3) and figure 8.4(K). The structure of the discriminator for the cycle was kept mainly the same, a discriminator based on the PatchGAN architecture such that the final layer is not fully connected allowing for back-propagation to select areas. A generator architecture that favoured a RESNET model over the previous U-NET. In this RESNET model, residual connections are used in the bottleneck but no skip connections exist between the encoder/decoder layers of equivalent dimensions [43].

The CycleCGAN total loss can be given by the following

$$L_{\text{total}} = \underbrace{L_{(D1)}(G_1, D_1, X, Y)}_{\text{Discriminator 1 loss}} + \underbrace{L_{(id1)}(G_1, D_1, X)}_{id\text{ loss}} + \underbrace{\lambda L_{(\text{cycf})}(G_1, G_2)}_{\text{Forward Cycle Consistency}} + \underbrace{\lambda L_{(\text{cycb})}(G1, G2)}_{\text{Backwards Cycle Consistency}} \tag{8.3}$$

In this formulation the H&E domain discriminator loss is once again defined as the mean squared error between the discriminator predictions of authenticity and their corresponding inverted accuracy. Inspired by the conditional GAN an *id* loss term is added; however, this time no ground truth is required as the *id* loss calculates mean squared difference between the input image and generated image, thus guarding against changes of the image content. The forward cycle consistency measures the mean squared difference between an input image and a cyclical generation of the same domain. That is to say, a nonlinear microscopy image will be compared with the translation of the H&E generated by the first generator after it has been regenerated by the second generator back into a nonlinear microscopy image, and the same for the backwards cycle consistency with the domains inverted. These cycle consistency terms ensure that the information required to translate from one domain to another is preserved.

8.4.3 Stimulated Raman CycleGan—the Ji group [4]

While the previous methods used frozen H&E samples for training and validation, formalin-fixed and paraffin embedded (FFPE) H&E staining is currently considered the gold standard for histopathology. This is because it is demonstrably better at preserving tissue architecture and cellular detail, it also allows for thinner samples that are more in line with the vertical focal area of nonlinear microscopy systems. However, frozen samples are often prefferred in surgical situations due to the foreshortened timeframe for analysis. The Frozen H&E staining process takes in the proximity of 45 min, while FFPE can take longer than 36 h. The Ji group developed a routine to produce FFPE appearing images using SRS in shorter time than either the frozen H&E or the FFPE staining methods. The acquisition time and subsequent style transfer of a nonlinear microscopy image taking in the vicinity of 3 min according to the author's estimates.

Image-to-image translation between SRS microscopy and FFPE H&E staining presents a significant challenge for paired networks. This difficulty arises from the interference of the paraffin Raman signal, which obscures the signals of interest and hinders the establishment of accurate ground truth for supervised training. To address these limitations, Ji *et al* developed a stimulated Raman CycleGAN (SRC-GAN) figure 8.5(a) based on a modified CycleGAN architecture. Their key innovation was the incorporation of a dynamic training domain that includes both strongly and weakly supervised elements.

As SRC-GAN is designed to map between two image domains, corresponding datasets were required for training. The SRS dataset was acquired using a dual-phase lock-in detection SRS system. A series of brain tissue lipid and protein (L&P) false colour composite images were generated using two-colour SRS microscopy at two Raman frequencies: 2845 cm^{-1} (CH_2 stretching vibration) and 2930 cm^{-1} (CH_3 stretching vibration). The H&E dataset was generated through two approaches. First, true FFPE H&E images were acquired using a bright-field microscope equipped with a CCD. Mosaic images were captured and stitched together to create large whole-slide images of the stained tissue. Second, virtual H&E images were generated by applying H&E look-up tables to the L&P false colour composites, providing strongly supervised training data.

Figure 8.5(a) Shows the basic structure of the CycleGAN network with the SRS lipid and protein false colour composites as the first domain, and the virtual FFPE images as the second domain. In the standard CycleGAN form there are two pairs of

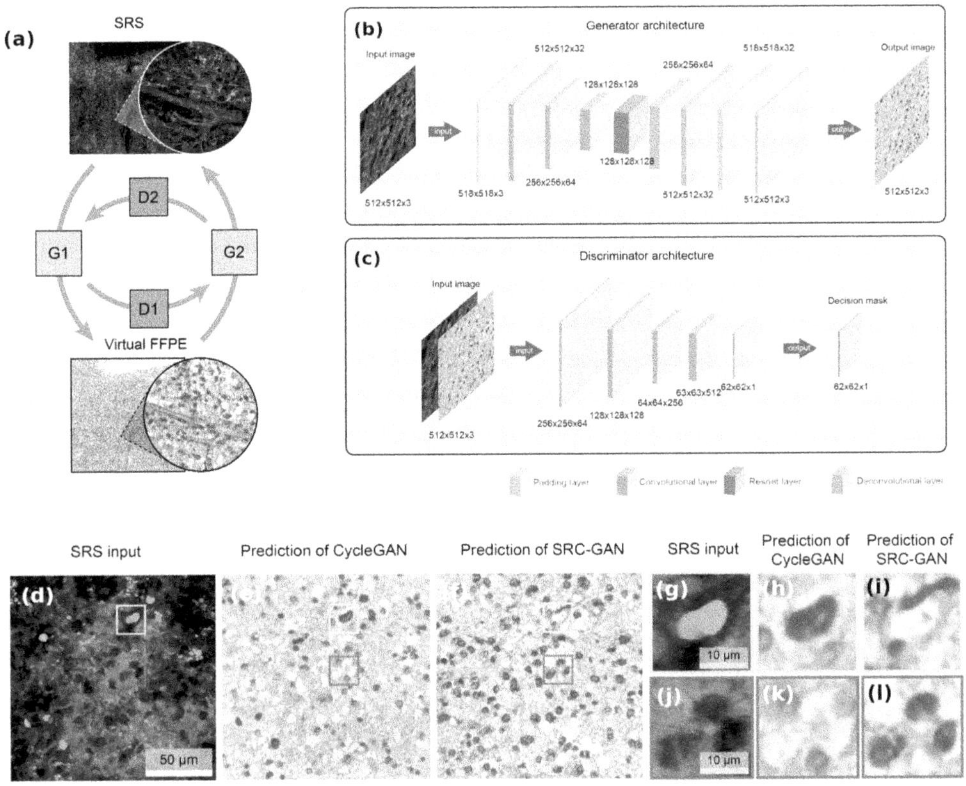

Figure 8.5. (a) An illustration of the CycleGAN structure between the SRS image domain and virtual FFPE domain. (b) A diagram of the generator CNN architecture. (c) Diagram of the discriminator architecture. (d) Lipid and protein false colour composite. (e) Traditional CycleGAN generated image. (f) SRC-GAN generated image. (g–l) Close-up of two mismap errors highlighted between source SRS image, CycleGan prediction and SRC-GAN prediction. Figure reproduced from figures 1 and 2 in [4], reprinted with permission from AAAS.

generators and discriminators. The first for mapping from the SRS domain to the H&E domain, the second to map the inverse. For each input H&E image the total loss is that of the generators' ability to overcome the discriminator and the total difference between the original image and the twice transformed image. Real H&E data from the second domain are treated similarly, translated to the SRS lipid and protein false colour composites and tested by the second discriminator, and cycled back through G1 where a cycle consistency loss is used to compare the newly generated H&E image with the initial input. As such, the loss can be formulated as below in equation (8.4).

$$\text{Loss}_{\text{Generator}_\text{A}} = \underbrace{\text{MSE}(D_B(G_A(X)), \text{real\_mask})}_{\text{Generated Image Classified as Original}} + \underbrace{\text{L1\_loss}(X, G_B(G_A(X)))}_{\text{Cycle Consistency Loss}} \tag{8.4}$$

$$\text{Loss}_{\text{Discriminator}_\text{A}} = \underbrace{\text{MSE}(D_a(G_B(Y)), \text{fake\_mask})}_{\text{Failure to Identify generated image}} + \underbrace{\text{MSE}(X, \text{real\_mask})}_{\text{Failure to identify real image}} \tag{8.5}$$

Where the ability of the generator is measured by the minimization of the mean squared error between the real mask and the discriminators' predicted mask for generated images. This is followed by a cycle consistency term, in this case the rectilinear distance between the generated image and its initial source. The discriminators' loss is given as the mean squared error between the discriminators' prediction of the generated images and the false mask summed with the mean squared error of the original images and the true mask. Generator B follows the same logic with the opposite domains and generator/discriminator pairs. Unlike for the GAN developed by the Blocklitz group, no *id* loss term was used for regularization.

The structure of the generator and discriminator architectures are illustrated in figure 8.5(b) and (c), Where the generator is an autoencoder comprised of an initial padded layer followed by three convolutional layers, each with a 3×3 kernel. The padding layers were incorporated to assist with poor edge mapping. A residual architectural layer was used before deconvolution to enable the network to map both linearly and nonlinearly. This is particularly useful in the context of style transfer where the nonlinear transformations are likely to capture complex relationships and the linear mappings allow for preservation of image content. The discriminator is a classifier based on PatchGAN [41]. This discriminator is fully convolutional with 4×4 kernels. Decision labels and output dimensions are kept the same to allow varying dimensions to the input images. This discriminator provides an output array of values rather than a single scalar, enabling the discriminator to pay closer attention to more refined segments.

To aid the network in learning correct mapping despite the lack of real ground truth, a dynamic training set was used to set the initial direction of the networks learning in a strongly supervised manner. These strongly supervised samples are slowly dominated by additional weakly supervised data until eventually they are completely phased out. The strongly supervised samples used are SRS images and virtually stained H&E images. The weakly supervised samples contain true SRS false colour composites and FFPE H&E images. The authors highlight that this dynamic training set was utilized to address a common pitfall of traditional CycleGANs whereby incorrect mappings can be learned due to the significant difference in colour styles and contrast mechanisms between the two modalities. Two common examples of these mapping errors are highlighted in figures 8.5(g)–(l); lipid droplets being mismapped to cell nuclei and nuclei mismapped to common voids.

As can be seen in figures 8.5(g–l), the SRC-GAN predictions (i) and (l) appear to be significantly better than the traditional CycleGAN predictions (h) and (k). While true FFPEs were diagnosed equally accurately or more accurately by histologists in the study, the stimulated Raman virtual histology generated from the SRC-GAN significantly outperformed the frozen H&E in terms of accurate diagnosis and approached close to that of the FFPE.

8.5 Automated diagnosis with SRH

8.5.1 Overview

The virtual staining methods explored earlier hold great utility for enabling intra-operative pathological tissue imaging. This is achieved by mitigating time-consuming bottlenecks and providing FFPE-H&E (like) gold standard images using frozen tissue. However, the pathologist is still required to interpret these virtually stained images and there currently exists a global shortage in the number of histopathologists. In intra-operative scenarios it is also preferable to avoid the need for an additional on-site clinician, additionally another concern is that it is well known that pathologists can produce variable diagnostics. For these reasons, a growing corpus of work has been built to not only reduce time required to generate usable imagery for diagnosis, but also to automate the diagnosis process itself based on these images. In this section we review several recently proposed methods to do this. The question of automated diagnosis can generally be viewed as a classification problem and as such there are many viable machine learning methods that can be utilized to address it, including, multilayer perceptrons (MLPs), random forests, and support vector machines. These methods can be applied to the virtually stained imagery generated with the previously explored methods and/or the relevant spectra themselves without the need to produce RGB images. Research has been carried out in a wide number of examples.

8.5.2 Multi-layer perceptrons [1]

The intra-operative image data required for diagnosis and clinical decision making can be produced using Raman-based virtual staining methods, as described in earlier sections. However the interpretation of this data can still be costly in terms of time and prone to variability of diagnosis by different histopathologists. To produce more quantitative analysis of tissue attributes, the Orringer group proposed the use of a MLP for interpreting and classifying the SRS microscopy images automatically with an appropriate diagnosis. MLPs are feed forward neural networks with a minimum of three layers, an input layer, one or more hidden layers and an output layer. Each node except for those in the input layer, are neurons that utilize a nonlinear activation function. The inputs to the activation functions are updated with weights and biases throughout training, where the weights control how sensitive each neuron is to changes in the input and the biases control the threshold for activation. In an MLP, attempting to classify between more than two classes, the output layer has as many nodes as there are classes. The neurons in this layer utilize a softmax activation function (equation (8.6)) to transform the raw output values into a probability distribution, ensuring that all neurons have values between 0 and 1, and their sum adds to 1. In a supervised manner the network is trained to produce these probability values for each of the final nodes based on the loss between the output probabilities and the known labels for each input by back-propagation the difference between the supervised label of an input with the predicted output neuron.

$$\sigma(\mathbf{z})_i = \frac{e^{z_i}}{\sum_{j=1}^{K} e^{z_j}} \qquad \text{for } i = 1, \ldots, N \tag{8.6}$$

The Orringer group generated a labelled dataset of SRH images. This dataset was generated by imaging biopsies from neurosurgical patients undergoing tumour resection, imaged immediately following removal, via an SRS microscopy system at the 2845 cm^{-1} and 2930 cm^{-1} wavenumbers. SRH images were generated following the procedural methods developed by the Xie group for virtual staining explored in section 8.3.2. The data for training the MLP was a subset of the total 101 neurosurgical patients with a total of 12,879 $400\mu \times 400\mu$ SRH fields of view (FOVs). Of these, 30 patients were used for training the MLP. A sample of a mosaic with visible FOV grid lines can be seen in figure 8.6(a).

The Orringer group utilized a well-known image processing library 'WND-CHRM' to extract a total of 2919 image attributes from each FOV. These features (included statistical features such as the mean and variance), texture features

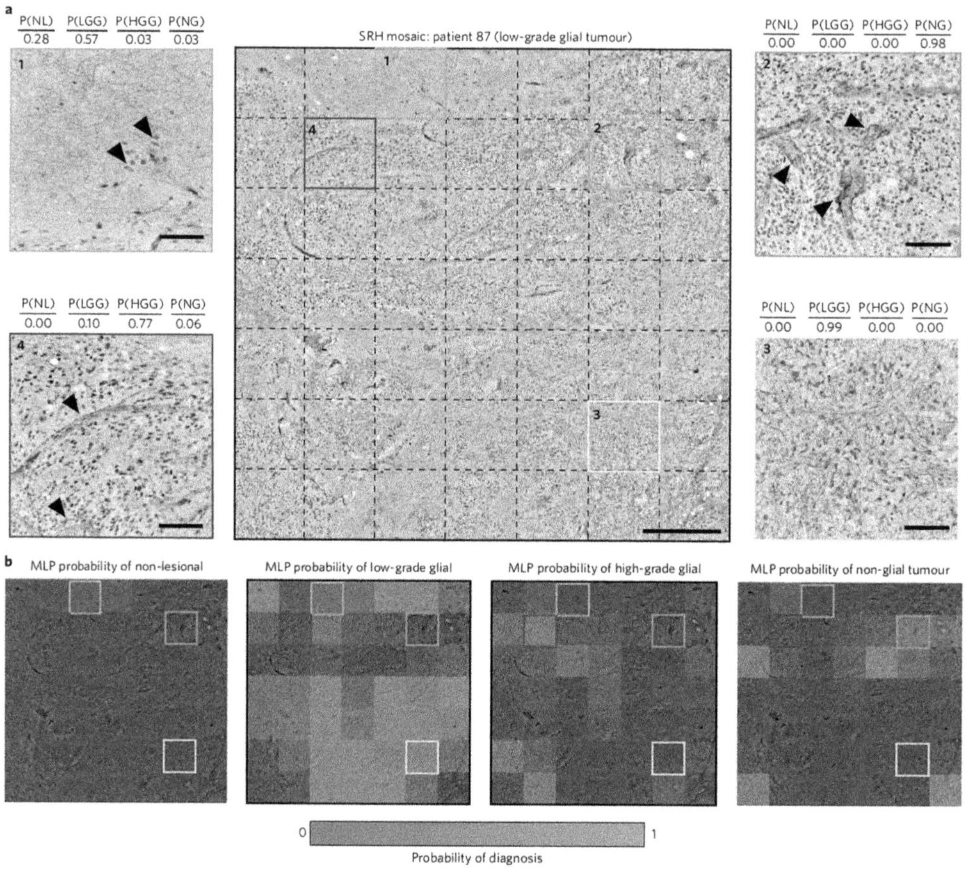

Figure 8.6. (a) An SRH mosaic with its corresponding field of view (FOV) grid lines. Four enlarged, colour-coded sample FOVs (1–4) are shown either side of the mosaic, highlighting specific regions of interest. Each enlarged FOV is accompanied by the diagnostic class probabilities: P(NL) for non-lesional, P(LGG) for low-grade glial, P(HGG) for high-grade glial, and P(NG) for non-glial tumours. (b) The four heatmaps represent the overall diagnostic classification probabilities across the entire SRH mosaic. The four colour-coded FOVs from (a) are also indicated on each heatmap. In this particular case, the modal diagnosis can be seen by the eye and is correct as a low-grade glial tumour. This figure was reproduced from figure 6 in [1], reprinted by permission from Springer Nature Customer Service Centre GmbH: Springer Nature, Nature Biomedical Engineering, copyright 2017.

calculated from co-occurence matrices (including contrast, correlation, energy and homogeneity), geometric features (such as area, perimeter and compactness of an image region), and wavelet features (that capture frequency information at different scales). Normalized image attributes were fed to the MLP for training which utilized the leave-one-out approach, thus maximizing the size of the training set and mitigating risks of overfitting. The final output of the MLP was a probability vector where each neuron in the output layer gave a value for the learned probability that the input data belonged to the diagnostic classes: non-lesional, low-grade glial, high-grade glial or non-glial tumour. The authors highlight these four classes in particular as being particularly significant in decision making during brain tumour surgeries. Figure 8.6(a) Displays the probabilities of four FOVs extracted from a larger stimulated Raman histology mosaic with associated probability values for each of the four key diagnoses. In this instance the SRH is taken from a sample with low-grade glial tumour. Where some patches show significant probabilities of the low-grade glial tumour diagnosis, such as figure 8.6(a-3), some of the individual patches show strong confidences to the contrary, for example figure 8.6(a-2), indicating a strong probability of non-glial tumour, while figure 8.6(a-4) indicates a strong probability of a high-grade glial tumour. To ensure accurate diagnoses after all patches are classified by the MLP, those with a probability of less than 25% are discarded, following which the modal diagnosis is used to determine the diagnosis for the overal mosaic. Figure 8.6(b) Shows the heatmap for a low-grade glial tumour sample with respect to each of the four diagnostic classes. While there are patches classified with high probabilities of being non-glial or high-grade and some lower probabilities of non-lesional, it is apparent by the heatmap that the low-grade glial is the dominant diagnosis in this case.

Overall this study provided a compelling proof of concept on the applicability of MLPs for automated diagnosis, with an accuracy of 100% in classifying lesional from non-lesional samples, and 90% in classifying glial from non-glial tumours. The predictions of the MLP were well in accordance with that of the pathologists survey with a 90% correspondence. The MLP did misclassify a number of cases due to subtle differences in tissue, or limited tumour presence in the analyzed FOVs. These examples highlight the challenge in accurately classifying cases with minimal abnormalities, or where there is an uneven distribution of diagnostically relevant features across all FOVs. Nevertheless, this work represents a significant first step in automated SRH diagnosis, with further machine learning methods to follow.

8.5.3 Random forests decision trees [5]

While MLPs have proven valuable in diagnostic applications, their inherent 'black-box' nature presents a challenge for interpretability. The complex interplay of interconnected nodes and weighted connections within MLPs often obscures the underlying decision-making process, making it difficult to understand how specific inputs contribute to the 'diagnosis'. In contrast to this, decision trees offer a transparent model of the decision making process. They achieve this by providing a visual representation of the tree structure clearly delineating the decision nodes and the specific conditions employed at each step to arrive at a classification. Decision trees are supervised learning algorithms often used for either classification or regression. They work by partitioning data into subsets based on the attribute values, with the end goal of homogeneity within each subset. The partitioning process is represented as a tree with nodes and branches, each branch representing the outcome of a decision and the final leaf nodes representing the predicted outcome. While simpler decision trees are readily interpretable, random forest comprises multiple decision trees in which each tree is trained on a subset of the data, generated by using a method called bootstrapping, in which a new dataset is constructed by randomly sampling the initial dataset, thus allowing for duplicates and missing data points. The average output value from all trees in a random forest is used to calculate the final prediction (modal for discrete predictions and arithmetic mean for continuous). This can lead to intricate interactions between the trees, potentially obscuring the overall decision logic. However, random forests still offer insights into the model's behaviour by revealing the relative importance of different features and the general patterns used for classification. Recently random forest decision trees have been applied to SRH images.

Orringer *et al* acquired 25 SRH images at two wavenumbers (2845 cm^{-1} and 2930 cm^{-1}). Computational staining was performed using the methods described in section 8.3.2. 'CellProfiler' software was employed to segment individual nuclei and tumour-associated macrophages (TAMs) in the SRH images based on morphological features such as size, shape, and intensity. Following segmentation, CellProfiler was further utilized to extract key histological features, examples of which are illustrated in figure 6(a)[1] of [5]. These features included nuclear density, TAM density, and a variety of nuclear morphology descriptors: area, perimeter, eccentricity, minimum and maximum Feret diameter, compactness, solidity, form factor, extent, orientation, and maximum radius.

The authors used these extracted features to train two random forest classifiers; the first for classifying whether a sample is normal or lesional tissue, and the second for classifying between high-grade and low-grade tissue. In total 25 full SRH images were used for the model development and validation using 10-fold cross-validation, whereby the data is divided into 10 equal parts and a model is trained on nine parts of these and tested on the remaining part. This process is repeated 10 times, with each part used for testing once. The 'caret' package in R was used for model training and the 10-fold cross-validation. The 'mtry' parameter in a random forest controls how many features are randomly considered at each node while building a decision tree. It is tuned by evaluating the out-of-bag accuracy, i.e. by testing each tree's prediction on the data that was not included in the bootstrapped dataset used to train it. Of the two finalized random forest models, the normal/lesional classifier had a 93.8%±2.2% accuracy, and the low-grade/high-grade classifier had a 89.4%±1.9%. Once each patch was classified, the predicted diagnosis for a whole slide was calculated based on the modal diagnosis across all FOVs. An example of this is given

[1] Could not be reproduced due to copyright concerns.

in figure 7 (a)[2] where the heatmaps for both predictive decisions are given with 53.1% of FOVs classified as lesional tissue, correctly predicting the given slide.

While the classifications themselves have utility for differentiating diagnostic categories, the authors also exploited the interpretability of the random forest models. By analyzing feature importance, they identified the most significant features contributing to the classification process. This information can guide further analysis or the development of new machine learning methods. Gini impurity was employed as the metric to calculate node impurity. The most salient features identified were nuclear density, TAM density, nuclear compactness, and maximum radius.

8.5.4 Deep convolutional networks [6]

Similar to the Blocklitz CycleCGAN generators discussed in section 8.4.2, which facilitated the transformation of 2–3 channel Raman/SHG data into histologically relevant H&E-appearing images, Ji *et al* employed a similarly inspired U-net autoencoder architecture. Their objective was to translate between two Raman modalities, specifically converting single-shot femto-SRS spectral images to dual-channel pico-SRS images. This conversion effectively recovers chemical contrast without necessitating complex optical engineering modifications. This process is illustrated in figures 8.7(a) and (b), which presents amplitude graphs and side-by-side comparisons of ground truth and predicted values.

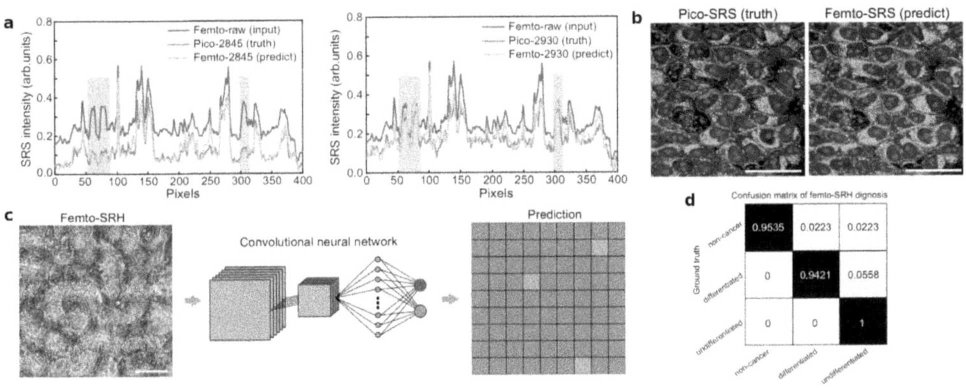

Figure 8.7. (a) Comparison of pixel intensity profiles for a single row: 2845 cm^{-1} (left) and 2930 cm^{-1} (right). The profiles correspond to the raw femtosecond SRS image (blue), the picosecond SRS ground truth (red), and the predicted values from the femtosecond SRS (yellow). (b) Comparison of the picosecond SRS false colour composite ground truth (left) and the image generated from the autoencoder-predicted values for the femtosecond SRS image (right). (c) Schematic illustration of the classification process, where a SRH image is fed into a deep CNN ending in a softmax dense layer to generate predictions. (d) Confusion matrix summarizing the performance of the classification model. This figure was reproduced from figures 2–5 in [6] CC BY 4.0.

[2] Could not be reproduced due to copyright concerns.

It is important to understand the distinction between these two modalities. Femto-SRS, employing a faster laser pulse, captures a broad range of wavenumbers and compresses them into a single intensity value. This provides a composite but less specific view of the sample's chemical composition. Conversely, pico-SRS acquires hyperspectral images by recording intensities at specific wavenumbers (e.g., 2845 cm^{1} and 2930 cm^{-1}). These wavenumbers correspond to distinct molecular vibrations, enabling the extraction of detailed chemical information and the generation of separate images for each channel. The U-net model developed by Ji *et al* was trained on paired femto-SRS and pico-SRS images of live HeLa cells and fresh gastric tissues. This training enabled the model to effectively recover chemical contrast from the femto-SRS images.

The U-net generated two-channel femto-SRS predicted image, along with a separately recorded SHG image, was used to procedurally generate an SRH image employing methods similar to those described in sections 8.3.3 and 8.2. This SRH image was primarily intended for validation by histopathologists, as the U-net outputs were used without this transformation in the training of the deep CNNs.

The Ji group employed the Inception-ResNet-v2 architecture for classification tasks. This architecture represents an advancement over the Inception family by integrating residual connections within the parallel inception modules, inspired by the ResNet architecture. These residual connections effectively address the vanishing gradient problem commonly encountered in training deep neural networks by facilitating smoother gradient flow throughout the network. This characteristic is particularly beneficial for the Inception-ResNet-v2, which consists of 572 layers, organized into distinct blocks. The input layer initially receives the raw data, which is subsequently processed by the stem layer performing initial convolution operations for feature extraction. The first significant block encountered is the Inception-ResNet-A, designed to conduct a series of parallel convolution operations, the outputs of which are concatenated. A reduction layer follows, downsampling the extensive feature set via pooling layers. This sequence is succeeded by the Inception-ResNet-B and a reduction block, leading into the Inception-ResNet-C block. Subsequently, an average pooling layer is applied to aggregate the learned features spatially before feeding these values to the fully connected layer, which comprises 1536 neurons. Although not explicitly stated by the authors, it is plausible that the final layer consisted of a single neuron with a sigmoid activation function for binary classification or two neurons with a softmax function for the two classes.

For the training step, the Ji group trained two separate classification networks on femto-SRS images from 279 patients. These images were split into 300 × 300 FOVs and fed to the network returning a classification at the FOV level, as illustrated in figure 8.7(c). The image dataset was split into training/validation and testing with a 7:3 ratio, where the training/validation set was further split into a 4:1 ratio for training to validation. The model employed five-fold cross-validation for training and validation with cross entropy loss as the loss function. Whole-slide images were classified based on thresholds from the predictions on the FOVs, with a threshold of 0.476 for cancer/non-cancer and 0.505 for differentiated/undifferentiated each determined by Youdens index.

The final confusion matrix for these networks is given in figure 8.7(d), showing that no false negatives were returned for the cancer diagnosis and a respectable number of false positives at a rate of 2.23%. Similarly for differentiated/undifferentiated cancer, the more aggressive undifferentiated cancer was never labelled as differentiated and a small proportion of the differentiated were misclassified at a rate of 5.58%. The CNNs were near-perfect in determining cancerous lesions with an accuracy of 96.4%, and of particular note were capable of outperforming the pathologists at differentiating subtypes with a 94.1% accuracy compared to an 85.3% mean accuracy for the pathologists.

8.6 The future is broadband

As we look ahead, this section presents a vision for the future of hyperspectral Raman imaging and histology. Reflecting on previous chapters, most discussions have centred around SRH, focussing on high-speed imaging using one or two SRS wavenumbers to generate H&E-like images. These images were either interpreted directly by pathologists or used as inputs for machine learning classifiers, bypassing the need for a traditional histopathological review. This significant capability, derived from just two wavenumbers, sets the stage for a broader application spectrum.

There have been some recent advancements in hyperspectral Raman imaging that enable more chemical information to be recorded, extending beyond the two-wavenumber model. This additional information could potentially enhance the SRH approach for improved automated diagnostics. One method is to scan the SRS pump wavelength during acquisition enabling multiple Raman wavenumbers to gather a broad spectral dataset quickly. This approach allows for the rapid acquisition of a hyperspectral cube where each pixel contains a full spectrum. The Graham group have applied phasor analysis to simplify this complex data into a more manageable form by transforming the time-consuming multi-dimensional spectral data into a two-dimensional graphical representation [44]. This transformation aids in the quick identification of chemical components within the tissue, enhancing drug and disease diagnosis by pinpointing specific cellular interactions and metabolic processes.

While the pump scanning approach is innovative, it has the disadvantage of requiring both scanning in wavelength and space, which significantly limits the overall scan time. Recently, the introduction of parallel LIAs, as pioneered by the Polli group, [17] marks another breakthrough in the field. By employing 32 parallel LIAs, the system can simultaneously acquire signals across multiple channels, dramatically reducing scan times while covering a broad bandwidth. This setup not only speeds up the imaging process but also broadens the range of chemical information that can be captured in a single scan. The ability to process multiple wavelengths concurrently allows for a more detailed and comprehensive analysis, facilitating a deeper understanding of tissue chemistry at a much faster rate than previously possible.

Raman-based diagnostics have been explored for decades across various diseases but have thus far failed to penetrate into the clinic [45–49]. In this context the recent success of SRH in terms of clinical application cannot be overstated. The principle of traditional Raman diagnostics involves recording a broad Raman spectrum from one or more points on known diseased and healthy tissues or cells, typically spanning both the fingerprint and the high-wavenumber CH-band. Due to slow acquisition times, only a few spectra are recorded per sample and these spectra have traditionally been used to train machine learning models—commonly PCA/LDA, partial least squares, or support vector machines—to create multivariate classification systems that can predict diseases from a single spectrum. Despite the successful demonstration of this approach in numerous studies, it has yet to gain clinical traction, primarily due to slow acquisition times, the expense of the equipment, and difficulties in cross-instrument calibration. However, recent advancements have significantly mitigated these issues, particularly in calibration and cost.

This brings us to an important distinction: traditional H&E pathology—and by extension, current SRH methods as reviewed above—rely primarily on spatial, morphological classification, whereas the full spectrum Raman approach offers a chemical classification of disease. The potential to combine these methodologies opens up exciting new possibilities for integrated diagnostic platforms.

Looking forward, we envision a hybrid approach where single or dual wavenumber SRH is used to rapidly produce a virtually stained image. Simple spatial-based algorithms (such as random forests, MLP, or CNN as described earlier) could then highlight areas likely affected by disease, and these regions could subsequently be analyzed using point-based Raman spectroscopy for detailed chemical classification. This method would leverage the speed of SRH for initial screening and the chemical specificity of Raman spectroscopy for precise diagnostics. Given that the SRH system could easily be adapted to include the spontaneous Raman modality, this approach seems particularly viable.

Similarly, another forward-looking approach could involve using SRH for initial high-speed imaging followed by broadband CARS hyperspectral scanning of suspect areas. As described in section 8.2 BCARS (ms acquisition time) offers a compromise between the slow acquisition speeds of traditional Raman spectroscopy (s acquisition time) and the rapid imaging capabilities of SRS microscopy (μs acquisition time). With acquisition times measured in milliseconds and the ability to record a full broadband spectrum (0–4000 cm^{-1}), BCARS is well-suited for detailed hyperspectral imaging of smaller regions of interest which could first be identified using SRH. These regions could then be analyzed using advanced multivariate classification models, potentially utilizing 3D CNNs, to provide a comprehensive diagnostic assessment that incorporates both morphological and chemical insights.

8.7 Conclusion

Hyperspectral imaging and histology with Raman spectroscopy is a transformative technology in medical diagnostics, which enables non-invasive, rapid pathological assessments. The advancements in this field underscore a significant shift towards precise, molecular-level medical diagnostics. The advent of virtual staining techniques in particular stands out as a pivotal innovation, eliminating the need for chemical stains in tissue analysis. This method preserves tissue integrity while providing critical morphological insights. It has proven to be a valuable tool in surgical settings, offering real-time guidance to surgeons and pathologists, thus enhancing the precision of surgical interventions and potentially improving patient outcomes.

The integration of machine learning algorithms with hyperspectral imaging technologies further advances this field. These algorithms can analyze complex datasets, identifying patterns and features that are not readily visible, thereby augmenting the diagnostic capabilities of medical professionals and supporting the rapid decision-making required in clinical environments. Future directions in this field are likely to focus on refining these technologies and exploring their integration into routine clinical practice. This could involve the development of more sophisticated and less expensive imaging systems that offer even higher resolution and deeper tissue penetration, or algorithms that can provide more nuanced interpretations of hyperspectral data.

It is the opinion of these authors that the future of hyperspectral imaging and histology lies in the seamless integration of morphological and chemical diagnostics, harnessing the strengths of SRH and Raman spectroscopy. This integrated approach could revolutionize pathology by providing rapid, accurate, and detailed diagnostic information, paving the way for more personalized and effective medical treatments.

Acknowledgments

We acknowledge the support of Research Ireland under (Grant Numbers 15/CDA/3667, 19/FFP/7025, and 16/RI/3399).

References

[1] Orringer D A, Pandian B, Niknafs Y S, Hollon T C, Boyle J, Lewis S, Garrard M, Hervey-Jumper S L, Garton H J L, Maher C O *et al* 2017 Rapid intraoperative histology of unprocessed surgical specimens via fibre-laser-based stimulated Raman scattering microscopy *Nat. Biomed. Eng.* **1** 0027

[2] Sarri B, Canonge R, Audier X, Simon E, Wojak J, Caillol F, Cador C, Marguet D, Poizat F, Giovannini M *et al* 2019 Fast stimulated Raman and second harmonic generation imaging for intraoperative gastro-intestinal cancer detection *Sci. Rep.* **9** 10052

[3] Pradhan P, Meyer T, Vieth M, Stallmach A, Waldner M, Schmitt M, Popp J and Bocklitz T 2021 Computational tissue staining of non-linear multimodal imaging using supervised and unsupervised deep learning *Biomed. Opt. Express* **12** 2280–98

[4] Liu Z, Chen L, Cheng H, Ao J, Xiong J, Liu X, Chen Y, Mao Y and Ji M 2024 Virtual formalin-fixed and paraffin-embedded staining of fresh brain tissue via stimulated Raman cyclegan model *Sci. Adv.* **10** eadn3426

[5] Hollon T C *et al* 2018 Rapid intraoperative diagnosis of pediatric brain tumors using stimulated Raman histology *Cancer Res.* **78** 278–89

[6] Liu Z *et al* 2022 Instant diagnosis of gastroscopic biopsy via deep-learned single-shot femtosecond stimulated Raman histology *Nat. Commun.* **13** 4050

[7] Ando J, Palonpon A F, Sodeoka M and Fujita K 2016 High-speed Raman imaging of cellular processes *Curr. Opin. Chem. Biol.* **33** 16–24

[8] Muddiman R, Harkin S, Butler M and Hennelly B 2024 Broadband CARS hyperspectral classification of single leukemia cells ChemRxiv. https://chemrxiv.org/engage/chemrxiv/article-details/66c49442a4e53c4876f068d3

[9] Cheng J X and Xie X S 2016 *Coherent Raman Scattering Microscopy Series in Cellular and Clinical Imaging* (Boca Raton, FL: CRC Press)

[10] Ma L, Luo K, Liu Z and Ji M 2024 Stain-free histopathology with stimulated Raman scattering microscopy *Anal. Chem.* **96** 7907–25

[11] Nishiyama R, Furuya K, Tamura T, Nakao R, Peterson W, Hiramatsu K, Ding T and Goda K 2024 Fourier transform coherent anti-Stokes Raman scattering spectroscopy: a comprehensive review *Anal. Chem.* **96** 18322–36

[12] Kerr L T and Hennelly B M 2016 A multivariate statistical investigation of background subtraction algorithms for Raman spectra of cytology samples recorded on glass slides *Chemometr. Intell. Lab. Syst.* **158** 61–8

[13] Vanna R *et al* 2024 High-resolution Raman imaging of> 300 patient-derived cells from nine different leukemia subtypes: a global clustering approach *Anal. Chem.* **96** 9468–77

[14] Kerr L T, Byrne H J and Hennelly B M 2015 Optimal choice of sample substrate and laser wavelength for Raman spectroscopic analysis of biological specimen *Anal. Methods* **7** 5041–52

[15] Mochizuki K *et al* 2023 High-throughput line-illumination Raman microscopy with multislit detection *Biomed. Opt. Express* **14** 1015–26

[16] Cheng J-X and Xie X S 2015 Vibrational spectroscopic imaging of living systems: an emerging platform for biology and medicine *Science* **350** aaa8870

[17] De la Cadena A *et al* 2022 Broadband stimulated Raman imaging based on multi-channel lock-in detection for spectral histopathology *Apl. Photon.* **7** 076104

[18] Camp C H, Lee Y J, Heddleston J M, Hartshorn C M, Hight Walker A R, Rich J N, Lathia J D and Cicerone M T 2014 High-Speed coherent Raman fingerprint imaging of biological tissues *Nat Photon.* **8** 627–34

[19] Wang Z, O'Dwyer K, Muddiman R, Ward T, Camp C H and Hennelly B M 2022 Vector: very deep convolutional autoencoders for non-resonant background removal in broadband coherent anti-Stokes Raman scattering *J. Raman Spectrosc.* **53** 1081–93

[20] Muddiman R, O'Dwyer K, Camp C H and Hennelly B 2023 Removing non-resonant background from broadband cars using a physics-informed neural network *Anal. Methods* **15** 4032–43

[21] Tamamitsu M, Sakaki Y, Nakamura T, Krishna Podagatlapalli G, Ideguchi T and Goda K 2017 Ultrafast broadband Fourier-transform cars spectroscopy at 50,000 spectra/s enabled by a scanning Fourier-domain delay line *Vib. Spectrosc.* **91** 163–9

[22] Francis A, Berry K, Chen Y, Figueroa B and Fu D 2017 Label-free pathology by spectrally sliced femtosecond stimulated Raman scattering (srs) microscopy *PLoS One* **12** e0178750

[23] Li Y, Xiao X and Yang C 2017 Spectral-compressed fiber laser source for broadband-cars microspectroscopy *2017 16th Int. Conf. on Optical Communications and Networks (ICOCN)* pp 1–3

[24] Liu D and Hennelly B M 2024 Wavenumber calibration protocol for Raman spectrometers using physical modelling and a fast search algorithm *Appl. Spectrosc.* **78** 790–805

[25] Barton S J and Hennelly B M 2019 An algorithm for the removal of cosmic ray artifacts in spectral data sets *Appl. Spectrosc.* **73** 893–901

[26] Hollon T C *et al* 2020 Near real-time intraoperative brain tumor diagnosis using stimulated Raman histology and deep neural networks *Nat. Med.* **26** 52–8
[27] Freudiger C W, Min W, Saar B G, Lu S, Holtom G R, He C, Tsai J C, Kang J X and Xie X S 2008 Label-free biomedical imaging with high sensitivity by stimulated raman scattering microscopy *Science* **322** 1857–61
[28] Jiang C *et al* 2022 Rapid automated analysis of skull base tumor specimens using intraoperative optical imaging and artificial intelligence *Neurosurgery* **90** 758–67
[29] Sarri B *et al* 2021 Observation of the compatibility of stimulated Raman histology with pathology workflow and genome sequencing *Transl. Biophoton.* **3** e202000020
[30] Sarri B, Poizat F, Heuke S, Wojak J, Franchi F, Caillol F, Giovannini M and Rigneault H 2019 Stimulated Raman histology: one to one comparison with standard hematoxylin and eosin staining *Biomed. Opt. Express* **10** 5378–84
[31] Sarri B *et al* 2024 In vivo organoid growth monitoring by stimulated Raman histology *npj Imaging* **2** 18
[32] Pekmezci M *et al* 2021 Detection of glioma infiltration at the tumor margin using quantitative stimulated Raman scattering histology *Sci. Rep.* **11** 12162
[33] Orringer D A *et al* 2017 Rapid intraoperative histology of unprocessed surgical specimens via fibre-laser-based stimulated Raman scattering microscopy *Nat. Biomed. Eng.* **1** 0027
[34] Eichberg D G *et al* 2019 Stimulated Raman histology for rapid and accurate intraoperative diagnosis of CNS tumors: prospective blinded study *J. Neurosurg.* **134** 137–43
[35] Hollon T C *et al* 2018 Rapid intraoperative diagnosis of pediatric brain tumors using stimulated Raman histology *Cancer Res.* **78** 278–89
[36] Einstein E H *et al* 2022 Stimulated Raman histology facilitates accurate diagnosis in neurosurgical patients: a one-to-one noninferiority study *J. Neuro-Oncol.* **159** 369–75
[37] Williams R M, Zipfel W R and Webb W W 2005 Interpreting second-harmonic generation images of collagen I fibrils *Biophys. J.* **88** 1377–86
[38] Jing Y, Yang Y, Feng Z, Ye J, Yu Y and Song M 2019 Neural style transfer: a review *IEEE Trans. Vis. Comput. Graphics* **26** 3365–85
[39] Gatys L A 2015 A neural algorithm of artistic style *a*rXiv preprint ArXiv:1508.06576
[40] Zhu J-Y, Park T, Isola P and Efros A A 2017 Unpaired image-to-image translation using cycle-consistent adversarial networks *Proc. of the IEEE Int. Conf. on Computer Vision* pp 2223–32
[41] Isola P, Zhu J-Y, Zhou T and Efros A A 2017 Image-to-image translation with conditional adversarial networks *Proc. of the IEEE Conf. on Computer Vision and Pattern Recognition* pp 1125–34
[42] Ronneberger O, Fischer P and Brox T 2015 U-net: convolutional networks for biomedical image segmentation *Medical Image Computing and Computer-Assisted Intervention–MICCAI 2015: 18th International Conference, Munich, Germany, October 5–9, 2015, proceedings, part III 18* (Springer) pp 234–41
[43] He K, Zhang X, Ren S and Sun J 2016 Deep residual learning for image recognition *Proc. of the IEEE Conf. on Computer Vision and Pattern Recognition* pp 770–8
[44] Tipping W J, Wilson L T, An C, Leventi A A, Wark A W, Wetherill C, Tomkinson N C O, Faulds K and Graham D 2022 Stimulated Raman scattering microscopy with spectral phasor analysis: applications in assessing drug-cell interactions *Chem. Sci.* **13** 3468–76
[45] Ellis D I and Goodacre R 2006 Metabolic fingerprinting in disease diagnosis: biomedical applications of infrared and Raman spectroscopy *Analyst* **131** 875–85

[46] Ellis D I, Cowcher D P, Ashton L, O'Hagan S and Goodacre R 2013 Illuminating disease and enlightening biomedicine: Raman spectroscopy as a diagnostic tool *Analyst* **138** 3871–84

[47] Stone N and Matousek P 2008 Advanced transmission Raman spectroscopy: a promising tool for breast disease diagnosis *Cancer Res.* **68** 4424–30

[48] Kerr L T, Domijan K, Cullen I and Hennelly B M 2014 Applications of raman spectroscopy to the urinary bladder for cancer diagnostics Photon *Lasers Med.* **3** 193–224

[49] Jermyn M, Mok K, Mercier J, Desroches J, Pichette J, Saint-Arnaud K, Bernstein L, Guiot M-C, Petrecca K and Leblond F 2015 Intraoperative brain cancer detection with Raman spectroscopy in humans *Sci. Transl. Med.* **7** 274ra19

IOP Publishing

Spectroscopic Techniques for Cancer Diagnostics

Inbarasan Muniraj and Bryan Hennelly

Chapter 9

Serum Raman spectroscopy-based biomedical diagnostics

Piyush Kumar and Aditi Sahu

List of Abbreviations

ANN	Artificial neural network
CNN	Convoluted neural network
FDA	Factorial discriminant analysis
KNN	K-nearest neighbor
LDA	Linear discriminant analysis
NNLM	Neural network language model
PCA	Principal component analysis
PC-LDA or PCA-LDA	Principal component-based LDA
PLS-DA	Partial least square discriminant analysis
QDA	Quadratic discriminant analysis
RF	Random forest
SVM	Support vector machine

Raman spectroscopy offers a rapid, nondestructive, and label-free diagnostic method. Serum Raman spectroscopy is becoming increasingly popular due to the ease of serum collection, storage, and transportation, the small volume of serum required for spectra collection, and the potential for repeated patient monitoring. This chapter highlights the explorations and advancements in serum Raman spectroscopy for diagnosing both cancerous and non-cancerous health conditions.

9.1 Introduction

Serum is one of the most commonly used samples for disease diagnosis and monitoring owing to a minimally invasive and almost pain-free sample collection, metabolically rich biochemical profile, and ease of storage and transportation. While the major component of serum is water, several metabolites present in serum make it a matrix rich in biomarkers for several health conditions. While plasma can also be

doi:10.1088/978-0-7503-5949-8ch9

used for biochemical profiling, this chapter focuses solely on serum-based studies. New diagnostic assays using serum are continually being developed, and advancements in artificial intelligence, nanotechnology, and biophotonics promise to enhance future diagnoses with lower costs and improved sensitivity and specificity [1].

Although some serum tests and assays are economical and easily available, some are still costly (e.g. serum ammonia and cancer antigen tests) and/or may involve complicated biochemical reactions. In the late 1990s, Raman spectroscopy (RS) caught the attention of biomedical researchers as a simple, rapid and label-free method that did not require any sample preparation, staining or other reagents for data acquisition. Historically, serum-based Raman studies have moved in two directions: (i) fundamental studies on chemical profiling of serum [2–4] towards improving the current understanding of serum composition, (ii) serum-based investigations to explore biomedical diagnostic potential using a small volume of serum towards diagnosing and monitoring several diseases including cancers. These are described in later sections.

9.1.1 Raman spectroscopy in serum chemical profiling

Initial studies estimated concentration of biochemicals such as cholesterol, urea, glucose, lactic acid and creatinine in saline to confirm potential of RS in detection of these aqueous analytes using chemometric methods such as partial least squares [5]. These were followed by studies on calibration and prediction of serum components, such as glucose, cholesterol and urea on a 66-patient data set using Raman spectra acquired with an 830 nm diode laser [6]. Another study utilized a 785 nm laser to estimate total protein, albumin, triglyceride, and glucose in human serum samples with prediction error ranging from 1% to 10% [7]. These and more such studies [8, 9] paved the way for future studies that ranged from detection of serum ultrafiltrates [2], high (globulins and albumins) and low molecular weight (urea, glucose) fractions [4], antibody phases [10], ferritin [11] and detection of infiltrates, pharmaceuticals, drugs and substance of abuse, paving the way for serum RS for disease diagnoses.

9.1.2 Raman spectroscopy-based disease diagnosis

RS has been explored for detecting several diseases including asthma, atherosclerosis, neurological disorders and several cancers [12–39, 65]. Especially, cancers have been the focus of several Raman researchers as RS is capable of identifying early biochemical changes that can help detect cancers at an early stage; as is well known, most cancers are diagnosed late due to lack of distinct clinical features, which leads to delayed treatment and poor survival rates.

RS has been extensively studied in the context of cancer, with tissue-based studies conducted both *in vivo* and *ex vivo* [29, 40–55]. Raman has been used to gain insights from relatively accessible cancers like oral and skin cancers to non-accessible tissues in gastrointestinal tract using endoscope-assisted Raman [56–59]. For more information on *ex vivo* and *in vivo* Raman studies, readers are encouraged to consult the cited publications, which are also summarized in this recent review [60]. Additionally, surface-enhanced Raman spectroscopy (SERS), an advancement of RS, has gained popularity in recent years and has been applied to serum samples from various disease conditions. However, discussing SERS is beyond the scope of this chapter; for more details, we recommend this recent review [61]. In the following subsections, we have highlighted methodology for Raman spectra acquisition, Raman data processing and analysis, and the progress in disease diagnosis using RS and serum samples.

9.1.3 Serum Raman spectra acquisition protocols

As mentioned earlier, any specific treatment of samples prior to Raman spectra collection is not required by most protocols. However, care should be taken in maintaining uniformity in serum extraction and storage conditions to avoid any unwanted variable that may skew sensitivity or specificity. Serum, either freshly extracted or frozen and thawed, can be aliquoted on substrates such as calcium fluoride and aluminum. Good Raman signal can be obtained with as little as 30 μl of sample. In most cases, drying/concentration of serum is not required, although this approach has also been explored as well (drop-coating deposition Raman, DCDR) [62]. Most serum-based Raman studies use near infrared wavelengths for spectra acquisition, typically near 785 nm while a few studies have also employed 532 nm laser for sample excitation. An interesting observation in the case of 532 nm has been resonance due to biochemical compounds like beta-carotene, leading to additional features in comparison to 785 nm excitation.

9.1.4 Raman spectra preprocessing and analysis

The raw Raman spectra often need to be corrected for cosmic rays, tissue autofluorescence, contributions from optical elements and intensity related variations before analysis. Additionally, spectra may be truncated in desired wavenumber regions. These preparatory steps are collectively known as 'preprocessing' in the field of RS. Most of these corrections can be carried out in the vendor-provided software. Alternatively, the raw spectra can be extracted and imported into commercially available software such as Unscrambler and MATLAB or free packages in R/Python for preprocessing. Following preprocessing, several research groups carry out dimension reduction before using machine learning tools for identifying trends in data, model building, validation and evaluation. Table 9.1 provides a list of the most commonly used preprocessing steps while table 9.2 provides a list of software packages used for preprocessing and/or analysis. For further reading on preprocessing and analysis methods, please check these cited references [63–67].

9.2 Raman serum spectroscopy in cancers

9.2.1 Oral cancers

Oral cancers have a high incidence in South Asia, and as such have been extensively explored through RS in India. Optical fiber-based handheld probes have been applied to study features in oral cancer patients, while Raman microspectroscopy has been used to study serum, plasma and exfoliated cells at several centers [60]. One of the earliest Raman based explorations of blood samples was published in 2009 by

Table 9.1. Commonly employed preprocessing steps.

Preprocessing step	Utility
Cosmic ray removal	Removes sharp peaks/noise
Baseline correction	Reduces autofluorescence component
Smoothing	Reduces noise
Interpolation (truncation)	Selection of desired wavenumber region for analysis
Normalization	Overcomes intensity related variations

Table 9.2. Commonly employed software for preprocessing and analysis.

Software package	Open source/commercial	Vendor/contact person
Wire	C	Renishaw
Project	C	WITec/Oxford
Cytospec	C	Peter Lasch
Spectragryph	C	Friedrich Menges
Labspec	C	Jobin Yvon
Hyperspec (R package)	O	Claudia Beleites
Chemometric Suite (MATLAB)	C	Mathwork Inc
Unscrambler	C	AspenTech
Raman SPY (Python library)	O	Mauricio Barahona

Harris *et al* [119]. This exploratory study acquired spectra from 20 head and neck cancer patients to achieve 65% accuracy of classification using linear discriminant analysis and inspired a lot of research groups to pursue blood/serum-based Raman studies. The Raman spectroscopy group (Chilakapati Laboratory) at Tata Memorial Centre's ACTREC (Navi Mumbai, India) became a pioneer of serum-based oral cancer diagnosis in the next decade with major initiatives led by Sahu *et al* (coauthor of this chapter). Near Infrared excitation at 785 nm was successfully applied on sera from 36 buccal mucosa cancer patients, 33 tongue cancer patients and 17 healthy volunteers, leading to an accuracy of 78% between healthy and cancer serum and 68% between buccal mucosa and tongue cancer sera [68]. Simultaneously, a 532 nm laser was also employed to investigate resonance Raman on serum samples from 14 buccal mucosa and 40 tongue cancer patients while serum from 16 healthy volunteers was used as control. The common spectral features in both these studies include contribution from proteins, aromatic amino acids and DNA, while due to resonance effect, intense β-carotene bands are also observed in the latter study. Another conclusion from these studies was that utilizing a subject/patient-wise approach for analysis rather than serum-wise approach irrespective of subjects should be a preferred mode to minimize bias introduced by sample heterogeneity [22]. A large scale study on 328 subjects comprising healthy controls, premalignant and cancer cases using the patient-wise approach was conducted and the classification was achieved with specificity of 80% suggesting utility of Raman spectroscopy as an adjunct for early detection of oral precancers and cancers [69].

Another interesting potential application of RS is in recurrence prediction in oral cancers. Employing a retrospective approach in patients who underwent surgery for oral cancers, serum Raman could classify recurrent and non-recurrent cases. Such studies can be very useful in monitoring recurrence-prone patients and formulating a dynamic treatment plan after the surgery [70]. Recurrence prediction while monitoring patients over a longer duration (7-year follow-up) with added complexities such as 'suspicious lesions' in patients who failed to follow up was studied recently [71]. The overall accuracy of distinguishing recurrence and non-recurrence cases was 84%. While these studies explored prediction potential of Raman spectroscopy, the probable causes for the spectral differences should be further explored.

9.2.2 Breast cancer

Breast cancer is the most common cancer in women. As per Globocan data, about 2.3 million new female breast cancer cases were detected worldwide in 2022 [72]. Some exhaustive reviews that have highlighted Raman studies in breast cancers are by Hanna *et al* [33] and Lazaro–Pacheco *et al* [73].

Serum RS for breast cancers was first explored by Pichardo–Molina *et al*, on serum from 11 patients and 12 healthy controls from Mexico to provide a proof-of-concept. PCA and LDA was utilized to achieve a sensitivity of 97% while specific band ratio was also utilized to explore discriminatory features [74]. Invasive ductal carcinoma has been explored through several classification models to achieve rapid diagnosis, with LDA, SVM and NNLM leading to 100% accuracy [75]. However, a perfect accuracy obtained in this study could have been a result of overestimation as per a comment by Bratchenko *et al* [76]. Nevertheless, studies such as those by Bratchenko *et al* are important and highlights that appropriate statistical approaches are extremely crucial for better fit.

Studies have also tried to explore differences between benign and malignant conditions. Benign (n = 91) and malignant cases (n = 129) and healthy controls (n = 113) were explored using SVM with 98% accuracy [77]. The classification of triple-negative breast cancer (n = 23), HER2-positive breast cancer (n = 22), and healthy controls was achieved with deep learning algorithms with a classification accuracy of 91% achieved using CNN [78]. Mean spectra of triple-negative, HER2-positive breast cancers and healthy subjects is shown in figure 9.1. Another recent study classified HER-2 positive and negative serum samples (total n = 459) using SVM [32]. In another recent study, a combination of complex molecular subtyping to classify breast cancer samples using ER/PR, Ki67 and HER2 expression status was used to classify breast cancer samples into four categories and subjected to SVM for classification. The area under the curve (AUC) values of the combination of classification models varied between 0.85 and 0.9273 [79].

Another utility of serum RS in breast cancer can be in monitoring patients during cancer treatment. A study continuously monitored six patients during therapy with a

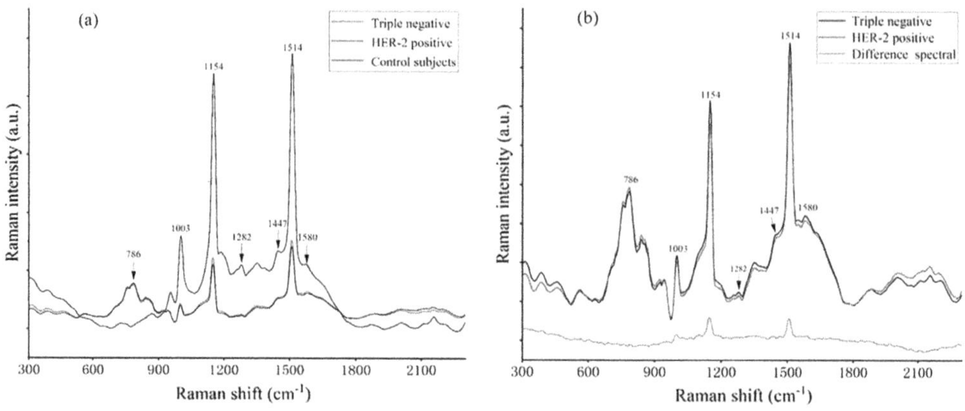

Figure 9.1. (a) Comparison of serum Raman spectra of patients with triple-negative, HER2-positive breast cancers and healthy subjects. (b) Comparison of serum Raman spectra between triple-negative, HER2-positive breast cancers. Adapted from [78], copyright 2022, with permission from Elsevier B.V. All rights reserved.

specific focus on 450 cm^{-1} Raman band (corresponding to glutathione) as a potential marker for treatment, and observed that cancer patients' spectra profile seemed to get closer to control group characteristics as treatment progressed [80]. In an attempt to decipher pre- and post-surgery differences in serum from tumor-specific molecular alterations, Sprague–Dawley rat models of adenocarcinoma showed differences attributed to tumor- associated factors in serum [81]. In line with oral studies on recurrence prediction, such studies can pave way for treatment monitoring as well as predicting treatment outcome at an early phase for suitable intervention and course correction.

9.2.3 Gynecological cancers

Cervical cancer is a leading cancer in women in developing countries. Shrivastava *et al* performed studies using confocal Raman for diagnosis and monitoring of treatment response. They achieved a sensitivity and specificity of 93% and 86% from controls and cancer sera [29]. As compared to healthy sera, increased glycogen, tryptophan, phenylalanine, nucleic acids and amide III bands were seen in cancer sera, while lower β carotene and glutathione were observed. Another study by González–Solís *et al* [82] also demonstrated that β carotene, tryptophan, glutathione, and amide III were the major spectral differences between sera from healthy and cervical cancer patients.

For monitoring treatment, longitudinally collected samples from patients at three time-points (pre-treatment, on-treatment and 6 months post-treatment) have been utilized. Chemical changes related to chemoradiation were identified by a decrease in proteins and nucleic acid signatures with elevated phospholipid, amide III and glutathione signatures [29]. These spectral differences need to be further explored to understand if these observations are attributable to chemoradiation treatment or persistent disease. Similarities between spectra from post-treatment and healthy sera also need validation through large follow-up studies.

Owens *et al* explored RS for ovarian cancer samples, however, in this study, their major focus was on plasma samples; only four serum samples were employed [83].

9.2.4 Gastro-intestinal cancers

Colorectal cancers (CRCs) are among the high incidence cancers worldwide. Serum Raman spectroscopy on samples from 30 normal, 46 colon cancer and 44 rectum cancer patients performed by Li *et al* using Raman peaks (intensity and width) and baseline coefficients as input parameters and comparing performance of principal component regression (PCR) and partial least square regression (PLSR), followed by LDA on the principal components to obtain an accuracy of 88% [84, 85]. Li *et al* further utilized serum samples from 65 preoperative and 60 postoperative colon cancer patients along with 75 healthy volunteers (514.5 nm laser wavelength). A diagnostic accuracy of 91% was achieved after PCA and KNN, attributed to differences in nucleic acids, amino acids and chromophores [86].

Ito *et al* [87] worked on serum from 184 cases who were scheduled for colonoscopy and utilized a boosted tree model for predicting colorectal cancers after categorizing the spectral regions into 15 groups. The authors used generalized R^2 values as a measure of classification with CRC yielding a value of 0.9982. However, of these, only 12 cases were clinically CRC and the sample size for some other cases were also low and a further larger dataset is needed for validation. Another study developed high throughput platforms for CRC detection using both, liquid and dry serum. This approach was applied on cancer ($n = 30$) and matched control patients ($n = 30$). Statistical analysis performed using PLS-DA achieved a sensitivity as well as specificity up to 83% [88].

Serum RS of gastric cancers provides a diagnosis comparable to traditional enzymatic tests. In a study on samples from 20 gastric cancer patients and 40 healthy subjects, PLS regression correctly classified 87.5% samples and correlation with enzymatic assays was around 94% [89].

9.2.5 Hepatocellular cancer (HCC)

Liver cancers are one of the major killers and the majority of primary liver cancers are known to be HCC [90]. In a proof-of-concept study by Taleb *et al*, micro-RS successfully discriminated serum samples from patients with ($n = 37$) and without HCC ($n = 34$) in the 600–1800 cm^{-1} wavenumber region [91]. Interestingly, the authors did not observe classification with PCA but SVM yielded a good result. Recently, Leng *et al* showed that RS can distinguish Hepatitis A, Hepatitis B and thyroid abnormalities. Hepatitis A and Hepatitis B which are both risk factors for liver cancers can also be distinguished using serum RS, as shown recently by Leng *et al* [92]. They compared eight different classifiers and obtained promising results.

9.2.6 Brain cancers

Several different types of brain/nervous system cancers have been explored using RS [20]. In comparison to healthy serum, meningioma serum spectra showed higher levels of proteins, DNA, lipids, and β-carotene in a study by Mehta *et al* ($n = 35$

each for meningioma and control serum). Using patient-wise approach, PC-LDA led to a classification efficiency 80% for meningioma [23]. The authors were also successful in classifying different grades of meningioma. A serum-derived extracellular vesicle (EV) has also been used to diagnose central nervous system tumors, as shown by Bukva *et al* [93].

9.2.7 Prostate cancer

EVs in serum can be a good candidate for several biomarkers and this is under investigation by several research groups [94, 95]. In conjunction with CNN, RS of serum-derived EVs has shown promising results in prostate cancer identification with more than 90% classification efficiency. This study by Lee *et al* also showed that CNN outperformed the traditional classification models such as PC-LDA [96].

9.2.8 Other cancers

In recent years, RS of serum has provided promising results for detection of several cancers. A pilot study on testicular cancers has used serum samples from nine patients and 10 controls to obtain encouraging results [97]. Lung cancer and benign lesions ($n = 45$ each) have been explored with SVM-based models on serum samples with more than 90% accuracy while benign and cancer cases were classified with 80% accuracy by Yan *et al* [98].

To evaluate classification models with increasing complexity, many groups are simultaneously investigating more than one type of cancer in the same study. Du *et al* demonstrated that CNN can be used to distinguish between gastric ($n = 38$), rectal ($n = 72$), colon ($n = 23$) and lung cancers ($n = 71$) along with healthy controls ($n = 69$) with over 94% accuracy [99]. The mean spectra of the serum samples are shown in figure 9.2.

To simultaneously classify cervical and breast cancers, 225 spectra from patients with cervical cancer ($n = 87$), breast cancer ($n = 60$), and 78 healthy individuals, Cao *et al* applied PC-LDA to achieve good classification [100].

9.3 Serum Raman spectroscopy in non-cancer conditions

9.3.1 Malaria and dengue

Tropical diseases like malaria and dengue are a menace [101]. Malaria diagnosis depends on the identification of *Plasmodium* species, the causative agent. Often the results are subjective with a risk of false negative diagnosis [102] leading to repeated blood smears for confirmation. Using healthy ($n = 34$), dengue ($n = 29$), and malaria ($n = 27$) serum samples, Patel *et al* achieved good classification for malaria versus healthy, dengue versus healthy, and malaria versus dengue versus healthy models through PC-LDA [103].

Serum samples from dengue infected ($n = 40$) and healthy controls ($n = 25$) have shown unique Raman features, such as a band at 750 cm^{-1} (adenosine diphosphate) and 1306 cm^{-1} (IgM) [104]. RS and SVM-based analysis of 31 positive and 53 negative samples yielded 85% accuracy in a study by Khan *et al* [105]. In another

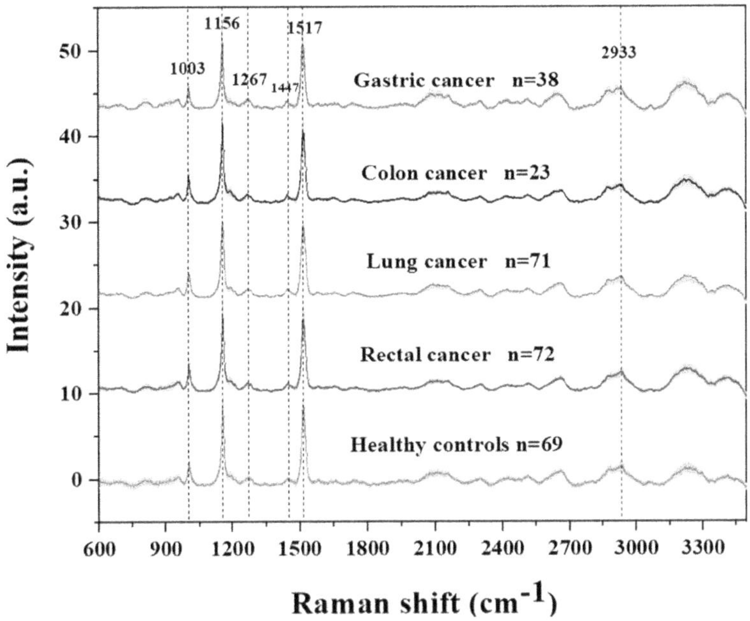

Figure 9.2. The mean normalized Raman spectra of healthy controls, rectal cancer, lung cancer, colon cancer, and gastric cancer. The shaded area represents the standard deviation. The letter *n* represents the sample number of each category. Reproduced from [99], copyright 2023, with permission from Elsevier B.V. All rights reserved.

study, Khan *et al* utilized random forest method with 91% accuracy on 100 samples [106]. Unique spectral signatures contributing to a high accuracy of 97% were shown by Amin *et al* [107].

9.3.2 Asthma

Asthma is a chronic condition and early risk prediction is important for effective management. Sahu *et al* obtained asthma serum samples from asthma ($n = 44$) of different grades such as mild, moderate and severe, and controls ($n = 15$) and achieved separation of the subgroups [108]. Asthma ($n = 80$) and healthy volunteer ($n = 30$) serum Raman spectra could be classified with 100% sensitivity by Ullah *et al* [109]

9.3.3 Neurological/neurodegenerative disorders

RS of serum has been successfully employed to diagnose several neurological and neurodegenerative conditions, including Alzheimer's (AD) and Parkinson's disease [110]. Serum Raman data from AD patients ($n = 20$), other neurodegenerative dementias (OD, $n = 18$) and healthy controls ($n = 10$) could be classified with 95% sensitivity and specificity by employing ANN models [111]. In another study 26 healthy and 31 AD patient serum samples were analyzed using PC-LDA, PC-QDA and RF methods [112]. Serum-derived EVs have been explored in Parkinson's patients [113]. Amyotrophic lateral sclerosis (ALS), a motor neuron disease of adulthood that leads to progressively severe symptoms including muscle atrophy and spasms. Alix *et al* followed up ALS patients at baseline and after 4 months and identified differences in spectral patterns between these time periods [114]. Attention deficit and hyperactivity disorder (ADHD) is a neurodevelopmental condition impacting a large number of children worldwide. In a recent study, patients with ADHD, bipolar disorder, and healthy controls could be differentiated with 97.4% accuracy. These studies indicate greater role of serum Raman spectroscopy in detection of neurological disorders in the future [115].

9.3.4 COVID

Covid needs no introduction. In view of false negative diagnosis through rapid methods, potential of Raman spectroscopy coupled with machine learning as a non-invasive diagnostic method for COVID-19 is being explored actively. Yin *et al* investigated serum samples from 63 COVID-19, 59 suspected cases, and 55 healthy control group and applied SVM for analysis [116]. Goulart *et al* used serum from 10 Covid and 10 healthy subjects for another preliminary study to detect COVID [117]. In a study of 47 COVID-19 patients, antibody levels were measured at 1, 3, and 6 months post-infection using serological methods and Raman spectra were also acquired. RS, particularly in specific spectral ranges, achieved nearly 100% sensitivity in distinguishing patients at different stages post-infection [118].

9.4 Conclusion

Serum Raman Spectroscopy holds great promise in the field of diagnosis due to the unique advantages and capabilities offered by this minimally invasive approach. The spectroscopic measurements require a very small quantity of blood sera (typically few microliters), making it a minimally invasive procedure compared to traditional biopsy or tissue sampling and consequently is ideal for early diagnosis, regular monitoring, and mass screening of diseases. Raman spectral signatures provide detailed information about the biochemical composition of serum and allow identification of specific biomarkers and disease-related molecular changes. Often, subtle sub-clinical molecular changes precede clinical observations, making Raman spectroscopy of serum an excellent avenue for early disease detection. Studies on some cancers have also confirmed the ability of serum to detect recurrence or disease progression at a much earlier stage. This technique has applications across a wide spectrum of diseases, including cancer, cardiovascular, neurological and infectious diseases. The versatility of the approach allows for the potential development of a universal diagnostic tool that can be applied to different health conditions by identifying characteristic molecular fingerprints in serum. Although setting up a Raman system can be expensive, once set up, the assay is relatively fast and cost-effective. Minimal sample preparation is normally involved, as opposed to other diagnostic methods, making it an efficient tool for real-time diagnostics. Lastly, the detailed and highly informative spectral data that is generated can be used to develop reliable diagnostic models using machine learning, further enhancing its diagnostic potential. Looking to the future, advanced data analysis techniques using AI and machine learning, are expected to play a critical role in unlocking the full potential of serum Raman spectroscopy. AI algorithms can be trained to recognize subtle molecular changes, improving the accuracy and speed of diagnosis. By integrating AI, serum Raman spectroscopy could evolve into a powerful predictive tool, capable of monitoring disease progression, response to treatment, and even offering prognostic insights.

References

[1] Liotta L A, Ferrari M and Petricoin E 2003 Clinical proteomics: written in blood *Nature* **425** 905

[2] Rohleder D, Kiefer W and Petrich W 2004 Quantitative analysis of serum and serum ultrafiltrate by means of Raman spectroscopy *Analyst* **129** 906–11

[3] Barman I, Singh G P, Dasari R R and Feld M S 2008 Transcutaneous measurement of blood analyte concentration using Raman spectroscopy *Perspect. Vib. Spectrosc.* **1075** 33–7

[4] Parachalil D R, Bruno C, Bonnier F, Blasco H, Chourpa I, McIntyre J and Byrne H J 2019 Raman spectroscopic screening of high and low molecular weight fractions of human serum *Analyst* **144** 4295–311

[5] Berger A J, Wang Y and Feld M S 1996 Rapid, noninvasive concentration measurements of aqueous biological analytes by near-infrared Raman spectroscopy *Appl. Opt.* **35** 209–12

[6] Berger A J, Koo T-W, Itzkan I, Horowitz G and Feld M S 1999 Multicomponent bloodanalysis by near-infrared Raman spectroscopy *Appl. Opt.* **38** 2916–26

[7] Qu J Y, Wilson B C and Suria D 1999 Concentration measurements of multiple analytes in human sera by near-infrared laser Raman spectroscopy *Appl. Opt.* **38** 5491–8

[8] Rohleder D, Kocherscheidt G, Gerber K, Kiefer W, Köhler W, Möcks J and Petrich W 2005 Comparison of mid-infrared and Raman spectroscopy in the quantitative analysis of serum *J. Biomed. Opt.* **10** 31108–10

[9] Enejder A M, Koo T-W, Oh J, Hunter M, Sasic S, Feld M S and Horowitz G L 2002 Blood analysis by Raman spectroscopy *Opt. Lett.* **27** 2004–6

[10] Baker A E, Mantz A R and Chiu M L 2014 Raman spectroscopy characterization of antibody phases in serum *MAbs* **6** 1509–17

[11] Ruvalcaba-López J M, Córdova-Fraga T, de la Rosa-Alvarez G, Murillo-Ortiz B O, Martínez-Espinosa J C, Guzmán-Cabrera R and Bernal-Alvarado J 2019 Qualitative evaluation of ferritin in serum samples by Raman spectroscopy and principal component analysis *Lasers Med. Sci.* **34** 35–40

[12] Zhang K, Liu R A, Wei X, Wang Z Y and Huang P 2024 Use of Raman spectroscopy to study rat lung tissues for distinguishing asphyxia from sudden cardiac death *RSC Adv.* **14** 5665–74

[13] Yang Y J *et al* 2024 Detection of SARS-CoV-2 in patient specimens by surface enhanced Raman spectroscopy and deep learning *Proc. SPIE 12999, Optical Sensing and Detection VIII* 12999 129991I

[14] Yang M G, Wang J J, Quan S Y and Xu Q Q 2024 Minireview: advances in spectral-based machine deep learning algorithms for thyroid function diagnosis *Anal. Lett.* **57** 138–61

[15] Yanagiya S, Honda T, Takanari H, Sogabe K, Nakamura S, Bando Y, Tsuneyama K, Abe M and Miki H 2024 Raman microspectroscopy for label-free diagnosis of amyloid light-chain amyloidosis in various organs *J. Raman Spectrosc.* **55** 753–60

[16] Tipatet K, Du Boulay I, Muir H, Davison-Gates L, Ellederová Z and Downes A 2024 Raman spectroscopy of brain and skin tissue in a minipig model of Huntington's disease *Anal. Methods* **16** 253–61

[17] Sun Z J, Wang Z and Jiang M Q 2024 RamanCluster: a deep clustering-based framework for unsupervised Raman spectral identification of pathogenic bacteria *Talanta* **275** 126076

[18] Qi Y P *et al* 2024 Applications of Raman spectroscopy in clinical medicine *Food Front.* **5** 392–419

[19] Zhao Q N *et al* 2024 Bilateral efforts to improve SERS detection efficiency of exosomes by Au/ $Na_7PMo_{11}O_{39}$ combined with phospholipid epitope imprinting *Biosens. Bioelectron.* **258** 116349

[20] Kumar P 2017 Raman spectroscopy as a promising noninvasive tool in brain cancer detection *J Innov. Opt. Heal. Sci.* **10** 1730012

[21] Sahu A, Dalal K, Naglot S, Aggarwal P and Krishna C M 2013 Serum based diagnosis of asthma using Raman spectroscopy: an early phase pilot study *PLOS One* **8** e78921

[22] Sahu A, Sawant S, Mamgain H and Krishna C M 2013 Raman spectroscopy of serum: an exploratory study for detection of oral cancers *Analyst* **138** 4161–74

[23] Mehta K, Atak A, Sahu A, Srivastava S and C M K 2018 An early investigative serum Raman spectroscopy study of meningioma *Analyst* **143** 1916–23

[24] Bhattacharjee T, Kumar P, Maru G, Ingle A and Krishna C M 2014 Swiss bare mice: a suitable model for transcutaneous *in vivo* Raman spectroscopic studies of breast cancer *Lasers Med. Sci.* **29** 325–33

[25] Hole A, Bhujbal M, Bendale K, Kumar P, Gera P, Krishna C M and Chaudhari P 2019 Preliminary study of canine oral cancer by Raman spectroscopy *InOtics and Biophotonics in Low-Resource Settings V* 1086917

[26] Kumar P, Ingle A and Krishna C M 2019 *In vivo* Raman spectroscopy: monitoring cancer progression post carcinogen withdrawal *Otical Imaging, Therapeutics, and Advanced Technology in Head and Neck Surgery and Otolaryngology 2019* 108530K

[27] Kumar P and Murali Krishna C 2019 Optical techniques: investigations in oral cancers *Oral Cancer Detection: Novel Strategies and Clinical Impact* (Springer) pp 167–87

[28] Austin C, Kumar P, Carter E A, Lee J, Smith T M, Hinde K, Arora M and Lay P A 2023 Stress exposure histories revealed by biochemical changes along accentuated lines in teeth *Chemosphere* **329** 138673

[29] Shrivastava A, Aggarwal L M, Krishna C M, Pradhan S, Mishra S P, Choudhary S, Patel C B, Singla S and Singh R K 2021 Diagnostic and prognostic application of Raman spectroscopy in carcinoma cervix: a biomolecular approach *Spectrochim. Acta* A **250** 119356

[30] Timchenko E, Timchenko P, Zybin M, Cherny-Tkach K, Frolov O and Dolgushov G 2020 Raman spectroscopy for studying the tissues of teeth infected by periodontitis *Proc. SPIE 11363, Tissue Optics and Photonics* 113632C

[31] Talari A C S, Movasaghi Z, Rehman S and Rehman I U 2015 Raman spectroscopy of biological tissues *Appl. Spectrosc. Rev.* **50** 46–111

[32] Li L, Li J, Wang X, Lu S, Ji J, Yin G, Luo H, Ting W, Xin Z and Wang D 2024 Convenient determination of serum HER-2 status in breast cancer patients using Raman spectroscopy *J. Biophotonics* **17** e202300287

[33] Hanna K, Krzoska E, Shaaban A M, Muirhead D, Abu-Eid R and Speirs V 2022 Raman spectroscopy: current applications in breast cancer diagnosis, challenges and future prospects *Br. J. Cancer* **126** 1125–39

[34] Kang J W, Park Y S, Chang H, Lee W, Singh S P, Choi W, Galindo L H, Dasari R R, Nam S H and Park J 2020 Direct observation of glucose fingerprint using *in vivo* Raman spectroscopy *Sci. Adv.* **6** eaay5206
[35] Gurushankar K, Gohulkumar M, Kumar P, Krishna C M and Krishnakumar N 2016 Raman spectroscopy detects biomolecular changes associated with nanoencapsulated hesperetin treatment in experimental oral carcinogenesis *Laser Phys. Lett.* **13** 035901
[36] Buschman H P, Motz J T, Deinum G, Römer T J, Fitzmaurice M, Kramer J R, van der Laarse A, Bruschke A V and Feld M S 2001 Diagnosis of human coronary atherosclerosis by morphology-based Raman spectroscopy *Cardiovasc. Pathol.* **10** 59–68
[37] Brauchle E, Sevgi F, Berrio D C, Schenke-Layland K, Casadei N, Riess O, Salker M S and Singh Y 2019 Raman imaging of α-synuclein aggregates in a rat model of Parkinson's disease *Proc. SPIE 10881, Imaging, Manipulation, and Analysis of Biomolecules, Cells, and Tissues XVII* 10881
[38] Sharma M, Tsai C L, Li Y C, Lee C C, Hsieh Y L, Chang C H, Chen S W and Chang L B 2024 Utilizing Raman spectroscopy for urinalysis to diagnose acute kidney injury stages in cardiac surgery patients *Ren. Fail.* **46** 2375741
[39] Huang Z F, Cao G, Sun Y, Du S R, Li Y Z, Lin J Q, Feng S Y and Lei J P 2016 Studies of male fertility with Raman spectroscopy *Spectrosc. Spect. Anal.* **36** 2818–22
[40] Sahu A, Deshmukh A, Ghanate A, Singh S, Chaturvedi P and Krishna C M 2012 Raman spectroscopy of oral buccal mucosa: a study on age-related physiological changes and tobacco-related pathological changes *Technol. Cancer Res. Treat.* **11** 529–41
[41] Singh S, Deshmukh A, Chaturvedi P and Krishna C M 2012 Raman spectroscopy in head and neck cancers: toward oncological applications *J. Cancer Res. Ther.* **8** 126
[42] Singh S, Deshmukh A, Chaturvedi P and Krishna C M 2012 *In vivo* Raman spectroscopy for oral cancers diagnosis *Proc. SPIE 8219, Biomedical Vibrational Spectroscopy V: Advances in Research and Industry* 82190K–K–6
[43] Singh S, Sahu A, Deshmukh A, Chaturvedi P and Krishna C M 2013 *In vivo* Raman spectroscopy of oral buccal mucosa: a study on malignancy associated changes (MAC)/cancer field effects (CFE) *Analyst* **138** 4175–82
[44] Kumar P, Bhattacharjee T, Ingle A, Maru G and Krishna C M 2016 Raman spectroscopy of experimental oral carcinogenesis: study on sequential cancer progression in Hamster Buccal pouch model *Technol. Cancer Res. Treat.* **15** 60–72
[45] Kumar P, Bhattacharjee T, Pandey M, Hole A, Ingle A and Murali Krishna C 2016 Raman spectroscopy in experimental oral carcinogenesis: investigation of abnormal changes in control tissues *J. Raman Spectrosc.* **47** 1318–26
[46] Sahu A, Deshmukh A, Hole A R, Chaturvedi P and Krishna C M 2016 *In vivo* subsite classification and diagnosis of oral cancers using Raman spectroscopy *J. Innov. Opt. Heal. Sci.* **9** 1650017
[47] Ramya A N, Arya J S, Madhukrishnan M, Shamjith S, Vidyalekshmi M S and Maiti K K 2021 Raman Imaging: an impending approach towards cancer diagnosis *Chem.-Asian. J.* **16** 409–22
[48] Stone N, Stavroulaki P, Kendall C, Birchall M and Barr H 2000 Raman spectroscopy for early detection of laryngeal malignancy: preliminary results *Laryngoscope* **110** 1756–63
[49] Faoláin E O, Hunter M B, Byrne J M, Kelehan P, Byrne H J and Lyng F M 2005 Potential of vibrational spectroscopy in the early detection of cervical cancer:: an exciting emerging field Opto-Ireland 2005 *Opt. Sens. Spectrosc.* **5826** 25–36

[50] Mo J H, Zheng W, Low J, Ng J, Ilancheran A and Huang Z W 2008 *In vivo* diagnosis of cervical precancer using high wavenumber Raman spectroscopy *Optics in Health Care and Biomedical Optics* **Iii** 6826

[51] O'Brien C M, Vargis E, Rudin A, Slaughter J C, Thomas G, Newton J M, Reese J, Bennett K A and Mahadevan-Jansen A 2018 *In vivo* Raman spectroscopy for biochemical monitoring of the human cervix throughout pregnancy *Am. J. Obstet. Gynecol.* **218** P528.E1–E18

[52] Fendel S and Schrader B 1998 Investigation of skin and skin lesions by NIR-FT-Raman spectroscopy *Fresen. J. Anal. Chem.* **360** 609–13

[53] Nijssen A, Maquelin K, Santos L F, Caspers P J, Schut T C B, den Hollander J C, Neumann M H and Puppels G J 2007 Discriminating basal cell carcinoma from perilesional skin using high wave-number Raman spectroscopy *J. Biomed. Opt.* **12** 34004–7

[54] Zhao J H, Lui H, McLean D and Zeng H S 2008 Real-time raman spectroscopy for noninvasive skin cancer detection—preliminary results *2008 30th Annual Int. Conf. of the Ieee Engineering in Medicine and Biology Society* Vols 1–8 *pp* 3107–9

[55] Wu M, Gao B B and Wei X B 2023 Recent advances in Raman spectroscopy for skin diagnosis *J Innov. Opt. Heal. Sci.* **16** 2330003

[56] Almond L M *et al* 2014 Endoscopic Raman spectroscopy enables objective diagnosis of dysplasia in Barrett's esophagus *Gastrointest. Endosc.* **79** 37–45

[57] Fraser-Miller S J, Rooney J S, Lau M, Gordon K C and Schultz M 2021 Can coupling multiple complementary methods improve the spectroscopic based diagnosis of gastro-intestinal illnesses? A proof of principle study using celiac disease as the model illness *Anal. Chem.* **93** 6363–74

[58] Wang J F, Lin K, Zheng W, Ho K Y, Teh M, Yeoh K G and Huang Z W 2016 Endoscope-based beveled and volume fiber-optic Raman probes for *in vivo* diagnosis of gastric dysplasia: a comparative study *Proc. SPIE 9704, Biomedical Vibrational Spectroscopy 2016: Advances in Research and Industry* 97040D

[59] Ding H, Dupont A W, Singhal S, Scott L D, Guha S, Younes M and Bi X H 2017 Analysis of mucosal lipids reveals histological disease activity in ulcerative colitis using endoscope-coupled Raman spectroscopy *Biomed. Opt. Express* **8** 3426–39

[60] Hanna K, Asiedu A-L, Theurer T, Muirhead D, Speirs V, Oweis Y and Abu-Eid R 2024 Advances in Raman spectroscopy for characterising oral cancer and oral potentially malignant disorders *Expert Rev. Mol. Med.* **26** e25

[61] Jin S, Lednev I K and Jung Y M 2024 Recent trends in surface-enhanced raman spectroscopy-based biosensors: label-free early disease diagnosis *J. Phys. Chem.* C **128** 8861–73

[62] Rath S, Sahu A, Gota V, Martínez-Torres P, Pichardo-Molina J and Murali Krishna C 2015 Raman spectroscopy for detection of imatinib in plasma: a proof of concept *J. Innov. Opt. Heal. Sci.* **8** 1550019

[63] Byrne H J, Knief P, Keating M E and Bonnier F 2016 Spectral pre and post processing for infrared and Raman spectroscopy of biological tissues and cells *Chem. Soc. Rev.* **45** 1865–78

[64] Ryabchykov O, Guo S and Bocklitz T 2019 Analyzing Raman spectroscopic data *Phys. Sci. Rev.* **4** 20170043

[65] Butler H J, Ashton L, Bird B, Cinque G, Curtis K, Dorney J, Esmonde-White K, Fullwood N J, Gardner B and Martin-Hirsch P L 2016 Using Raman spectroscopy to characterize biological materials *Nat. Protoc.* **11** 664–87

[66] Guo S, Popp J and Bocklitz T 2021 Chemometric analysis in Raman spectroscopy from experimental design to machine learning–based modeling *Nat. Protoc.* **16** 5426–59
[67] Anjikar A, Rao N P, Paneerselvam R, Jayaramulu K, Narayana C, Yamamoto T and Noothalapati H 2024 *Biomedical Imaging: Advances in Artificial Intelligence and Machine Learning* (Berlin: Springer) pp 209–47
[68] Sahu A, Sawant S, Talathi-Desai S and Murali Krishna C 2015 Raman spectroscopy of serum: a study on oral cancers *Biomed. Spectrosc. Imaging* **4** 171–87
[69] Sahu A K, Dhoot S, Singh A, Sawant S S, Nandakumar N, Talathi-Desai S, Garud M, Pagare S, Srivastava S and Nair S 2015 Oral cancer screening: serum Raman spectroscopic approach *J. Biomed. Opt.* **20** 115006
[70] Sahu A, Nandakumar N, Sawant S and Krishna C M 2015 Recurrence prediction in oral cancers: a serum Raman spectroscopy study *Analyst* **140** 2294–301
[71] Saha P, Sawant S, Deshmukh A, Hole A and Murali Krishna C 2023 Serum Raman spectroscopy: Prognostic applications in oral cancers *Head Neck* **45** 1244–54
[72] Sung H, Ferlay J, Siegel R L, Laversanne M, Soerjomataram I, Jemal A and Bray F 2021 Global cancer statistics 2020: GLOBOCAN estimates of incidence and mortality worldwide for 36 cancers in 185 countries *CA Cancer J. Clin.* **71** 209–49
[73] Lazaro-Pacheco D, Shaaban A M, Rehman S and Rehman I 2020 Raman spectroscopy of breast cancer *Appl. Spectrosc. Rev.* **55** 439–75
[74] Pichardo-Molina J, Frausto-Reyes C, Barbosa-García O, Huerta-Franco R, González-Trujillo J, Ramírez-Alvarado C, Gutiérrez-Juárez G and Medina-Gutiérrez C 2007 Raman spectroscopy and multivariate analysis of serum samples from breast cancer patients *Lasers Med. Sci.* **22** 229–36
[75] Li H, Wang S, Zeng Q, Chen C, Lv X, Ma M, Su H, Ma B, Chen C and Fang J 2022 Serum Raman spectroscopy combined with multiple classification models for rapid diagnosis of breast cancer *Photodiagn. Photodyn. Ther.* **40** 103115
[76] Bratchenko I A and Bratchenko L A 2023 Comment on 'Serum Raman spectroscopy combined with multiple classification models for rapid diagnosis of breast cancer' *Photodiagn. Photodyn. Ther.* **41** 103215
[77] Lin R, Peng B, Li L, He X, Yan H, Tian C, Luo H and Yin G 2023 Application of serum Raman spectroscopy combined with classification model for rapid breast cancer screening *Front. Oncol.* **13** 1258436
[78] Zeng Q, Chen C, Chen C, Song H, Li M, Yan J and Lv X 2023 Serum Raman spectroscopy combined with convolutional neural network for rapid diagnosis of HER2-positive and triple-negative breast cancer *Spectrochim. Acta* A **286** 122000
[79] Jiang J, Li L, Yin G, Luo H and Li J 2024 A molecular typing method for invasive breast cancer by serum raman spectroscopy *Clin. Breast Cancer* **24** 376–83
[80] Torre-Gutiérrez L G D l, Martínez-Zérega B E, Oseguera-Galindo D O, Aguilar-Lemarroy A, Jave-Suárez L F, Torres-González L A and González-Solís J L 2022 Breast cancer chemotherapy treatment monitoring based on serum sample Raman spectroscopy *Lasers Med. Sci.* **37** 3649–59
[81] Bhattacharjee T, Khan A, Kumar P, Ingle A, Maru G and Krishna C M 2015 Raman spectroscopy of serum: a study on 'pre'and 'post'breast adenocarcinoma resection in rat models *J. Biophotonics* **8** 575–83
[82] González-Solís J L, Martínez-Espinosa J C, Torres-González L A, Aguilar-Lemarroy A, Jave-Suárez L F and Palomares-Anda P 2014 Cervical cancer detection based on serum sample Raman spectroscopy *Lasers Med. Sci.* **29** 979–85

[83] Owens G L, Gajjar K, Trevisan J, Fogarty S W, Taylor S E, Da Gama-Rose B, Martin-Hirsch P L and Martin F L 2014 Vibrational biospectroscopy coupled with multivariate analysis extracts potentially diagnostic features in blood plasma/serum of ovarian cancer patients *J. Biophotonics* **7** 200–9

[84] Li X, Yang T and Li S 2012 Discrimination of serum Raman spectroscopy between normal and colorectal cancer using selected parameters and regression-discriminant analysis *Appl. Opt.* **51** 5038–43

[85] Li X, Yang T, Yu T and Li S 2011 Discrimination of serum Raman spectroscopy between normal and colorectal cancer *Euroean Conf. on Biomedical Optics* p 808727

[86] Li X, Yang T, Li S, Wang D, Song Y and Zhang S 2016 Raman spectroscopy combined with principal component analysis and k nearest neighbour analysis for non-invasive detection of colon cancer *Laser Phys.* **26** 035702

[87] Ito H *et al* 2020 Highly accurate colorectal cancer prediction model based on Raman spectroscopy using patient serum *World J. Gastrointest. Oncol.* **12** 1311–24

[88] Jenkins C A, Jenkins R A, Pryse M M, Welsby K A, Jitsumura M, Thornton C A, Dunstan P R and Harris D A 2018 A high-throughput serum Raman spectroscopy platform and methodology for colorectal cancer diagnostics *Analyst* **143** 6014

[89] Bahreini M, Hosseinzadegan A, Rashidi A, Miri S R, Mirzaei H R and Hajian P 2019 A Raman-based serum constituents' analysis for gastric cancer diagnosis: *in vitro* study *Talanta* **204** 826–32

[90] Foglia B, Turato C and Cannito S 2023 Hepatocellular carcinoma: latest research in pathogenesis, detection and treatment *Int. J. Mol. Sci.* **24** 12224

[91] Taleb I, Thiéfin G, Gobinet C, Untereiner V, Bernard-Chabert B, Heurgué A, Truntzer C, Hillon P, Manfait M and Ducoroy P 2013 Diagnosis of hepatocellular carcinoma in cirrhotic patients: a proof-of-concept study using serum micro-Raman spectroscopy *Analyst* **138** 4006

[92] Leng H, Zhang Z, Chen C and Chen C 2024 A class-imbalanced hybrid learning strategy based on Raman spectroscopy of serum samples for the diagnosis of hepatitis B, hepatitis A, and thyroid dysfunction *Spectrochim. Acta t* A **320** 124581

[93] Bukva M, Dobra G, Gomez-Perez J, Koos K, Harmati M, Gyukity-Sebestyen E, Biro T, Jenei A, Kormondi S and Horvath P 2021 Raman spectral signatures of serum-derived extracellular vesicle-enriched isolates may support the diagnosis of CNS tumors *Cancers* **13** 1407

[94] Nieuwland R and Siljander P R M 2024 A beginner's guide to study extracellular vesicles in human blood plasma and serum *J. Extracell. Vesicles* **13** e12400

[95] Palviainen M, Saraswat M, Varga Z, Kitka D, Neuvonen M, Puhka M, Joenväärä S, Renkonen R, Nieuwland R and Takatalo M 2020 Extracellular vesicles from human plasma and serum are carriers of extravesicular cargo—Implications for biomarker discovery *PLoS One* **15** e0236439

[96] Lee W, Lenferink A T, Otto C and Offerhaus H L 2020 Classifying Raman spectra of extracellular vesicles based on convolutional neural networks for prostate cancer detection *J. Raman Spectrosc.* **51** 293–300

[97] Lakpour N, Sadeghi M R, Jafarzadeh N, Henkel R, Hajiparvaneh A, Fathi Z, Ghods R, Gilany K and Madjd Z 2024 Metabolic fingerprinting of serum and seminal plasma of testicular cancer patients using Raman spectroscopy: a pilot study *J. Reprod. Infertil.* **25** 3–11

[98] Yan L, Su H, Liu J, Wen X, Luo H, Yin Y and Guo X 2024 Rapid detection of lung cancer based on serum Raman spectroscopy and a support vector machine: a case-control study *BMC Cancer* **24** 791

[99] Du Y, Hu L, Wu G, Tang Y, Cai X and Yin L 2023 Diagnoses in multiple types of cancer based on serum Raman spectroscopy combined with a convolutional neural network: gastric cancer, colon cancer, rectal cancer, lung cancer *Spectrochim. Acta* A **298** 122743

[100] Cao Y, Xiong J, Du Y, Tang Y and Yin L 2024 Raman spectroscopy combined with multivariate statistical algorithms for the simultaneous screening of cervical and breast cancers *Lasers Med. Sci.* **39** 68

[101] Paz-Bailey G, Adams L E, Deen J, Anderson K B and Katzelnick L C 2024 Dengue *Lancet* **403** 667–82

[102] Hänscheid T, Egan T J and Grobusch M P 2007 Haemozoin: from melatonin pigment to drug target, diagnostic tool, and immune modulator *Lancet Infect. Dis.* **7** 675–85

[103] Patel S K, Rajora N, Kumar S, Sahu A, Kochar S K, Krishna C M and Srivastava S 2019 Rapid discrimination of malaria-and dengue-infected patients sera using raman spectroscopy *Anal. Chem.* **91** 7054–62

[104] Khan S, Ullah R, Saleem M, Bilal M, Rashid R, Khan I, Mahmood A and Nawaz M 2016 Raman spectroscopic analysis of dengue virus infection in human blood sera *Optik* **127** 2086–8

[105] Khan S, Ullah R, Khan A, Wahab N, Bilal M and Ahmed M 2016 Analysis of dengue infection based on Raman spectroscopy and support vector machine (SVM) *Biomed. Opt. Express* **7** 2249–56

[106] Khan S, Ullah R, Khan A, Sohail A, Wahab N, Bilal M and Ahmed M 2017 Random forest-based evaluation of Raman spectroscopy for dengue fever analysis *Appl. Spectrosc.* **71** 2111–7

[107] Amin A, Ghouri N, Ali S, Ahmed M, Saleem M and Qazi J 2017 Identification of new spectral signatures associated with dengue virus infected sera *J. Raman Spectrosc.* **48** 705–10

[108] Sahu A, Dalal K, Naglot S, Aggarwal P and Murali Krishna C 2013 Serum based diagnosis of asthma using Raman spectroscopy: an early phase pilot study *PLoS One* **8** e78921

[109] Ullah R, Khan S, Farman F, Bilal M, Krafft C and Shahzad S 2019 Demonstrating the application of Raman spectroscopy together with chemometric technique for screening of asthma disease *Biomed. Opt. Express* **10** 600–9

[110] Chen C, Qi J, Li Y, Li D, Wu L, Li R, Chen Q and Sun N 2024 Applications of Raman spectroscopy in the diagnosis and monitoring of neurodegenerative diseases *Front. Neurosci-Switz.* **18** 1301107

[111] Ryzhikova E, Kazakov O, Halamkova L, Celmins D, Malone P, Molho E, Zimmerman E A and Lednev I K 2015 Raman spectroscopy of blood serum for Alzheimer's disease diagnostics: specificity relative to other types of dementia *J. Biophotonics* **8** 584–96

[112] Carota A G, Campanella B, Del Carratore R, Bongioanni P, Giannelli R and Legnaioli S 2022 Raman spectroscopy and multivariate analysis as potential tool to follow Alzheimer's disease progression *Anal. Bioanal. Chem.* **414** 4667–75

[113] Gualerzi A, Picciolini S, Carlomagno C, Terenzi F, Ramat S, Sorbi S and Bedoni M 2019 Raman profiling of circulating extracellular vesicles for the stratification of Parkinson's patients *Nanomed. Nanotechnol. Biol. Med.* **22** 102097

[114] Alix J J P, Verber N S, Schooling C N, Kadirkamanathan V, Turner M R, Malaspina A, Day J C C and Shaw P J 2022 Label-free fibre optic Raman spectroscopy with bounded simplex-structured matrix factorization for the serial study of serum in amyotrophic lateral sclerosis *Analyst* **147** 5113–20

[115] Dogan G Y, Halimoglu G, Kaplanoglu D, Aksoy U M, Kandeger A, Yavuz E, Kartal S, Fausto R and Ildiz G O 2024 Raman spectra of blood serum as holistic biomarker for differential auxiliary diagnoses of Attention Deficit and Hyperactivity Disorder (ADHD) in adults *Spectrosc. J.* **2** 53–67

[116] Yin G, Li L, Lu S, Yin Y, Su Y, Zeng Y, Luo M, Ma M, Zhou H and Orlandini L 2021 An efficient primary screening of COVID-19 by serum Raman spectroscopy *J. Raman Spectrosc.* **52** 949–58

[117] Goulart A C C, Silveira L, Carvalho H C, Dorta C B, Pacheco M T T and Zângaro R A 2022 Diagnosing COVID-19 in human serum using Raman spectroscopy *Lasers Med. Sci.* **37** 2217–26

[118] Guleken Z, Tuyji Tok Y, Jakubczyk P, Paja W, Pancerz K, Shpotyuk Y, Cebulski J and Depciuch J 2022 Development of novel spectroscopic and machine learning methods for the measurement of periodic changes in COVID-19 antibody level *Measurement* **196** 111258

[119] Harris A T, Lungari A, Needham C J, Smith S L, Lones M A, Fisher S E, Yang X B, Cooper N, Kirkham J, Smith D A and Martin-Hirsch D P 2009 Potential for Raman spectroscopy to provide cancer screening using a peripheral blood sample *Head Neck Oncol* **1** 34

IOP Publishing

Spectroscopic Techniques for Cancer Diagnostics

Inbarasan Muniraj and Bryan Hennelly

Chapter 10

Innovative phototherapy approaches for cancer diagnosis with surface-enhanced Raman scattering guidance

P Sanoop, Jyothi B Nair and Manu M Joseph

Phototherapy (PT) has emerged as a promising treatment modality for various cancers, leveraging the precise targeting of cancerous tissues while minimizing damage to surrounding healthy cells. This chapter examines novel phototherapy techniques that make use of surface-enhanced Raman scattering (SERS) technology to improve treatment monitoring and cancer diagnostics. Molecular-level insights into the tumour microenvironment are provided by SERS, a very sensitive spectroscopic technology that allows for real-time guidance and efficacy monitoring of PT. The chapter explores the most recent developments in SERS-based PT, such as the creation of multifunctional nanoparticles (NPs) that operate as SERS-active probes and therapeutic agents. These dual-purpose NPs make it possible to do *in situ* molecular imaging and PT at the same time. The chapter also highlights the potential for these combination approaches to improve therapeutic outcomes by integrating SERS with other phototherapeutic procedures like photodynamic therapy (PDT) and photothermal therapy (PTT). This chapter seeks to highlight the revolutionary potential of SERS-guided PT techniques in improving cancer treatment by offering a thorough summary of the latest research and technology advancements in the field. By improving cancer therapy's accuracy and effectiveness, the methodologies under discussion hold the potential to provide more individualized and successful treatment paradigms.

10.1 Introduction

Owing to its exceptional sensitivity and specificity, SERS has completely changed the field of molecular detection and imaging. SERS makes it possible to detect traces of biomolecules and provides rich structural information by improving the Raman scattering signals of molecules adsorbed on nanostructured metallic surfaces.

doi:10.1088/978-0-7503-5949-8ch10

Because of this, SERS is a handy tool in biological applications, especially for treatment monitoring and disease diagnostics. Various scientific reports connect the effective coupling of SERS with other therapeutic techniques, and they have received great attention in the medical field. Among these, two important phototherapeutic techniques are PDT and PTT, collectively known as PT. PDT and PTT are two types of phototherapies that use light to produce therapeutic effects. PDT uses photosensitizing chemicals to kill targeted cells by producing reactive oxygen species (ROS) activated by light. PTT, on the other hand, produces localized hyperthermia and cell death by converting light energy into heat using compounds that absorb light. Both methods minimize harm to the nearby healthy tissues by providing exact spatial and temporal control over the course of the therapy. SERS and PT together create a potent synergistic strategy that combines the best features of both techniques, especially for the diagnosis of tumours with its ability to provide accurate localization of therapeutic chemicals and real-time molecular information [1–5]. Future research could focus on optimizing the integration of SERS with phototherapies like PDT and PTT to enhance the precision and efficacy of treatment. Additionally, exploring the potential for real-time monitoring and feedback during therapy could further improve patient outcomes and reduce side effects.

10.1.1 Phototherapy

Phototherapy, also referred to as light therapy, has shown promise in providing novel approaches to the treatment of various diseases, especially different cancers. With the least amount of harm to the surrounding healthy tissues, this treatment approach targets and destroys cancer cells by utilizing light wavelengths. Using photosensitive agents that are delivered topically or systemically to the afflicted areas, phototherapy for cancer is based on its capacity to selectively activate these agents [6, 7]. PDT and PTT are the two main processes of PT. Using light-sensitive substances known as photosensitizers (PSs), photodynamic treatment produces ROS that cause cell death when they are activated by light with a certain wavelength. In contrast, PTT uses light energy to produce heat, which causes localized hyperthermia and the eventual death of tumour cells. The capacity of PT to offer a targeted treatment modality while lowering the systemic adverse effects frequently connected to conventional cancer treatments like radiation and chemotherapy is one of its main advantages. PTT is a rapidly advancing technique that leverages the ability of certain photothermal agents (PTAs) to convert near-infrared (NIR) light into localized heat, thereby inducing cell death in targeted tissues. Among the most commonly used agents are gold NPs, carbon-based materials like graphene oxide and carbon nanotubes, metal sulfides such as copper sulfide (CuS), and conjugated polymers including polypyrrole and polyaniline [8–11]. These materials are chosen for their strong NIR absorbance, high photothermal conversion efficiency, and biocompatibility, making them ideal for precise and effective treatments. The development of these agents has the potential to significantly enhance the efficacy of PTT, offering a non-invasive alternative for cancer therapy and other medical applications, with minimal damage to surrounding healthy tissues. Additionally, PT is carefully controlled and repeatable as needed, meaning that a treatment plan that is customized and flexible to meet the needs of each patient can be implemented. The effectiveness of PT has been significantly improved by recent developments in nanotechnology. The introduction of PTAs and PSs based on NPs has enhanced the delivery and activation of therapeutic agents, leading to a decrease in off-target effects and an increase in specificity. Furthermore, real-time monitoring of treatment progress and results has been made easier by the integration of imaging technologies with PT, which has improved the accuracy and efficacy of cancer care [9, 12–14]. An exciting development in this field is the integration of SERS for therapeutic monitoring. SERS, known for its diverse applications in diagnosis, imaging, chemical analysis, and detection, can be employed alongside PTT to provide real-time, molecular-level monitoring of the therapeutic process. This dual approach not only enhances the precision and effectiveness of PTT but also enables clinicians to track treatment progress and make adjustments as needed, ensuring optimal patient outcomes with minimal harm to surrounding healthy tissues. Additionally, the use of a single NIR laser for both SERS and PT presents a promising approach by enabling dual functionality within a single platform, enhancing treatment precision and efficiency. This integration could streamline the therapeutic process, reducing the need for multiple devices and minimizing patient discomfort. Furthermore, the combined application may allow for real-time monitoring of therapeutic effects, potentially leading to better-controlled and more effective treatments.

10.1.2 Surface-enhanced Raman scattering

Raman spectroscopy was discovered in 1928 by Indian scientist Sir C V Raman, and now it has become an essential tool in many scientific fields. It is a non-destructive, label-free technique for molecular investigation that offers insightful information about the vibrational and rotational modes of molecules. It depends on molecules scattering monochromatic light in an inelastic manner. Most incident photons in a laser beam that strikes a sample experience elastic scattering, while a tiny percentage experience inelastic scattering, which causes a wavelength shift known as the Raman effect. The energy levels linked to the rotational and vibrational modes of the molecules in the sample are reflected in this shift. The acquired Raman spectrum offers distinct fingerprint details regarding the molecular makeup of the specimen, facilitating both qualitative and quantitative examination. Every peak in the spectrum represents a distinct vibrational mode that reveals details about the molecular structure and chemical interactions. Raman spectroscopy has been used in many different scientific domains over the years, including chemistry, biology, material science, pharmaceuticals, forensics, and so on. Nevertheless, despite all its benefits, conventional Raman spectroscopy frequently has poor sensitivity, which restricts its use, particularly when working with trace amounts of analytes. To get over this restriction, SERS was introduced. SERS has noticeably higher sensitivity and makes it possible to identify analytes at much lower concentrations. At the most basic level, SERS is a surface-sensitive technique that enhances the Raman signal by adsorbing molecules on corrugated metal nano surfaces. It has various applications in the fields of diagnosis and imaging, chemical and compositional analysis, food and pharmaceutical industries, narcotics, and explosive detection [15–22]. Nowadays, the integration of SERS into phototherapies, such as PTT and PDT, offers a powerful tool for real-time therapeutic monitoring. SERS, with its established applications in diagnosis, imaging, chemical analysis, and various industries, provides molecular-level sensitivity that can be harnessed to track the efficacy of phototherapies. By monitoring the biochemical changes in tissues during treatment, SERS enables precise adjustments to be made on the fly, ensuring optimal therapeutic outcomes. This combination not only enhances the effectiveness of phototherapies but also minimizes damage to healthy tissues, offering a more controlled and personalized treatment approach.

10.1.3 Cancer treatment modalities

Over time, cancer treatment approaches have changed dramatically, taking advantage of advances in medical research, technology, and a better understanding of the biology of the disease. The main objectives of cancer treatment are to eradicate cancer cells, stop them from spreading, and reduce the number of harmful effects on healthy tissues. The type and stage of the cancer, the patient's general health, and their preferences are some of the elements that influence the treatment decision. Surgery, radiation therapy, chemotherapy, targeted therapy, immunotherapy, hormone therapy, and newer forms of care like gene therapy and precision medicine are the primary methods used to treat cancer. One of the most traditional and widely used cancer treatments is surgery. It entails the surgical removal of the tumour along with, occasionally, the lymph nodes and surrounding tissues. Minimally invasive treatments like laparoscopy and robotic-assisted surgery shorten the recovery periods and increase results. High-energy particles such as gamma rays, proton beams, or x-rays, are used in radiation therapy to kill or harm cancer cells. When it comes to reducing tumour size before surgery or getting rid of cancer cells that remain after surgery, this method can be utilized either alone or in combination with other therapies. Radiation therapy is now more precisely administered, reducing the amount of harm to nearby healthy tissues with the help of imaging and delivery methods. Using medications to destroy cancer cells that divide quickly is known as chemotherapy. These medications can be injected intravenously, orally, or directly into the afflicted areas. Chemotherapy is useful in killing cancer cells, but it can also harm healthy, quickly proliferating cells and cause adverse effects. Targeted therapy targets chemicals or pathways that are essential to the development and survival of cancer cells. Through disruption of certain targets, these treatments can effectively impede the advancement of cancer and may have fewer adverse effects than conventional chemotherapy. Immunotherapy is a fast-growing field of study and development that has demonstrated amazing success in curing several forms of cancer. Breast and prostate cancer are two examples of malignancies that respond well to hormone therapy. This therapy slows or stops the proliferation of cancer cells by either interfering with hormone receptors on the cells or by inhibiting the body's ability to manufacture hormones. On the cutting edge of cancer treatment are novel techniques including gene therapy, precision medicine, and the application of artificial intelligence in treatment planning. Gene therapy seeks to rectify genetic flaws in cancer cells, whereas precision medicine customizes treatment according to the patient's and the tumour's genetic profiles. Predicting treatment outcomes and customizing therapeutic programs are made easier with the use of artificial intelligence. Similarly, phototherapies including PDT and PTT have great attention for the effective diagnosis of diseases, especially cancers. Once these PTs are applied with suitable monitoring techniques such as Raman spectroscopy, fluorescence spectroscopy shows enhanced outcomes for the overall diagnostics and treatment [23–27]. Integrating SERS over fluorescence for monitoring cancer therapy offers a significant advantage due to its higher sensitivity and ability to detect subtle molecular changes in the tumour microenvironment. SERS provides more detailed and specific information, enabling earlier detection of therapeutic responses and resistance. This enhanced monitoring capability could lead to more personalized and effective cancer treatments by allowing clinicians to make timely adjustments based on real-time molecular feedback.

10.1.4 Rationale for combining SERS and PT

In the realm of medical diagnosis and treatment, SERS and PT represent cutting-edge methodologies. The synergistic benefits of combining these techniques improve therapeutic efficacy and diagnostic accuracy. Real-time molecular changes during PT can be tracked by SERS, which enables quick modifications to treatment plans. SERS's great sensitivity makes it possible to identify early molecular alterations that may be signs of the treatment's effectiveness. When PT and SERS are combined, it becomes easier to implement a theranostic strategy, in which treatment and diagnosis are combined into one operation. This can shorten the period between diagnosis and intervention and, finally enhance treatment results. Therapeutic compounds can be engineered into the NPs used in SERS. PT can cause these compounds to be released once they reach the target region, resulting in localized treatment and a reduction in systemic adverse effects. With the use of quantitative data on biomolecular changes provided by SERS, detailed tracking of illness development and therapy efficacy is made possible. Through dynamic feedback enabled by the integration, light dosage, and treatment duration can be optimally tailored based on real-time molecular information during PT sessions. The combination of SERS and PT offers a compelling rationale by merging the strengths of both techniques to create a highly effective and precise treatment approach. SERS provides unparalleled molecular sensitivity, enabling real-time monitoring of therapeutic progress at the biochemical level, while PT, through methods like photothermal and photodynamic therapy, delivers targeted destruction of cancerous cells with minimal damage to surrounding healthy tissues. This synergy not only enhances the accuracy and efficacy of the treatment but also allows for dynamic adjustments during therapy, leading to improved patient outcomes and reduced side effects. Precise PT treatment can be used to destroy germs and real-time monitoring of bacterial infections [7, 9, 28–30].

10.2 Fundamentals of phototherapy

The medical procedure of PT uses artificial or natural light to treat a patient's illness. Light-emitting diodes (LEDs), sunlight, halogen lights, and ultraviolet (UV) fluorescent light bulbs can all be used as forms of treatment. This method is used to treat a range of medical conditions, such as malignancies, skin wound infections, circadian rhythm sleep-wake problems, and seasonal affective disorder (SAD).

10.2.1 Photodynamic therapy and photothermal therapy

PDT is a type of PT that targets diseased and malignant cells by producing toxic ROS using non-toxic light-sensitive compounds or PSs selectively exposed to light at a controlled wavelength, laser intensity, and irradiation time. Because oxygen is necessary for function, it is less effective in hypoxic conditions and highly established tumours. Because ROS are radicals, it is challenging to cause selective apoptosis in sick cells. However, this can be achieved by controlling membrane potential, other cell-type-specific features that affect permeability, or photoimmunotherapy. The phototoxicity of the treatment wavelength should be considered while developing any phototherapeutic agent [12, 14, 31].

PTT is another type of PT that uses non-toxic substances known as PTAs that directly convert light energy to heat energy when exposed to a certain wavelength of light. The amount of light converted to heat is determined by the photothermal conversion efficiency, which can also determine the required laser intensity and irradiation time for treatments. NIR spectra, which are further subdivided into NIR-I (760–900 nm), NIR-II (900–1880 nm), and NIR-III (2080–2340 nm) windows, are typically used for PTT treatments. These regions' wavelengths are usually less phototoxic than UV or intense visible light. Furthermore, it has been noted that NIR-II wavelengths penetrate deeper than NIR-I wavelengths, making it possible to treat malignancies, infections, and deeper wounds. The creation of a PTA requires careful consideration of various factors, such as photothermal conversion efficiency, phototoxicity, laser intensity, irradiation period, and the temperature range between 46 °C and 60 °C at which human cell viability is compromised. Currently, indocyanine green which is effective against both tumour and bacterial cells is the only FDA-approved photothermal agent [5, 32, 33].

Because of its heat-based mode of action, PDT is more selective than PTT; nevertheless, PTT is also less likely to induce drug resistance than the majority of currently available treatments, if not all of them. Furthermore, because PTT uses a greater wavelength of light than PDT, it can be used for deeper wounds, infections, and tumours as well as hypoxic settings. Because PTT is active in hypoxic conditions, it can be applied to cancers that are more advanced than PDT. Because heat is proportionate to membrane permeability, low-temperature PTT ($\leqslant$45 °C) for the treatment of infections is potentially a possibility when paired with an antibiotic agent. Increased membrane permeability brought on by a hotter environment permits the medication to enter the cell. This would remove the effect on the survival of human cells, and promoting the accumulation of antibiotics within the target cell might help restore the activity of antibiotics to which infections have grown resistant [34, 35].

10.2.2 Mechanisms of action

PDT is a medical treatment that utilizes a combination of a photosensitizing agent, light, and oxygen to induce cell death, primarily in cancer cells. A PS is administered to the patient. This agent can be given intravenously, orally, or applied topically, depending on the location and type of lesion being treated. The PS accumulates more in cancer cells than in normal cells. There is a waiting period to allow the PS to be preferentially absorbed by the targeted cells. This interval can vary from a few hours to a couple of days. The targeted area is exposed to a specific wavelength of light, usually delivered through a laser or a light-emitting diode. Upon activation by light, the PS undergoes a chemical change and transfers energy to molecular oxygen, producing ROS, particularly singlet oxygen (figure 10.1). These ROS are highly reactive and can damage cellular components. The ROS generated by the activated PS can cause direct damage to cellular structures such as membranes, mitochondria, and DNA, leading to cell death. This can occur through various mechanisms including programmed cell death (apoptosis), uncontrolled cell death (necrosis), or self-digestion (autophagy). PDT can also induce an immune response. The cellular debris and altered tumour microenvironment created by PDT can stimulate an immune response against the remaining cancer cells, providing an additional therapeutic effect [36–38].

PTT is a minimally invasive treatment method that uses light usually NIR light to generate heat to destroy cancer cells or other pathological tissues. Common

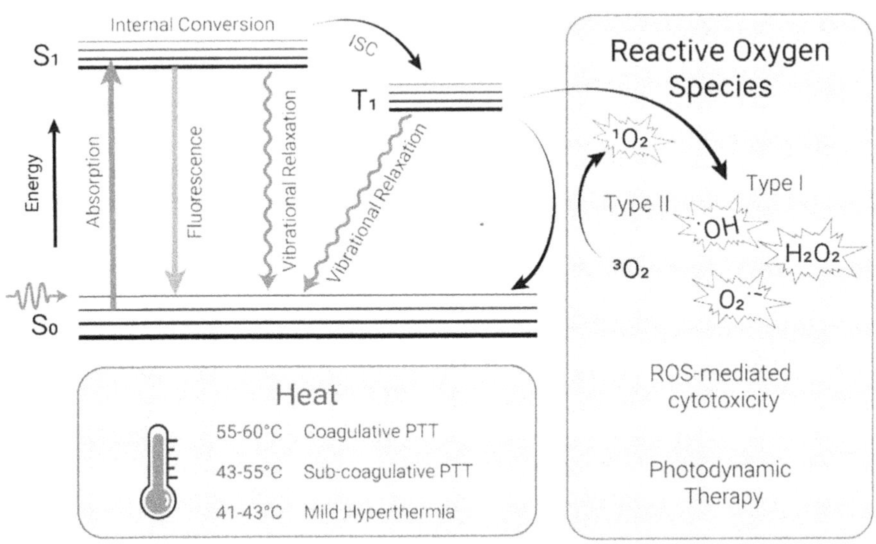

Figure 10.1. Simplified Jablonski diagram depicting the photophysical and photochemical mechanisms underlying PDT and PTT, adapted with permission from [9]; copyright 2023, American Chemical Society.

materials include gold NPs, carbon nanotubes, and other nanomaterials. These materials have strong absorption in the NIR region and convert absorbed light into heat. The NPs or (PTAs are typically administered into the body and accumulate in the tumour tissue due to the enhanced permeability and retention (EPR) effect. Alternatively, they can be conjugated with targeting ligands that bind specifically to cancer cells. After accumulation at the target site, the area is exposed to NIR light. NIR light is preferred because it can penetrate deeper into tissues compared to visible light, ensuring that the therapy can reach deeper tumours. The NPs or PTAs absorb the NIR light and convert it into heat through non-radiative processes. The temperature at the target site rises significantly, typically in the range of 42 °C–45 °C, which is sufficient to damage or destroy cancer cells. The localized heating leads to the denaturation of cellular proteins, disruption of cell membranes, and ultimately cell death. The heat can also induce programmed cell death(apoptosis) or uncontrolled cell death(necrosis) in cancer cells. In some cases, PTT can stimulate an immune response against the tumour, aiding in the recognition and destruction of cancer cells by the immune system. The remnants of the NPs or PTAs are eventually cleared from the body through natural excretory pathways, depending on the material properties and the size of the NPs [5, 11, 39].

10.2.3 Photosensitizers and photothermal agents: types and functions

PDT is an experimental medicine mostly used to treat cancer and other illnesses. It uses light-sensitive substances called PSs in combination with oxygen and light to cause cell death. There are first-, second-, and third-generation PSs based on the nature of PT activity. The most widely used first-generation PS is porphyrins, which are naturally occurring substances with structural similarities to haemoglobin. The porphyrin that is most frequently utilized in PDT is photofrin, which is the pure version of hematoporphyrin derivative (HPD). Examples of the second generation include derivatives of benzoporphyrin, phthalocyanines, and chlorins. In comparison to first-generation PSs, second-generation PSs have higher specificity, fewer adverse effects, and greater light absorption qualities. Third-generation PSs are made with fewer side effects and improved targeting capabilities. Frequently, they undergo modifications such as conjugation to peptides, antibodies, or NPs to improve their selective accumulation within the intended tissue. PSs serve a multitude of purposes, for instance, they exhibit selective accumulation, meaning that malignant cells preferentially absorb them over healthy cells. To minimize injury to healthy tissue, this selective buildup is essential. A certain wavelength of light activates the PS once it has been collected in the target tissue. The PS's absorption properties influence the wavelength selection. The PS releases energy into molecular oxygen when it is exposed to light, producing ROS like free radicals and singlet oxygen. These ROS cause cellular constituents to suffer oxidative damage, which results in cell death. In similar ways, PTAs can cause localized hyperthermia and cell death because they absorb light and transform it into heat. Examples of these agents include gold NPs, carbon nanotubes, and other nanomaterials. For efficient heating, these agents are made to have a high absorption in the NIR spectrum [14, 33, 40, 41].

10.2.4 Phototherapy in clinical practice: applications and outcomes

PT includes both PDT and PTT diagnostics techniques. The most well-known application of PDT is in the treatment of malignancies, such as those of the skin, head, and neck regions, lungs, and gastrointestinal tract. PDT is useful in treating non-melanoma skin malignancies such as squamous cell carcinoma and basal cell carcinoma. When topical PSs and light exposure are used together, malignant cells can be specifically destroyed while healthy tissue is left intact. PDT is also used for recurring malignancies in the head and neck area as well as early-stage cancers. It provides a less intrusive substitute for radiation and surgery. PDT can be used to relieve symptoms in advanced stages of non-small cell lung cancer as well as treat it in its early stages. For patients who are not candidates for surgery, it is especially helpful. Barrett's oesophagus, a condition that precedes oesophageal adenocarcinoma, and oesophageal cancer are treated using PDT. In addition to treating cancer, PDT is frequently used in dermatology to treat diseases like actinic keratosis, psoriasis, and acne. PDT works by attacking propionibacterium acnes and sebaceous glands to lessen severe acne. One alternate treatment for psoriasis is PDT, which works by regulating immune responses and decreasing skin cell growth. PDT lowers the chance of developing squamous cell carcinoma by effectively curing this precancerous condition. PDT is used to treat several eye diseases, most notably age-related macular degeneration (AMD). PDT targets aberrant blood vessels in the retina using verteporfin, a typical PS, which helps patients with wet AMD from losing their eyesight. Because PDT kills both bacteria and fungi, it has potential use in the treatment of microbial illnesses. For types of bacteria resistant to antibiotics, PSs which are activated by light offer an alternative to antibiotics by destroying microbial cells. The application of PDT for neurological disorders, such as gliomas and Alzheimer's disease, is still being studied. PDT, for instance, may be a less invasive approach than surgery for treating malignant brain tumours. PDT is being studied experimentally to lower brain amyloid plaques, which are linked to Alzheimer's disease [42–46].

Having several uses in contemporary medicine, photothermal treatment is a very adaptable and promising technology. It is very appealing for cancer therapy, bacterial infection control, and possibly other therapeutic fields because of its limited invasiveness and capacity to deliver localized treatment. The important use of PTT is in tumour ablation. Some nanomaterials such as graphene, carbon nanotubes, and gold NPs with a high photothermal conversion efficiency can be made to accumulate in tumours The NIR light that these NPs emit causes them to get heated, which in turn causes cancer cells to be destroyed locally by hyperthermia. The therapeutic efficacy of PTT can be increased by combining it with other cancer treatments such immunotherapy, radiation, and chemotherapy. PTT can also go after cancer cells that have spread. PTT can lessen the spread of cancer and enhance patient outcomes by focusing on circulating tumour cells or cells in the pre-metastatic microenvironment. Treatment of bacterial infections, especially those brought on by strains resistant to antibiotics, has showed potential with PTT. It is possible to combine PTAs with peptides or antibodies that target bacterial cells specifically. Through thermal damage, the heat produced by NIR irradiation can kill microorganisms. For instance, by getting rid of harmful bacteria and speeding up the healing process, PTT can be used to treat infected wounds. Wound dressings can benefit from the controlled and focused approach to infection management that photothermal NPs offer. PTT drugs offer both therapeutic and diagnostic benefits when used as contrast agents for photoacoustic imaging. Real-time monitoring of treatment progress and necessary adjustments to therapeutic parameters are made possible by this dual feature. According to recent studies, PTT may be utilized to treat specific neurological conditions. PTT has been investigated, for instance, in the ablation of epileptic foci and the control of neuronal activity in disorders like Parkinson's disease. PTT may be used in the field of ophthalmology, specifically for the ablation of aberrant blood vessels in diseases like AMD and the treatment of ocular malignancies [10, 11, 32, 33, 40, 47].

10.3 Surface-enhanced Raman scattering

SERS was introduced in the late 1970s as a technique to enhance the Raman signal by several orders of magnitude. The enhancement arises from the interaction of the analyte molecules with nanostructured metallic surfaces, typically gold or silver, which exhibit localized surface plasmon resonances. In SERS, when analyte molecules are adsorbed onto the surface of metal NPs or nanostructures, they experience an intense electromagnetic field enhancement due to the excitation of surface plasmons. This enhancement results in a dramatic increase in Raman scattering intensity, making it possible to detect even a single molecule. This extraordinary sensitivity has led to widespread applications of SERS in areas such as biomedical diagnostics, environmental monitoring, food safety, and homeland security. Raman spectroscopy and its surface-enhanced variant, SERS, have revolutionized the field of molecular analysis, offering powerful tools for chemical identification and characterization. While traditional Raman spectroscopy provides valuable information about molecular structure and composition, SERS extends its capabilities by offering unparalleled sensitivity and detection limits [48–51].

10.3.1 Principle of SERS

SERS is a powerful analytical technique that enhances the Raman scattering signal by several orders of magnitude through the interaction of molecules with nano-structured metallic surfaces (figure 10.2).

This enhancement enables the detection and characterization of analytes at extremely low concentrations, making SERS a valuable tool in various scientific disciplines and technological applications. The enhancement mechanism in SERS arises from two main phenomena such as electromagnetic enhancement, and chemical enhancement. SERS experiments typically involve several key steps, including substrate preparation, sample deposition, spectral acquisition, and data analysis. The choice of experimental parameters and methodologies can significantly impact the sensitivity and reproducibility of SERS measurements.

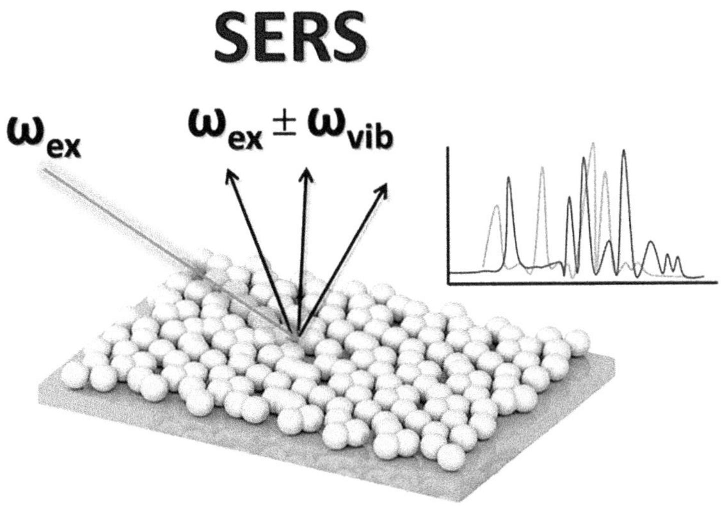

Figure 10.2. The overall schematic diagram of SERS, adapted with permission from [52], copyright 2020, American Chemical Society.

The first step in performing SERS experiments is the preparation of nanostructured metal substrates. These substrates can be fabricated using various techniques, such as nanosphere lithography, electron beam lithography, chemical synthesis, or electrodeposition. Once the substrates are prepared, the analyte molecules of interest are deposited onto the substrate surface. This can be achieved through methods such as drop casting, spin coating, or evaporation. Care must be taken to ensure uniform coverage of the substrate and to optimize the concentration of analyte molecules for maximum SERS signal enhancement. After sample deposition, the SERS spectra are acquired using a Raman spectrometer equipped with a laser excitation source. The acquired spectra contain information about the vibrational and rotational modes of the analyte molecules, allowing for qualitative and quantitative analysis. The final step in SERS experiments involves data analysis to extract relevant information from the acquired spectra. This may include peak assignment, spectral deconvolution, multivariate analysis, and comparison with reference spectra or databases. Advanced data processing techniques, such as chemometric methods and machine learning algorithms, can further enhance the accuracy and reliability of SERS-based molecular identification and quantification [53–56].

10.3.2 Enhancement mechanisms in SERS

Central to the success of SERS is the enhancement mechanisms that amplify the Raman signals of molecules adsorbed on nanostructured metal surfaces. Understanding these enhancement mechanisms is crucial for optimizing SERS performance and expanding its applications across various fields [57]. One of the primary enhancement mechanisms in SERS is electromagnetic enhancement, which arises from the interaction between the incident electromagnetic field and localized surface plasmon resonances (LSPRs) in the metal nanostructures. When a metal NP is irradiated with light at its resonance frequency, it induces collective oscillations of conduction electrons, known as surface plasmons. These plasmons generate intense electromagnetic fields localized around the NP surface, creating 'hot spots' where the Raman scattering of nearby molecules is significantly enhanced. The enhancement factor can be as high as 10^6–10^{14}, enabling the detection of single molecules [58, 59]. Chemical enhancement in SERS stems from the modification of the electronic and chemical properties of molecules upon interaction with the metal surface. This enhancement mechanism is particularly relevant for molecules with specific chemical functionalities, such as aromatic groups or unsaturated bonds. Adsorption of molecules onto the metal surface can lead to charge transfer processes, resonance effects, and changes in molecular orientation, resulting in enhanced Raman scattering [60, 61]. Chemical enhancement is often observed in conjunction with electromagnetic enhancement, further boosting the overall SERS signal [62]. Recent research efforts have focused on advancing our understanding of SERS enhancement mechanisms and developing novel strategies to further improve SERS performance. Hybrid nanostructures combining plasmonic metals with other materials, such as semiconductors or dielectrics, have been explored to achieve synergistic enhancement effects. Additionally, precise control over the spatial distribution of electromagnetic fields using techniques like tip-enhanced Raman spectroscopy (TERS) and gap-mode SERS has enabled sub-nanometre resolution imaging and spectroscopy of molecules. Furthermore, advances in theoretical modelling and simulation techniques have provided valuable insights into the complex interplay of factors governing SERS enhancement [63–65].

10.3.3 Applications of SERS in biomedicine

SERS's excellent sensitivity, molecular specificity, and capacity for real-time data have made it a potent tool in biomedical diagnostics. At very low concentrations, SERS can identify biomarkers linked to cancer. It has been used, for example, to pinpoint particular DNA sequences and protein markers that are suggestive of different types of cancer. By identifying cancerous cells, SERS can assist surgeons in defining the boundaries of tumours during surgery and guarantee that all malignant tissues are removed while leaving healthy ones intact. Clinical sample microorganisms have been identified and quantified using SERS. The method uses each strain's distinct Raman signature to identify it from others. SERS-based tests are capable of quickly diagnosing viral infections like COVID-19 and influenza by detecting viral particles and their genetic content. One essential use of SERS is non-invasive glucose monitoring. SERS can give diabetic patients with continuous glucose monitoring without requiring blood samples by measuring sweat or interstitial fluid. Personalized therapy can benefit from the remarkable sensitivity with which SERS can monitor medication concentrations in biological fluids. Forensic science also employs this approach to find evidence of illegal drug use in body fluids. Early biomarkers for neurodegenerative illnesses such as Parkinson's and Alzheimer's can be found using SERS. For example, SERS can be used to identify certain protein aggregations linked to various disorders. Early diagnosis and monitoring of cardiovascular illnesses can be aided by the identification of biomarkers in blood samples, such as triglycerides, cholesterol, and certain proteins. SERS technology and substrates will probably continue to progress, increasing its application in clinical diagnostics and enabling earlier disease identification and more individualized therapy [2, 66–69].

10.4 Integration of SERS and PT: concept and design

Theranostics is the fusion of therapeutic and diagnostic modalities that has drawn a lot of interest in contemporary medical research. The combination of PT and SERS provides a strong foundation for concurrent diagnosis and treatment. While PT, such as PDT and PTT, offers efficient treatment choices for a variety of disorders, particularly cancer, SERS offers incredibly sensitive detection capabilities. Metallic nanostructures that boost the Raman signal and offer a large surface area for molecule adsorption, such as gold or silver NPs. For efficient ROS formation, PSs with strong absorption in the therapeutic window of 650–900 nm should be chosen. There should be a coincidence between the PS's absorption peak for PT and the NPs' plasmon resonance for SERS. A better optimization study can achieve efficient PT and increase the SERS signal without resulting in thermal damage ensuring the effective and precise delivery of PSs and NPs to the intended location [70–72].

10.4.1 Synergistic potential of SERS-guided PT

There are several reports suggesting that SERS and PT will work in concert to improve treatment results. Targeted tissue molecular fingerprinting can be obtained in real-time with SERS. This makes it possible to distinguish between malignant and healthy cells with precision, directing to the precise location that needs care. Theranostic applications of simultaneous therapy and diagnostics are supported by the combination of SERS with PT. The dual roles of the SERS-active NPs are as imaging contrast agents and as carriers of PSs or PTAs. By functionalizing them to target cell receptors, NPs can promote the accumulation of phototherapeutic and SERS-active drugs in the tumour microenvironment. The local concentration of light-absorbing agents can be increased using SERS-active NPs, enhancing the effectiveness of both PDT and PTT. This focussed concentration can decrease negative effects and lower the dosage of PSs needed. SERS offers instantaneous feedback on the molecular alterations taking place in the tissue as a result of PT. This enables medical professionals to track the course of the treatment and alter as needed. The phototherapeutic dose can be adjusted to maximize therapy benefit while minimizing side effects by examining the SERS spectra. Understanding the pathophysiological alterations at the molecular level both during and after treatment can be facilitated by SERS-guided PT. This can help uncover possible biomarkers for more effective treatment approaches and provide insight into the mechanism's underlying resistance. Patients experience less trauma when non-invasive or minimally invasive diagnosis methods are possible thanks to SERS's excellent sensitivity. The combination minimizes systemic side effects and permits localized treatment, which lessens the influence on nearby healthy tissues (figure 10.3) [6, 30, 66, 73].

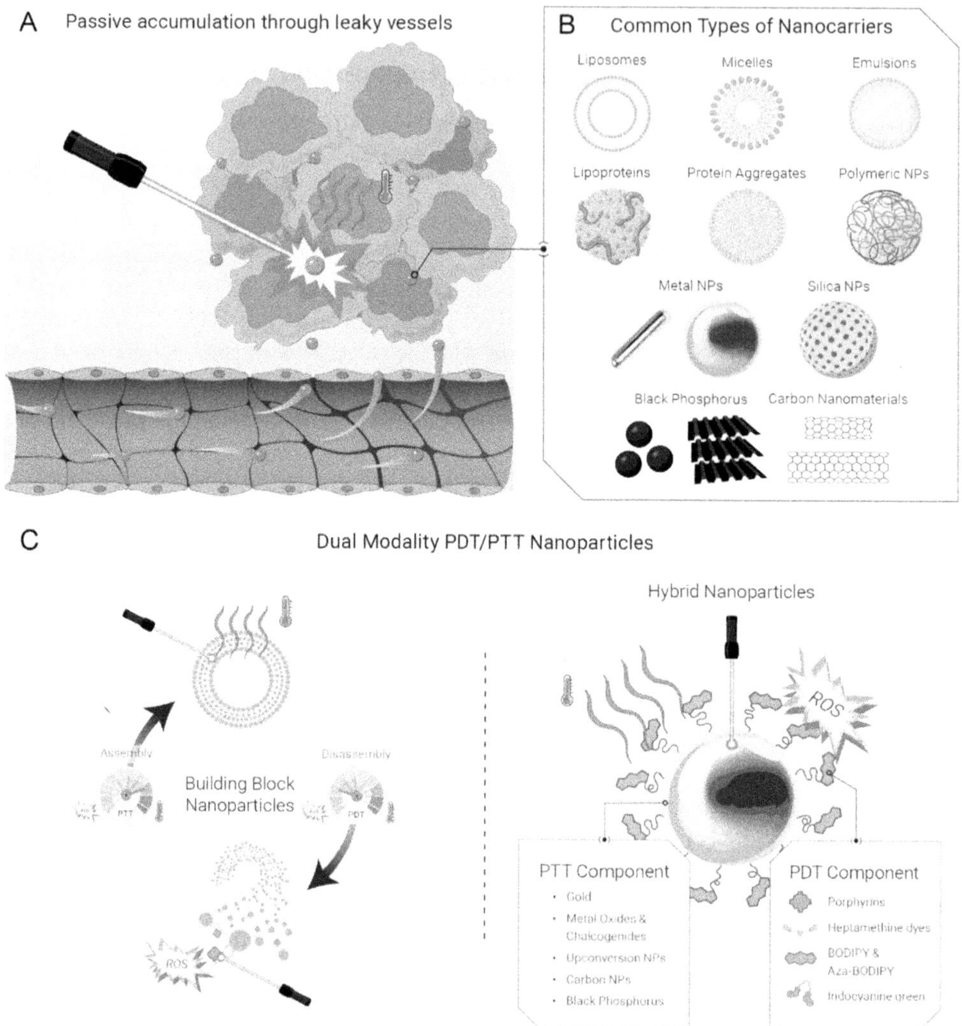

Figure 10.3. Use of NPs for dual PDT/PTT treatment. (A). NPs passively accumulate in tumours due to the EPR effect, where they can be activated with light to produce ROS or heat. (B). Common delivery vehicles include liposomes, micelles, nanoemulsions, lipoproteins and lipoprotein mimetics, protein-based NPs, polymeric NPs, metal, silica, black-phosphorus and carbon-based nanomaterials. (C). Left panel: PDT/PTT-active NPs can be designed with a single monomer that can act as a PTT agent within an intact nanostructure and a PS upon dissociation. Right panel: Hybrid PDT/PTT-active NPs can incorporate two or more photoactive agents, one of which acts as a PS, while another enhances heat generation, adapted with permission from [9], copyright 2020, American Chemical Society.

10.4.2 Design of multifunctional nanoparticles

Because multifunctional NPs can combine therapeutic and diagnostic functions on a single platform, they have become a potent tool in the field of nanomedicine. The use of these NPs in SERS-guided PT is one such potential application that provides a synergistic approach to cancer diagnosis and treatment. This approach makes use of NPs' special qualities to improve Raman signals for accurate molecular detection and to deliver phototherapeutic drugs to the intended locations. Since gold and silver NPs have a strong plasmonic resonance that greatly increases Raman scattering, they are frequently used in SERS applications. Magnetic materials such as iron oxide can be included to provide targeted delivery and magnetic resonance imaging (MRI). Surface functionalization can be achieved by combining the nanomaterials with polymer covering, ligands, or Raman reporter molecules. Strong Raman-signature molecules known as Raman reporter molecules are affixed to the NP surface to produce discernible spectroscopic signals. To enable specific attachment to cancer cells, chemicals like peptides, antibodies, or tiny molecules are affixed. It is possible to improve bloodstream circulation time and biocompatibility by using polymers like polyethylene glycol (PEG).[9, 29, 41, 42, 69, 72]

10.4.3 Light source and dosimetry

Lasers are the common light sources used in PDT, and PTT because lasers can give focussed energy at certain wavelengths. They can be used to provide more even lighting over bigger regions. Non-coherent light sources, like lamps with filters, can occasionally provide the required wavelength of light. The wavelength of light affects penetration depth because different light wavelengths permeate tissues to varying degrees. For deeper penetration, red and NIR light are typically utilized. In the case of PTT, to ensure that the targeted tissue gets the intended therapeutic temperature usually between 42 °C and 45 °C without endangering nearby healthy tissues, temperature monitoring is essential. PTT depends on the conversion of light energy into heat, whereas PDT depends on the production of ROS to destroy cells. For these treatments to be safe and successful, dosimetry, which involves precisely regulating the amount, duration, and intensity of light must be done with accuracy. In both PTT and PDT, selecting the right light source, wavelength, and treatment settings is essential to getting the intended therapeutic result with the fewest possible side effects [74–77].

The efficiency and dependability of SERS rely heavily on the selection of the light source and precise dosage measurement. The laser's wavelength, power stability, and spectral purity are some of the criteria that affect the choice of light source for SERS. Because of their great coherence, monochromaticity, and intensity, lasers are the light sources that are most frequently utilized in SERS. The SERS substrate's plasmonic characteristics and the particular application will determine the ideal laser wavelength. Wavelengths such as 488, 514, 532, and 633 nm are frequently utilized. These wavelengths can significantly boost surface plasmon excitation in silver and gold NPs. When working with biological material, NIR lasers with reduced fluorescence background and deeper tissue penetration like those at 785 and 1064 nm are the preferable choice. Stable laser power maintenance is essential for repeatability in SERS experiments. Variations in laser power can cause changes in the Raman signal's strength, which can impact how accurate quantitative analyses are. High local field increases can only be attained by tightly focusing the laser beam onto the SERS substrate, which is made possible by the lasers' spatial coherence. By ensuring that just the intended excitation wavelength is used, spectral purity reduces background signals and raises the signal-to-noise ratio. The sample or the SERS substrate may be harmed by photothermal effects that result from extended exposure or high-power density. Consistency in the experiments requires regular calibration of the laser power output and monitoring of the power density. Calibration can be performed using power meters and photodetectors [1, 67, 68, 73, 78].

10.4.4 Targeting and delivery strategies

Molecular recognition elements, environmental targeting, and ligand-receptor targeting are the targeting strategies for SERS-guided PT. For instance, in ligand-receptor targeting, overexpressed receptors on the surface of sick cells can be precisely targeted by conjugating antibodies and antibody fragments to SERS-active NPs. Aptamers are short sequences of DNA or RNA that can be engineered to attach selectively to target molecules or cells. NPs functionalized with aptamers have a high affinity and selectivity for cancer cells. Peptides and tiny compounds are utilized in the targeting of molecular recognition elements. Peptide sequences, for instance, can be designed to identify and attach to particular markers on target cells. For targeted delivery, these peptides can be coupled to NPs. SERS-active NPs can be directed to target cells by using particular small molecules that have a high affinity for particular cell receptors. Lastly, environmental targets such as situations that are redox or pH sensitive. Certain NPs, for instance, are engineered to discharge their payload in reaction to the acidic milieu of tumours, while other NPs are made to release their payload in response to the elevated concentrations of ROS present in cancerous cells [73, 79].

The delivery methods include polymer, liposome-micelle, and NP-based. Because of their superior plasmonic qualities, gold and silver NPs are frequently employed in SERS. In addition to enhancing the SERS signal and producing photothermal effects when exposed to near-infrared light, they can be functionalized with targeting ligands to achieve selective delivery to target cells. This helps facilitate the killing of target cells. Another approach is to encapsulate SERS-active NPs in liposomes or micelles, which can subsequently be functionalized with targeted ligands. The NPs' circulation duration and biocompatibility may be enhanced by this encapsulation. It is possible to construct dendrimers and polymer micelles to release their cargo in response to stimuli, such as temperature, pH, or enzyme activity. For targeted delivery, they can also be functionalized using targeting ligands [79–81].

10.4.5 Real-time monitoring and feedback

During treatment, combining SERS with PT offers a potent tool for real-time feedback and monitoring. SERS can quickly ascertain the physiological condition of the tissue being treated by detecting the presence and concentration of particular biomolecules or metabolites. The target area's molecular makeup can be ascertained using SERS prior to treatment, which aids in choosing the best PS type and dosage of light. SERS can provide real-time feedback on the efficacy of the treatment by continuously monitoring changes in the molecular composition during PT, such as the production of ROS or variations in biomarker levels. Real-time feedback allows for dynamic adjustments to the treatment. For instance, the light intensity or exposure duration might be extended if the SERS signal shows that not enough ROS is being generated. On the other hand, if the signal indicates elevated ROS, which could harm healthy tissue, the course of treatment can be adjusted. The phototherapic techniques are also incorporated with fluorescence spectroscopy. However, in comparison with SERS-guided PT, fluorescent dyes can degrade upon prolonged exposure to light, fluorescence signals can be weak in deeper tissues, and fluorescence spectroscopy is less sensitive than SERS in detecting low concentrations of biomarkers [82–84].

10.5 SERS-guided phototherapy in cancer treatment

Though there are still issues with targeting tumour cells while preserving healthy tissue, cancer treatment has come a long way. Using the great sensitivity of SERS for cancer detection and the accuracy of PT for treatment, SERS-guided PT is emerging as a potential approach. The goal of this combination is to increase treatment efficacy and diagnostic precision. Functionalized SERS-active NPs are made with targeting ligands such as antibodies that are particular to cancer cell markers. As these NPs attach themselves to cancer cells, they gather near the site of the tumour. The Raman-active molecules on the NPs are excited by a laser. The Raman signal is enhanced by the metal NPs, making it possible to detect cancer cells with great precision. The accumulation of SERS-active and phototherapeutic drugs in the tumour microenvironment can be enhanced by functionalizing NPs to target cell receptors. The effectiveness of PDT and PTT can be enhanced by SERS-active NPs by raising the local concentration of light-absorbing agents [23, 85].

10.5.1 Mechanisms of action: synergy between SERS and PT

By giving real-time molecular knowledge of the tumour microenvironment, SERS can direct PTT. Selectively targeting cancer cells is possible with NPs functionalized with PTAs and SERS-active compounds. While the PTAs cause localized heating and cell death, the SERS signal guarantees accurate localization. Similar to this, SERS can direct PDT by determining whether PSs are present in the tumour and at what concentration. This makes it possible to maximize the amount of light exposure and PS used, improving the therapeutic result while reducing harm to nearby healthy tissues. The targeting and accumulation of therapeutic drugs in cancer cells are improved by the combination of SERS and PT. To ensure selective accumulation, SERS-active NPs can be coupled with targeting ligands that identify particular cancer cell markers. Real-time feedback on the concentration and dispersion of medicinal substances is provided by SERS. This feature makes it possible to dynamically modify the settings of treatment, resulting in more efficient and individualized care. SERS's accurate targeting and in-the-moment monitoring capabilities improve PT's overall effectiveness. Through precise and effective delivery of therapeutic chemicals, this integrated strategy maximizes the death of cancer cells while reducing collateral damage [29, 86, 87].

10.5.2 Preclinical studies: experimental designs and outcomes

Murine models such as mice and rats implanted with human cancer cell lines, such as HeLa (cervical cancer), MCF-7 (breast cancer), and A549 (lung cancer), are frequently used animal models (figure 10.4). Cancer cells are injected subcutaneously or orthotopically to create tumours, providing a reliable and repeatable model for assessing treatment effects. Usually made of gold or silver, SERS NPs are functionalized with targeting ligands such as peptides or antibodies to enable targeted interaction with tumour cells. Using methods like dynamic light scattering (DLS), Raman spectroscopy, and transmission electron microscopy (TEM), NPs can be thoroughly characterized in terms of their size, shape, surface charge, and Raman enhancement capabilities. The wavelength, power density, and exposure duration of the laser are optimized to effectively activate phototherapeutic drugs without endangering nearby healthy tissues. Combining SERS NPs with PSs such as porphyrins, phthalocyanines, or PTAs such as gold nanorods to increase therapeutic efficacy. In addition to SERS, non-invasive imaging modalities like MRI, positron emission tomography (PET), and fluorescence imaging are utilized to track the

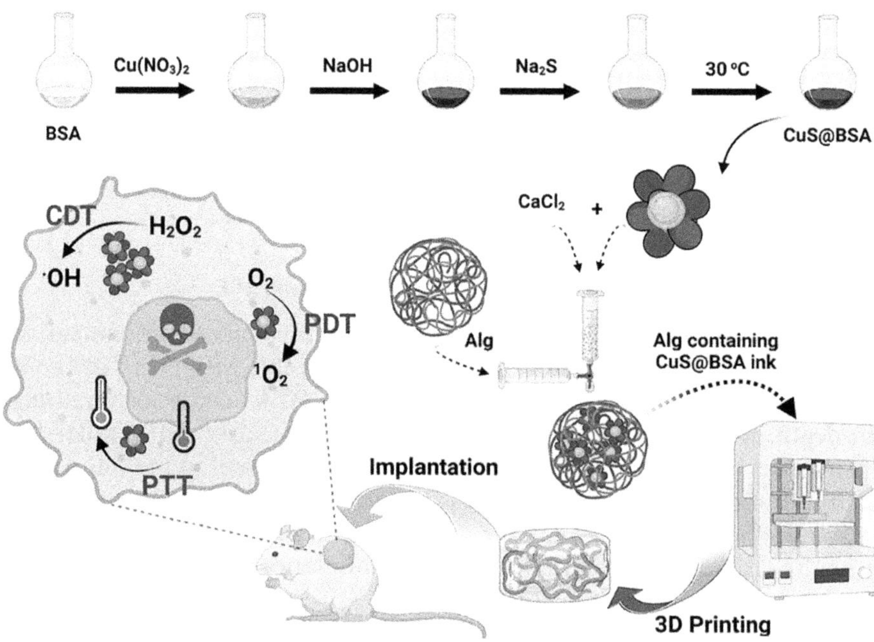

Figure 10.4. Schematic illustration of the synthesis of CuS/BSA NPs, in preparation, 3D printing, and the proposed anticancer mechanism, adapted with permission from [88] CC BY 4.0.

location of tumours, the dispersion of NPs, and the effectiveness of treatment. *Ex vivo* organ imaging and quantification of NP biodistribution analysis are performed to assess targeting effectiveness and off-target consequences. When it comes to identifying micrometastases and remaining tumour cells, SERS-guided PT shows excellent sensitivity and specificity in tumour detection and localization. The ability to make dynamic modifications to treatment procedures by real-time monitoring of the therapeutic response and NP distribution. When compared to controls, treated mice showed a significant reduction in both tumour volume and size, suggesting that PT was working, a longer period of tumour suppression, lower rates of recurrence, and improved survival rates in the treated groups. Because SERS-guided PT is focussed, there is a low occurrence of off-target effects and systemic toxicity. The safety of the treatment is confirmed by the histopathological investigation, which reveals no significant harm to the major organs [87, 89–92].

10.5.3 Clinical trials: current status and future prospects

Preclinical research has shown that SERS-guided PT is a powerful tool for identifying and eliminating cancer cells. Researchers have demonstrated that accurate localization of therapeutic drugs within tumours can be achieved by conjugating PSs to SERS-active NPs. In comparison to conventional PT techniques, animal research has shown that SERS-guided PT has a positive safety profile with few off-target effects. In the first phase of trials, the main objectives of these trials are to evaluate the safety, tolerability, and ideal dosage of SERS-guided PT in people. Promising first findings indicate that the treatment is well tolerated and can target tumour cells specifically while causing little harm to the surrounding healthy tissue. The purpose of these trials is to assess the effectiveness of SERS-guided PT on a broader patient population. Comparing early phase II trials to standard PT, better results were seen in terms of tumour shrinkage and patient survival rates. The goal of current research is to create SERS-active NPs of the next generation that are more stable, effective in targeting targets, and have improved stability. Theranostics, the fusion of therapeutic and diagnostic roles into a single NP platform has enormous potential for tailored cancer therapy. It may be possible to improve overall therapeutic outcomes and get around resistance mechanisms by combining SERS-guided PT with other therapeutic modalities like immunotherapy or chemotherapy. Large-scale, multicentre clinical trials will be essential to determining SERS-guided PT's therapeutic utility and safety profile. Regulatory approval and clinical adoption of SERS-active NPs will be aided by the development of standard operating procedures for their manufacture, characterization, and clinical application. Precision oncology has advanced significantly with the capacity to customize SERS-guided PT to the unique molecular and genetic profile of a patient's tumour [8, 91, 93–95].

10.5.4 Case studies: success stories and lessons learned

Combining SERS and PT allows for the selective destruction of cancer cells while also utilizing the diagnostic precision of SERS to locate and identify cancer cells.

This combined strategy promises decreased adverse effects and increased efficacy. The patient was treated for breast cancer using SERS-guided PT, which targeted cancer cells using gold NPs functionalized with a Raman reporter. A near-infrared laser was used to activate the PS after it was localized. Following four weeks of treatment, there was a noticeable decrease in the size of the tumour, little harm to the surrounding healthy tissues, and no serious side effects were noted [29, 96]. Gold–silver alloy NPs were employed as SERS substrates to target cancer cells in the treatment of prostate cancer. A low-power laser was used in PT to activate the PS. SERS-active NPs were administered topically to cure skin cancer, and then the PS was activated by laser. Following treatment, there was no adverse reaction, the carcinoma was completely eradicated in two weeks, and the cosmetic results were excellent with minimal scarring. Because of this, topical application of NPs enabled non-invasive treatment and demonstrated the effectiveness of SERS-guided PT for superficial tumours with a prompt reaction time [97, 98].

10.6 Challenges and limitations

A new method combines the curative advantages of PT with the great sensitivity of SERS for molecular identification. This strategy has a lot of potential to increase the accuracy and effectiveness of cancer treatment, but it also has several drawbacks and difficulties.

10.6.1 Complexity of SERS substrate design

The substrates' repeatability is one of the main issues with SERS. Reproducible and high-quality SERS substrates are essential for dependable and consistent signal amplification. Significant variations in the size, shape, and distribution of NPs can result in variations in the intensity of the SERS signal. Another problem is the SERS substrates' long-term stability. The aggregation or degradation of NPs might result in a reduction in signal amplification. Practical application of these substrates requires ensuring their long-term stability in biological settings. To target cells or tissues, SERS substrates frequently need to be functionalized with certain molecules. It is difficult to achieve effective and targeted functionalization without sacrificing the SERS activity. The efficiency of the method can be decreased by non-specific proteins and other biomolecules adhering to the SERS substrate and interfering with the technique's ability to target and detect targets [87, 99, 100].

10.6.2 Variability in biological environments

There are significant differences in pH, oxygen saturation, and the types of cells present in the tumour microenvironment. Inconsistent outcomes may arise from this variability's impact on the dispersion and accumulation of SERS NPs. Biological systems are dynamic, undergoing constant modifications to their molecular and cellular makeup. Due to its dynamic nature, reliable and real-time SERS readings may be difficult to obtain. NPs' possible toxicity and biocompatibility are brought up by their usage in SERS. For the NPs to be used in clinical settings, it is imperative that they do not have negative side effects on the body. Foreign NPs can be identified by the immune system, which can then target and eliminate them from the body before they can reach their intended location. SERS-guided PT may become less effective as a result of this immunological reaction [79, 101].

10.6.3 Difficulties for integration of SERS with PT

Precise timing and dosage of the therapeutic agents are necessary for the successful integration of SERS with PT. Making sure that the PT is precisely guided by the SERS signal is crucial to optimizing therapeutic effectiveness and reducing adverse effects. To precisely target particular cells or tissues, a high spatial resolution is needed. It can be difficult to achieve this resolution with SERS-guided PT, particularly in deep tissues. Light is frequently used in PT to activate medicinal substances. It is crucial to regulate the activation to prevent harm to the nearby healthy tissues. Precise SERS-guided activation is necessary to guarantee both safety and effectiveness. To destroy cancer cells, PT uses heat generation. While not enough heat may not be helpful, and large amount of heat generation can harm healthy tissues. It is a big challenge to balance these consequences [94, 102].

10.6.4 Potential for phototoxicity

If PT light usage is not adequately regulated, it can harm healthy tissues. A key problem is making sure that the light exposure is contained to the target area and does not result in phototoxicity. Cumulative phototoxic effects may result from repeated PT treatments. The treatment's long-term effectiveness depends on careful observation and management of these side effects. ROS are frequently produced during PDT to cause cell death. On the other hand, too much ROS can cause inflammation and harm to healthy tissues. Reducing ROS levels is essential for therapy to be both safe and successful. However, to reach the full potential of SERS-guided PT, several obstacles and restrictions must be overcome. Enhancing SERS substrate stability and reproducibility, controlling biological variability, guaranteeing biocompatibility, successfully combining SERS with PT, and reducing phototoxicity are a few of these. Future studies ought to concentrate on resolving these issues to progress the practical use of SERS-guided PT [103, 104].

10.7 Future directions

SERS guided by PT is a rapidly developing discipline that combines analytical chemistry, nanotechnology, and medical research. It makes use of SERS's incredibly sensitive and focussed molecular detection capabilities to direct and improve PT's effectiveness, especially when treating cancer disease. The development of NPs with enhanced stability, targeting effectiveness, and biocompatibility will be the focus of future research. This includes creating NPs that can break down into non-toxic byproducts after serving their purpose and combining SERS, imaging, and medicinal functions into a single NP. It is still difficult to distribute SERS-active NPs precisely to tumour locations. Potential future initiatives could involve creating NPs that release therapeutic drugs in response to particular tumour microenvironment variables like pH and enzyme activity, as well as using ligands, antibodies, or aptamers that bind selectively to cancer cell markers. SERS-assisted real-time PT monitoring can improve treatment efficacy and safety. To monitor NP dispersion and therapy response, for instance, it is important to improve the depth and resolution of *in vivo* SERS imaging. Additionally, methods for dynamically monitoring the therapeutic process and modifying treatment parameters in real time need to be developed. Results can be enhanced by combining SERS-guided PT with other therapeutic approaches. To obtain synergistic benefits, for instance, SERS-guided PT might be combined with established immunotherapies or chemotherapy methods. Additionally, SERS can be used with other imaging modalities, such as computed tomography (CT) scanning and MRI, for thorough monitoring. Resolving scalability and regulatory issues is essential for clinical translation. Using artificial intelligence will help conduct rigorous preclinical and clinical trials to prove safety and efficacy, as well as creating scalable and affordable manufacturing techniques for SERS-active NPs. To fully realize the promise of this unique method and overcome current hurdles, interdisciplinary and collaborative research will be essential.

10.8 Conclusions

SERS and PT techniques are possibly combined in this chapter to improve therapeutic results. SERS offers extremely specific and sensitive biomolecule detection, which can help with early disease diagnosis. With SERS, distinct molecular fingerprints of different disease markers can be identified, allowing for precise PT targeting. When PT and SERS are used together, sick cells can be precisely targeted, minimizing damage to healthy tissues. Real-time monitoring of the therapeutic process is possible with SERS, enabling changes for the best possible therapeutic outcomes. When PT and SERS-guided diagnostics are used together, therapeutic efficacy can be increased beyond what would be possible with either approach alone. PT side effects can be considerably decreased by more precisely focussed therapy. By utilizing NPs in SERS, PT can be made more effective and provide additional therapeutic options. The integration of SERS technology with is further enhanced by technological advancements like the creation of novel substrates and improvement methods. Potential uses for SERS-guided PT include treating various infections, neurological conditions, and different cancers. Sustained investigation is necessary to enhance SERS-guided PT methodologies, investigate novel applications, and guarantee secure and efficient clinical execution. It is necessary to address problems like the repeatability of SERS signals and the creation of biocompatible SERS substrates. Strict regulatory control and ethical considerations are needed to guarantee the safety and effectiveness of these cutting-edge treatments.

References

[1] Prochazka M 2016 Basics of surface-enhanced Raman scattering (SERS) *Surface-Enhanced Raman Spectroscopy* (Springer) pp 21–59

[2] Tahir M A, Dina N E, Cheng H, Valev V K and Zhang L J N 2021 Surface-enhanced Raman spectroscopy for bioanalysis and diagnosis *Nanoscale* **13** 11593–634

[3] Li P, Long F, Chen W, Chen J, Chu P K and Wang H J 2020 Fundamentals and applications of surface-enhanced Raman spectroscopy–based biosensors *Curr. Opin. Biomed. Eng.* **13** 51–9
[4] Van Straten D, Mashayekhi V, De Bruijn H S, Oliveira S and Robinson D J 2017 Oncologic photodynamic therapy: basic principles, current clinical status and future directions *Cancers (Basel)* **9** 19
[5] Melamed J R, Edelstein R S and Day E S 2015 Elucidating the fundamental mechanisms of cell death triggered by photothermal therapy *ACS Nano.* **9** 6–11
[6] Ng C W, Li J and Pu K J 2018 Recent progresses in phototherapy-synergized cancer immunotherapy *Adv. Funct. Mater.* **28** 1804688
[7] Shi H and Sadler P J 2020 How promising is phototherapy for cancer? *Br. J. Cancer* **123** 871–3
[8] Das A, Tsai H-C, Sen T and Moirangthem R S 2023 Plasmonic nanoparticle-based surface-enhanced Raman spectroscopy-guided photothermal therapy: emerging cancer theranostics *Nanomedicine* **18** 555–76
[9] Overchuk M, Weersink R A, Wilson B C and Zheng G 2023 Photodynamic and photothermal therapies: synergy opportunities for nanomedicine *ACS Nano* **17** 7979–8003
[10] Zhang Y, Zhang S, Zhang Z, Ji L, Zhang J, Wang Q, Guo T, Ni S, Cai R and Mu X 2021 Recent progress on NIR-II photothermal therapy *Front. Chem.* **9** 728066
[11] Zhi D, Yang T, O'hagan J, Zhang S and Donnelly R F 2020 Photothermal therapy *J. Control. Release.* **325** 52–71
[12] Algorri J F, Ochoa M, Roldán-Varona P, Rodríguez-Cobo L and López-Higuera J M 2021 Photodynamic therapy: a compendium of latest reviews *Cancers (Basel)* **13** 4447
[13] Barros N D M, Sbroglio L L, Buffara M D O, Baka J L C E S, Pessoa A D S and Azulay-Abulafia L 2021 Phototherapy *An. Bras. Dermatol.* **96** 397–407
[14] Correia J H, Rodrigues J A, Pimenta S, Dong T and Yang Z 2021 Photodynamic therapy review: principles, photosensitizers, applications, and future directions *Pharmaceutics* **13** 1332
[15] Krishnan R S and Shankar R K 1981 Raman effect: history of the discovery *J. Raman. Spectrosc* **10** 1–8
[16] Vandenabeele P 2013 *Practical Raman Spectroscopy: An Introduction* (New York: Wiley)
[17] Gardiner D J 1989 Introduction to Raman scattering *Practical Raman Spectroscopy* (Berlin: Springer) pp 1–12
[18] Ferraro J R 2003 *Introductory Raman Spectroscopy* (Amsterdam: Elsevier)
[19] Colthup N 2012 *Introduction to Infrared and Raman Spectroscopy* (Amsterdam: Elsevier)
[20] Rostron P, Gaber S and Gaber D J 2016 Raman spectroscopy, review *Laser* **21** 24
[21] Mulvaney S P and Keating C D 2000 Raman spectroscopy *Anal. Chem.* **72** 145–58
[22] Moon J, Li M, Ramirez-Cuesta A J and Wu Z 2023 Raman spectroscopy *Springer Handbook of Advanced Catalyst Characterization* (Berlin: Springer) pp 75–110
[23] Abbas Z and Rehman S J 2018 An overview of cancer treatment modalities *Neoplasm* (InTech Open) pp 139–57
[24] Nikolaou M, Pavlopoulou A, Georgakilas A G, Kyrodimos E J C and Metastasis E 2018 The challenge of drug resistance in cancer treatment: a current overview *Clin. Exp. Metastasis.* **35** 309–18
[25] Naser R, Dilabazian H, Bahr H, Barakat A and El-Sibai M 2022 A guide through conventional and modern cancer treatment modalities: a specific focus on glioblastoma cancer therapy *Oncol. Rep.* **48** 1–17

[26] Davies M 2014 New modalities of cancer treatment for NSCLC: focus on immunotherapy *Cancer Manag. Res.* **2014** 63–75
[27] McGunigal M, Lischalk J W, Randolph-Jackson P and Khaitan P G 2021 Radiation modalities used in lung cancer: an overview for thoracic surgeons *Semin. Thorac. Cardiovasc. Surg.* **33** 1114–21
[28] Czarnecka-Czapczyńska M, Aebisher D, Oleś P, Sosna B, Krupka-Olek M, Dynarowicz K, Latos W, Cieślar G and Kawczyk-Krupka A 2021 The role of photodynamic therapy in breast cancer–a review of *in vitro* research *Biomed. Pharmacother.* **144** 112342
[29] Narayanan N *et al* 2021 Nanotheranostic probe built on methylene blue loaded Cucurbituril [8] and gold nanorod: targeted phototherapy in combination with SERS imaging on breast cancer cells *J. Phys. Chem.* B **125** 13415–24
[30] Sujai P T, Joseph M M, Karunakaran V, Saranya G, Adukkadan R N, Shamjith S, Thomas R, Nair J B, Swathi R S and Maiti K K 2018 Biogenic cluster-encased gold nanorods as a targeted three-in-one theranostic nanoenvelope for SERS-guided photochemotherapy against metastatic melanoma *ACS Appl. Bio Mater.* **2** 588–600
[31] Niculescu A-G and Grumezescu A M 2021 Photodynamic therapy—an up-to-date review *Appl. Sci.* **11** 3626
[32] Ren Y, Yan Y and Qi H 2022 Photothermal conversion and transfer in photothermal therapy: from macroscale to nanoscale *Adv. Colloid Interface Sci.* **308** 102753
[33] Jori G and Spikes J D 1990 Photothermal sensitizers: possible use in tumor therapy *J. Photochem. Photobiol.* B **6** 93–101
[34] Yoo S W, Oh G, Ahn J C and Chung E 2021 Non-oncologic applications of nanomedicine-based photo-therapy *Biomedicines* **9** 113
[35] Lee J S, Kim J, Ye Y-S and Kim T-I 2022 Materials and device design for advanced phototherapy systems *Adv. Drug Deliv. Rev.* **186** 114339
[36] Kwiatkowski S, Knap B, Przystupski D, Saczko J, Kędzierska E, Knap-Czop K, Kotlińska J, Michel O, Kotowski K and Kulbacka J 2018 Photodynamic therapy–mechanisms, photosensitizers and combinations *Biomed. Pharmacother.* **106** 1098–107
[37] Sharma D, Singh S, Kumar P, Jain G K, Aggarwal G, Almalki W H and Kesharwani P 2023 Mechanisms of photodynamic therapy *Nanomaterials for Photodynamic Therapy* (Amsterdam: Elsevier) pp 41–54
[38] Yoo J-O and Ha K-S 2012 New insights into the mechanisms for photodynamic therapy-induced cancer cell death *Int. Rev. Cell Mol. Biol.* **295** 139–74
[39] Li J, Zhang W, Ji W, Wang J, Wang N, Wu W, Wu Q, Hou X, Hu W and Li L 2021 Near infrared photothermal conversion materials: mechanism, preparation, and photothermal cancer therapy applications *J. Mater. Chem. B.* **9** 7909–26
[40] Bhole R, Bonde C, Kadam P and Wavwale R 2021 A comprehensive review on photodynamic therapy (PDT) and photothermal therapy (PTT) for cancer treatment *Turk. J. Oncol.* **36** 125–32
[41] Nasseri B, Alizadeh E, Bani F, Davaran S, Akbarzadeh A, Rabiee N, Bahadori A, Ziaei M, Bagherzadeh M and Saeb M R 2022 Nanomaterials for photothermal and photodynamic cancer therapy *Appl. Phys. Rev.* **9** 011317
[42] Paszko E, Ehrhardt C, Senge M O, Kelleher D P, Reynolds J V and Therapy P 2011 Nanodrug applications in photodynamic therapy *Photodiagnosis Photodyn. Ther.* **8** 14–29
[43] Wan M T and Lin J Y 2014 Current evidence and applications of photodynamic therapy in dermatology *Clin. Cosmet Investig. Dermatol.* **21** 145–63

[44] Henderson B W 2020 *Photodynamic Therapy: Basic Principles and Clinical Applications* (Boca Raton, FL: CRC Press)

[45] Wang Z, Peng H, SHi W, Gan L, Zhong L, He J, Xie L, Wu P, Zhao Y and Deng Z 2021 Application of photodynamic therapy in cancer: challenges and advancements *Biocell* **45** 489

[46] Yang D *et al* 2021 Application of photodynamic therapy in immune-related diseases *Photodiagnosis Photodyn. Ther.* **34** 102318

[47] Fernandes N, Rodrigues C F, Moreira A F and Correia I J 2020 Overview of the application of inorganic nanomaterials in cancer photothermal therapy *Biomater. Sci.* **8** 2990–3020

[48] Ding S Y, Zhang X M, Ren B and Tian Z Q 2006 Surface-enhanced Raman spectroscopy (SERS): general introduction *Encyclopedia of Analytical Chemistry: Applications, Theory and Instrumentation* (Wiley) pp 1–34

[49] Fleischmann M, Hendra P J and McQuillan A J 1974 Raman spectra of pyridine adsorbed at a silver electrode *Chem. Phys. Lett.* **26** 163–6

[50] Dieringer J A, McFarland A D, Shah N C, Stuart D A, Whitney A V, Yonzon C R, Young M A, Zhang X and Van Duyne R P 2006 Introductory lecture surface enhanced Raman spectroscopy: new materials, concepts, characterization tools, and applications *Faraday Discuss.* **132** 9–26

[51] Cialla D, März A, Böhme R, Theil F, Weber K, Schmitt M and Popp J 2012 Surface-enhanced Raman spectroscopy (SERS): progress and trends *Anal. Bioanal. Chem.* **403** 27–54

[52] Langer J *et al* 2020 Present and future of surface-enhanced Raman scattering *ACS Nano.* **14** 28–117

[53] Lin Z and He L 2019 Recent advance in SERS techniques for food safety and quality analysis: a brief review *Curr. Opin. Food Sci.* **28** 82–7

[54] Lee H K, Lee Y H, Koh C S L, Phan-Quang G C, Han X, Lay C L, Sim H Y F, Kao Y-C, An Q and Ling X Y 2019 Designing surface-enhanced Raman scattering (SERS) platforms beyond hotspot engineering: emerging opportunities in analyte manipulations and hybrid materials *Chem. Soc. Rev.* **48** 731–56

[55] Betz J F, Yu W W, Cheng Y, White I M and Rubloff G W 2014 Simple SERS substrates: powerful, portable, and full of potential *Phys. Chem. Chem. Phys.* **16** 2224–39

[56] Tripp R A, Dluhy R A and Zhao Y 2008 Novel nanostructures for SERS biosensing *Nano Today* **3** 31–7

[57] Kruszewski S 1998 Enhancement mechanisms in the SERS phenomenon *Tenth Polish-Czech-Slovak Optical Conf.: Wave and Quantum Aspects of Contemporary Optics* pp 281–93

[58] Schatz G C, Young M A and Van Duyne R P 2006 Electromagnetic mechanism of SERS *Surface-Enhanced Raman Scattering: Physics and Applications* (Berlin: Springer) pp 19–45

[59] Otto A and Futamata M 2006 Electronic mechanisms of SERS *Surface-Enhanced Raman Scattering: Physics and Applications* (Berlin: Springer) pp 147–82

[60] Kim J, Jang Y, Kim N-J, Kim H, Yi G-C, Shin Y, Kim M H and Yoon S 2019 Study of chemical enhancement mechanism in non-plasmonic surface enhanced Raman spectroscopy (SERS) *Front. Chem.* **7** 582

[61] Trivedi D J, Barrow B and Schatz G C 2020 Understanding the chemical contribution to the enhancement mechanism in SERS: connection with Hammett parameters *J. Chem. Phys.* **153** 124706

[62] Valley N, Greeneltch N, Van Duyne R P and Schatz G C 2013 A look at the origin and magnitude of the chemical contribution to the enhancement mechanism of surface-enhanced Raman spectroscopy (SERS): theory and experiment *J. Phys. Chem. Lett.* **4** 2599–604
[63] Li M, Qiu Y, Fan C, Cui K and Zhang Y 2018 Design of SERS nanoprobes for Raman imaging: materials, critical factors and architectures *Acta Pharm. Sin.* B **8** 381–9
[64] Le Ru E C, Blackie E, Meyer M and Etchegoin P G 2007 Surface enhanced Raman scattering enhancement factors: a comprehensive study *J. Phys. Chem.* C **111** 13794–803
[65] Arbuz A, Sultangaziyev A, Rapikov A, Kunushpayeva Z and Bukasov R 2022 How gap distance between gold nanoparticles in dimers and trimers on metallic and non-metallic SERS substrates can impact signal enhancement *Nanoscale Adv.* **4** 268–80
[66] Joseph M M, Narayanan N, Nair J B, Karunakaran V, Ramya A N, Sujai P T, Saranya G, Arya J S, Vijayan V M and Maiti K K 2018 Exploring the margins of SERS in practical domain: an emerging diagnostic modality for modern biomedical applications *Biomaterials* **181** 140–81
[67] Chen Y, An Q, Teng K, Liu C, Sun F and Li G 2023 Application of SERS in in-vitro biomedical detection *Chem. Asian J.* **18** e202201194
[68] Zheng X-S, Jahn I J, Weber K, Cialla-May D, Popp J and Spectroscopy B 2018 Label-free SERS in biological and biomedical applications: recent progress, current challenges and opportunities *Spectrochim. Acta A Mol. Biomol. Spectrosc.* **197** 56–77
[69] Sinha S S, Jones S, Pramanik A and Ray P C 2016 Nanoarchitecture based SERS for biomolecular fingerprinting and label-free disease markers diagnosis *Acc. Chem. Res.* **49** 2725–35
[70] Shen Y, Yue J, Xu W and Xu S 2021 Recent progress of surface-enhanced Raman spectroscopy for subcellular compartment analysis *Theranostics* **11** 4872
[71] Liang X, Li N, Zhang R, Yin P, Zhang C, Yang N, Liang K and Kong B 2021 Carbon-based SERS biosensor: from substrate design to sensing and bioapplication *NPG Asia Mater.* **13** 8
[72] Cheng L, Wang C, Feng L, Yang K and Liu Z 2014 Functional nanomaterials for phototherapies of cancer *Chem. Rev.* **114** 10869–939
[73] Li Q, Huo H, Wu Y, Chen L, Su L, Zhang X, Song J and Yang H 2023 Design and synthesis of SERS materials for *in vivo* molecular imaging and biosensing *Adv. Sci. (Weinh)* **10** 2202051
[74] Finlay J C and Darafsheh A 2016 Light sources, drugs, and dosimetry *Biomedical Optics in Otorhinolaryngology* (Springer) pp 311–36
[75] Profio A E and Doiron D R 1981 Dosimetry considerations in phototherapy *Med. Phys.* **8** 190–6
[76] Vreman H J, Wong R J, Stevenson D K, Route R K, Reader S D, Fejer M M, Gale R and Seidman D S 1998 Light-emitting diodes: a novel light source for phototherapy *Pediatr. Res.* **44** 804–9
[77] Romano G, Insero G, Marrugat S N and Fusi F 2022 Innovative light sources for phototherapy *Biomol. Concepts* **13** 256–71
[78] Mirza J A, Park H, Park S Y and Ye S J 2016 Use of radiochromic film as a high-spatial resolution dosimeter by Raman spectroscopy *Med. Phys.* **43** 4520–8
[79] Wen C, Chen H, Guo X, Lin Z, Zhang S, Shen X-C and Liang H 2020 Lysosome-targeted gold nanotheranostics for *in situ* SERS monitoring pH and multimodal imaging-guided phototherapy *Langmuir* **37** 569–77

[80] Zhu W, Gao M-Y, Zhu Q, Chi B, Zeng L-W, Hu J-M and Shen A-G 2020 Monodispersed plasmonic Prussian blue nanoparticles for zero-background SERS/MRI-guided phototherapy *Nanoscale* **12** 3292–301

[81] Tang P, Xing M, Xing X, Tao Q, Cheng W, Liu S, Lu X and Zhong L 2021 Receptor-mediated photothermal/photodynamic synergistic anticancer nanodrugs with SERS tracing function *Colloids Surf. B Biointerfaces* **199** 111550

[82] Huang X, Sheng B, Tian H, Chen Q, Yang Y, Bui B, Pi J, Cai H, Chen S and Zhang J 2023 Real-time SERS monitoring anticancer drug release along with SERS/MR imaging for pH-sensitive chemo-phototherapy *Acta Pharm. Sin.* **B 13** 1303–17

[83] Li L, Yang J, Wei J, Jiang C, Liu Z, Yang B, Zhao B and Song W 2022 Applications, SERS monitoring of photoinduced-enhanced oxidative stress amplifier on Au@ carbon dots for tumor catalytic therapy *Light Sci. Appl.* **11** 286

[84] Horgan C C, Bergholt M S, Nagelkerke A, Thin M Z, Pence I J, Kauscher U, Kalber T L, Stuckey D J and Stevens M M 2021 Integrated photodynamic Raman theranostic system for cancer diagnosis, treatment, and post-treatment molecular monitoring *Theranostics* **11** 2006

[85] He J, Wei Q, Wang S, Hua S and Zhou M 2021 Bioinspired protein corona strategy enhanced biocompatibility of Ag-Hybrid hollow Au nanoshells for surface-enhanced Raman scattering imaging and on-demand activation tumor-phototherapy *Biomaterials* **271** 120734

[86] Błaszkiewicz P and Kotkowiak M 2018 Gold-based nanoparticles systems in phototherapy-current strategies *Curr. Med. Chem.* **25** 5914–29

[87] Pekkanen A M, DeWitt M R and Rylander M N 2014 Nanoparticle enhanced optical imaging and phototherapy of cancer *J. Biomed. Nanotechnol.* **10** 1677–712

[88] Colak B, Cihan M C and Ertas Y N 2023 3D-Printed, implantable alginate/CuS nanoparticle scaffolds for local tumor treatment via synergistic photothermal, photodynamic, and chemodynamic therapy *ACS Appl. Nano Mater.* **6** 16076–85

[89] Deng B, Wang Y, Bu X, Li J, Lu J, Lin L L, Wang Y, Chen Y and Ye J 2024 Sentinel lymph node identification using NIR-II ultrabright Raman nanotags on preclinical models *Biomaterials* **308** 122538

[90] Tian Y, Qiang S and Wang L 2019 Biotechnology, Gold nanomaterials for imaging-guided near-infrared *in vivo* cancer therapy *Front. Bioeng. Biotechnol.* **7** 398

[91] Sekar R, Basavegowda N, Thathapudi J J, Sekhar M R, Joshi P, Somu P and Baek K-H 2023 Recent progress of gold-based nanostructures towards future emblem of photo-triggered cancer theranostics: a special focus on combinatorial phototherapies *Pharmaceutics* **15** 433

[92] Dennahy I S, Han Z, MacCuaig W M, Chalfant H M, Condacse A, Hagood J M, Claros-Sorto J C, Razaq W, Holter-Chakrabarty J and Squires R 2022 Nanotheranostics for image-guided cancer treatment *Pharmaceutics* **14** 917

[93] Li X, Yang G, Zhang S and Ren H 2024 Advancing clinical cancer care: unveiling the power of surface-enhanced Raman spectroscopy *J. Raman Spectrosc.* **55** 429–44

[94] Chen H, Cheng Z, Zhou X, Wang R and Yu F 2021 Emergence of surface-enhanced Raman scattering probes in near-infrared windows for biosensing and bioimaging *Anal. Chem.* **94** 143–64

[95] Darrigues E, Dantuluri V, Nima Z A, Vang-Dings K B, Griffin R J, Biris A R, Ghosh A and Biris A S 2017 Raman spectroscopy using plasmonic and carbon-based nanoparticles for cancer detection, diagnosis, and treatment guidance. Part 2: treatment *Drug. Metab. Rev.* **49** 253–83

[96] Zeng L, Pan Y, Wang S, Wang X, Zhao X, Ren W, Lu G and Wu A 2015 Interfaces, Raman reporter-coupled Agcore@ Aushell nanostars for *in vivo* improved surface enhanced Raman scattering imaging and near-infrared-triggered photothermal therapy in breast cancers *ACS Appl. Mater. Interfaces.* **7** 16781–91
[97] Wang L 2021 *Synthesis and Their Theranostic Applications of Plasmonic Gold-Silver Alloy Nanoparticles and Porous Nanostructures* (Montreal (Canada): Ecole Polytechnique)
[98] Sultangaziyev A, Ilyas A, Dyussupova A and Bukasov R 2022 Trends in application of SERS substrates beyond Ag and Au, and their role in bioanalysis *Biosensors* **12** 967
[99] Solís D M, Taboada J M, Obelleiro F, Liz-Marzán L M and García de Abajo F 2017 Optimization of nanoparticle-based SERS substrates through large-scale realistic simulations *ACS photonics* **4** 329–37
[100] Li C, Huang Y, Li X, Zhang Y, Chen Q, Ye Z, Alqarni Z, Bell S E and Xu Y 2021 Towards practical and sustainable SERS: a review of recent developments in the construction of multifunctional enhancing substrates *J. Mater. Chem.* C **9** 11517–52
[101] Liu Y-Q, Zhu W, Hu J-M and Shen A-G 2021 Recent advances in plasmonic Prussian blue-based SERS nanotags for biological application *Nanoscale Adv.* **3** 6568–79
[102] Gollavelli G, Ghule A V and Ling Y-C 2022 Multimodal imaging and phototherapy of cancer and bacterial infection by graphene and related nanocomposites *Molecules* **27** 5588
[103] Coelho M M V and Apetato M 2016 The dark side of the light: phototherapy adverse effects *Clin. Dermatol.* **34** 556–62
[104] Vreman H J, Wong R J and Stevenson D K 2004 Phototherapy: current methods and future directions *Seminars in Perinatology* (Elsevier) pp 326–33

www.ingramcontent.com/pod-product-compliance
Ingram Content Group UK Ltd.
Pitfield, Milton Keynes, MK11 3LW, UK
UKHW051924100926
8556IPUK00021B/1352